BIOPSY INTERPRETATION:
THE FROZEN SECTION

BIOPSY INTERPRETATION SERIES

Series Editor: Jonathan I. Epstein, MD

BIOPSY INTERPRETATION SERIES

BIOPSY INTERPRETATION: THE FROZEN SECTION

Jerome B. Taxy, MD
Professor
Department of Pathology
University of Chicago Medical Center
Chicago, Illinois

Aliya N. Husain, MD
Professor
Department of Pathology
University of Chicago Medical Center
Chicago, Illinois

Anthony G. Montag, MD
Professor
Departments of Pathology and Surgery
University of Chicago Medical Center
Chicago, Illinois

Wolters Kluwer | Lippincott Williams & Wilkins
Health
Philadelphia · Baltimore · New York · London
Buenos Aires · Hong Kong · Sydney · Tokyo

Senior Executive Editor: Jonathan W. Pine, Jr.
Product Manager: Marian Bellus
Senior Marketing Manager: Angela Panetta
Creative Director: Doug Smock
Production Service: Aptara, Inc.

530 Walnut Street
Philadelphia, PA 19106 USA
LWW.com

Printed in China

Library of Congress Cataloging-in-Publication Data

Taxy, Jerome B.
  Biopsy interpretation : the frozen section / Jerome B. Taxy, Aliya N. Husain, Anthony G.
Montag. – 1st ed.
    p. ; cm. – (Biopsy interpretation series)
  Includes bibliographical references and index.
  ISBN 978-0-7817-6779-8 (alk. paper)
  1. Frozen tissue sections.   2. Biopsy.   I. Husain, Aliya N.   II. Montag, Anthony G.
III. Title.   IV. Series: Biopsy interpretation series.
  [DNLM: 1. Frozen Sections–methods.   2. Biopsy–methods. QY 95 T235b 2009]
  RB27.T39 2009
  616.07'58—dc22
                                                                    2009021303

10 9 8 7 6 5 4 3 2 1

CONTENTS

PREFACE

Surgical pathology including the practice of frozen section was conceived and developed by surgeons. However, the very first frozen section was accomplished by a pathologist. In 1891, at the newly established Johns Hopkins Hospital, William S. Halsted, the surgeon, requested a frozen section on a breast tumor. The procedure was carried out by the pathologist William H. Welch. The procedure went so well that Halsted did not request another frozen for 25 years. Nonetheless, over the last almost 120 years, frozen section has evolved from a novelty to an accepted, even mundane, part of the practice of what we now recognize as surgical pathology. While the advent of laparoscopic, robotic, and microsurgical techniques has changed the utilization of frozen section and the nature of the questions asked, the essentials are the same: a freezing apparatus to harden tissue, a microtome to shave off thin slices, a staining set-up, a microscope, and a pathologist.

While the general public may be unaware of the active role of the pathologist in the conduct of surgery, intraoperative consultations including frozen section are a mainstay of 21st century patient care and an inseparable aspect of any pathology training program. These consultations take several forms, including the triage of fresh tissue for special studies, gross specimen examination, imprints, or the actual appearance in the operating room by the pathologist to view the operative field and speak directly to the surgeon. Frozen section, despite its associated artifacts and potential sampling error, is regarded as the most definitive form of consultation, since it involves the microscopic examination of tissue designated by the surgeon as important. The consequences of these consultations, and especially frozen section, are potentially dramatic. It is essential that the pathologist know the clinical setting and gross findings as well as the treatment algorithm for a given disease.

Currently, resident training in pathology is centered on organ system specialization. Despite acknowledged organ-specific expertise, faculty members in many university departments regularly participate in the frozen section rotation, which frequently involves organs outside their comfort zone. The downsides of this circumstance are that intradepartmental specialist-consultants need to be available and that the pathologist faces potential credibility issues with surgeons and clinicians outside his or her specialty area. The potential awkwardness for specialists and the mixed educational message notwithstanding, it is in this context that the practice of general surgical pathology persists. There is thus an implied value for pathologists with broadly based clinical medical knowledge, a capacity for practical decision making, an ease in rapid communication, and the possession of excellent morphologic skills. The pathologist's confidence level is dependent on training and tempered by experience so that good medical judgment dictates what and how much to report, aspects of diagnostic pathology that are sometimes more important than specific lesion identification.

Pathologists regard a frozen section as an emergency requiring cessation of whatever the activity of the moment may be. This is true not only for the pathologist on call but also for any colleague from whom an intradepartmental consultation is sought. While most surgeons and pathologists do recognize that this is a cooperative effort of some gravity, friction is created when it is perceived by the pathologist that a frozen section is frivolously requested. Reporting a frozen section only to discover that the diagnosis had no potential to change what was done, that the surgeon is no longer in the room, or that the patient is already in recovery implies that the information was inherently irrelevant and the pathologist's effort inconsequential.

This book regards frozen section as a selective, clinically relevant interdisciplinary effort. The application of frozen section to all specimens is not mainstream practice and will not be addressed. Readers may wonder why certain topics are or are not included. The specifics of each pathologist's practice related to intraoperative consultations, the rationales for those consultations and specifically frozen sections do differ, possibly are institutionally driven. We acknowledge that the selection of topics is reflective of our respective experiences; however, we hope that at least some information will be applicable to the circumstances of individual readers.

This book is an outgrowth of a recently completed USCAP short course. It is not designed to be a comprehensive traditional listing of entities as would be encountered in a textbook of surgical pathology, nor the promotion of frozen section heroics in the diagnosis of rare conditions. Frozen section is the focus but the central idea is intraoperative consultation. Although unusual entities may be illustrated, the principal concern is the practical use of frozen section in the management of a clinical problem, mostly involving tumors. Emphasis is placed on the morphologic expertise of the surgical pathologist in standard hematoxylin and eosin evaluations. The histologic illustrations, insofar as possible, are actual, frozen sections, with artifacts. Immunostains are not routinely available in this setting and are not diagnostically relevant. It is hoped that this volume will contribute to an informed practice of frozen section and an appreciation of the physician role of the general surgical pathologist for the patients they serve.

Jerome B. Taxy, MD
Aliya N. Husain, MD
Anthony G. Montag, MD

CONTRIBUTORS

Adriana Acurio, MD
Fellow
Section of Surgical Pathology
University of Chicago Medical
    Center
Chicago, Illinois

Ilyssa O. Gordon, MD, PhD
Pulmonary Pathology Fellow
University of Chicago Medical
    Center
Chicago, Illinois

John Hart, MD
Professor
Sections of Surgical Pathology and
    Hepatology
University of Chicago Medical
    Center
Chicago, Illinois

Kelly A. Dakin Haché, MD, PhD
Fellow, Bone and Soft Tissue
    Pathology
University of Chicago Medical
    Center
    and
Department of Pathology
Queen Elizabeth II Health Sciences
    Centre
Halifax, Nova Scotia, Canada

Kimmo J. Hatanpaa, MD, PhD
Assistant Professor of Pathology
Division of Neuropathology
The University of Texas Southwestern
    Medical School
Dallas, Texas

Aliya N. Husain, MD
Professor
Department of Pathology
University of Chicago Medical Center
Chicago, Illinois

Christopher Kinonen, MD
Department of Pathology
Rush University Medical Center
Chicago, Illinois

Anthony G. Montag, MD
Professor
Departments of Pathology and
    Surgery
University of Chicago Medical Center
Chicago, Illinois

Amy Noffsinger, MD
Professor
Section of Surgical Pathology
University of Chicago Medical Center
Chicago, Illinois

Rish K. Pai, MD, PhD
Fellow, Gastrointestinal Pathology
University of Chicago Medical Center
    and
Assistant Professor
Department of Pathology
Washington University
St. Louis, Missouri

Ajit Paintal, MD
Department of Pathology
University of Chicago Medical Center
Chicago, Illinois

Jack Raisanen, MD
Associate Professor of Pathology
Division of Neuropathology
The University of Texas Southwestern
  Medical School
Dallas, Texas

Vijaya B. Reddy, MD
Professor, Department of Pathology
Rush University Medical Center
Chicago, Illinois

Kimiko Suzue, MD, PhD
Pulmonary Pathology Fellow
University of Chicago Medical Center
Chicago, Illinois

Jerome B. Taxy, MD
Professor
Department of Pathology
University of Chicago Medical Center
Chicago, Illinois

Charles L. White III, MD
Professor of Pathology
Director, Division of Neuropathology
The University of Texas Southwestern
  Medical School
Dallas, Texas

Rebecca Wilcox, MD
Fellow, Gastrointestinal and Liver
  Pathology
University of Chicago Medical
  Center
Chicago, Illinois
    and
Assistant Professor
Department of Pathology
University of Vermont
Burlington, Vermont

BIOPSY INTERPRETATION:
THE FROZEN SECTION

1

THE FROZEN SECTION: HISTORICAL BACKGROUND AND QUALITY ASSURANCE

ANTHONY G. MONTAG

HISTORY OF THE FROZEN SECTION

The history of the frozen section as intraoperative consultation is intertwined with the development of pathology as a clinical specialty. Prior to the late 19th century, pathology, or pathologic anatomy, was an exercise in the gross correlation of premortem symptoms and physical examination with postmortem findings. As pathology developed into a distinct specialty in the late 19th century, its focus was largely research oriented; the correlation of pathologic findings to clinical disease continued to be carried out by practicing clinicians, predominantly surgeons, well into the 20th century. The frozen section served a pivotal role in bringing microscopy into the clinical practice of medicine and the pathologist into the clinical management of patients.

Although autopsies were performed by ancient Greek and Egyptian physicians, the father of pathologic anatomy is regarded to be Giovanni Morgagni, who published his treatise, *The Seats and Causes of Disease*, in 1761, detailing clinical and gross pathological correlation of 700 autopsies (1). Morgagni correlated his autopsy findings with the clinical impressions of Antonio Valsalva, his physician collaborator, and recognized the association of clinical symptoms with a specific organ, such as jaundice with abnormalities of the liver. His treatise argued against the humoral theory of disease, which had been dominant since Galen.

The French morbid anatomist Marie Francois Xavier Bichat published *Treatise on Membranes in General and on Various Membranes in Particular* in 1800, followed in 1801 by *Physiological Researches on Life and Death* (2). Bichat realized that organs were themselves complex structures composed of tissues, or membranes, and described 21 separate types, including cartilage, fibrous tissue, serous membrane, glands, and hair. This reductionist approach to anatomy, breaking an organ into tissue components, led Bichat to be considered as the father of histology.

Ironically, his observations were made using only a hand lens; the microscopes available in the late 18th century had poor resolution and were regarded as unreliable novelties by most anatomists.

Pathology as an independent specialty of medicine has its origins in Vienna with Karl Rokitansky, who founded the first institute for pathology, and is said to have supervised 70,000 autopsies and performed 30,000 autopsies (3). Between 1842 and 1846, Rokitansky published his treatise *General Pathologic Anatomy*, putting forth a general classification of diseases, including blood dyscrasias, new growths, and congenital abnormalities. Rokitansky also made little use of the microscope, although he did publish one treatise with the help of microscopy: *On Connective Tissue Tumors of the Nervous System*.

Rudolf Virchow, Rokitansky's pupil working at the Charity Hospital in Berlin, popularized microscopy in the study of pathology and is regarded as the father of modern pathology (4). Virchow realized that at a more fundamental level cells, rather than Bichat's tissues, were the probable root of disease. In 1858, he published *Cellular Pathology as Based Upon Physiological and Pathological Histology*, which was widely accepted and established microscopic anatomy as integral to the understanding of pathology and medicine. His other major contribution was to refute the tenet of spontaneous generation of cells from inanimate material, which still lingered in the cell theory published in 1839 by Theodor Schwann and Matthias Schleiden. Virchow asserted "Omnis cellula e cellula," or that all cells come from cells. Ironically, in spite of the rise of cellular pathology as a concept, Virchow was primarily an experimental and autopsy pathologist, and the diagnosis of disease on living patients continued to be based on clinical impression and gross features as judged by the surgeon (5). Only rare attempts at diagnosis from a tumor fragment or biopsy had been attempted, and Virchow had his own reasons to be reluctant about the reliability of biopsy as a diagnostic technique. One of Virchow's first attempts at biopsy diagnosis occurred in 1887 on specimens from the German Emperor Frederick III, who had developed a laryngeal mass. Virchow rendered a benign diagnosis, however, Frederick died the following year from laryngeal carcinoma (6). Although the lesion was probably inoperable at the time of biopsy, Frederick's death led to the ascension of the more militaristic Wilhelm II, and may have contributed to the development of World War I. More directly, there was a lingering distrust of the technique of microscopic evaluation of biopsy specimens, which resulted in reluctance and disinterest in using microscopic pathology to direct the care of living patients.

Several technical developments in the field of microscopy in the latter half of the 19th century led to its adoption as a reliable technique (3). The microscope itself was improved with the introduction of achromatic and apochromatic lenses to correct distortion and by the invention of the substage condenser and oil immersion lens by Ernest Abbe. Consequently, German microscope manufacturers became the leaders in microscopy, and high-quality instruments were readily available. Histochemical stains from natural dyes were introduced in the mid-1800s, but the development of the aniline dye industry in Germany led to the introduction of many new stains between 1870 and 1900, including methylene blue, Gram, Congo red, and Mallory trichrome stains (7). Microtomes, including freezing microtomes, were introduced by the 1870s, and the introduction of formalin fixation and wax embedding led to more uniform histology.

Surgical practice also underwent a revolution in the late 19th century. In 1846, the first public demonstration of anesthesia using ether was carried out at the Massachusetts General Hospital. Oliver Wendell Holmes published his treatise on puerperal fever in 1847, establishing that it was frequently carried by the obstetrician from patient to patient, and called for more sanitation in hospitals and in the operating room. In 1867, Joseph Lister published on antisepsis, and proposed hand washing, gloves, and the use of carbolic acid. The result was that surgery became less painful, and the patient was more likely to survive. It also gave the surgeon the luxury of time, to better define the disease, and to tailor an operation that would not have been possible with a writhing patient.

By the end of the 19th century, all the elements were in place for surgical pathology to emerge as a clinical specialty, yet the use of biopsy to make a definitive diagnosis before surgery was seldom done. Pathology emerged as an academic pursuit, using microscopy to correlate gross and microscopic findings with clinical history and to classify disease, however in most cases only on autopsy or material from definitive surgeries. For most surgical cases, clinicopathologic evaluation was performed by the surgeon, often by gross examination only. This practice was reinforced by the tradition of academic surgeons spending a year or two in pathology departments in Europe, virtually none of which were handling biopsy material and most of which were grounded in autopsy pathology and experimental pathology. This dichotomy continued in academic centers past the middle of the 20th century with the tradition of having a separate group of research faculty involved in autopsy pathology. As a consequence, many of the advances in the application of pathology to living patients took place in departments of surgery or gynecology, or in clinically oriented private hospitals and clinics.

William Halsted, Chief of Surgery of the new Johns Hopkins hospital, requested the first intraoperative frozen section be done by the pathologist William Welch in 1891 (8). Welch had studied pathology extensively in Europe and had established the first hospital pathology laboratory in Bellevue Hospital Center, New York, prior to being recruited to Johns Hopkins. Halsted scheduled the frozen section on a suspected breast cancer case, and Welch prepared a slide using a carbon dioxide freezing microtome, but not before Halsted had concluded the case. Subsequently, Thomas Cullen, who had studied in Germany and learned a technique for freezing formalin fixed tissue, published a frozen section method in the Johns Hopkins' bulletin in 1895. The fixation step prior to freezing the tissue block meant the procedure still took nearly an hour to complete.

Although several other rapid frozen section methods were subsequently published in Europe, it is generally accepted that the standard cryostat method used today was first published in *JAMA* in 1905 by Louis Wilson of the Mayo Clinic (9). Wilson used a dextrin solution to embed the tissue and a carbon dioxide freezing microtome. By using methylene blue and reading the slides without permanent mounting the technique could be performed in a few minutes as opposed to an hour for Cullen's method. This method rapidly became a routine at the Mayo Clinic, and was adopted by other clinical centers. Most centers today include a brief fixation prior to staining in hematoxylin and eosin, followed by permanent mounting, but the essential technique is largely unchanged (10).

Unfortunately, standard textbooks of pathology in the early 20th century continued to feel that the rapid frozen section technique was unreliable, and the technique was not widely adopted until after the late 1920s. In many academic centers, pathologists continued to regard diagnostic pathology as outside the interest of the pathology department. The American Society of Clinical Pathology was formed in 1922 to elevate the status of the pathologist as a physician who provided clinical services for live patients, and the frozen section consultation was one of the first services promoted by the organization (11,12).

A strong proponent of the frozen section was Dr Joseph Bloodgood, a surgeon at Johns Hopkins. Prior to the 1920s, he had been skeptical of the frozen section technique, believing that an experienced surgeon could recognize the nature of a tumor with the naked eye (13). Beginning in 1927, Bloodgood began a campaign to promote the frozen section as a medical standard (14). He submitted editorials to major regional medical journals and, in an editorial in *JAMA* in 1927, extended the invitation to surgeons and pathologists to visit the laboratory at Johns Hopkins. Several times a year, approximately 40 people a day attended seminars on the technique. In a 1929 editorial, Bloodgood hinted that a growing public enlightenment required that the diagnosis of cancer be made on a frozen section. He also recognized the need to specifically train pathologists for diagnostic microscopy, stating "There is a greater demand today for pathologists . . . than for operators."

The acceptance of the frozen section as a diagnostic tool in the setting of a one-step surgical procedure eventually led to the acceptance of biopsy techniques to allow a presurgical diagnosis. Although today performed only on a small percentage of all surgical cases and representing a small fraction of the typical pathology laboratory's activity, the frozen section played a pivotal role in the acceptance of microscopy in the clinical management of patients and the development of modern surgical pathology.

INDICATIONS FOR FROZEN SECTION

Intraoperative consults, with or without frozen section, should be limited to the following indications (15,16):

1. Provide a diagnosis that will allow the surgeon to make an intraoperative decision regarding further surgery during that operative event. For example, a benign ovarian tumor requires no additional staging as opposed to a malignant ovarian tumor.
2. Assess margins when additional excision to attain a negative margin is an option.
3. Assess adequacy of diagnostic tissue in a biopsy specimen from an open or complicated procedure. For example, a bone biopsy in the operating room may yield only reactive bone, and a second biopsy procedure may be avoided with the frozen section.
4. Plan the workup of the specimen. The need for cytogenetics, flow cytometry, and other special studies should reasonably be evaluated prior to fixation. Tissue for protocols or banking may need to be sampled.
5. Plan for resources. Scheduling of operating room time for definitive procedure pending permanents may require faster diagnosis. For example, placement of chemotherapy catheters during initial biopsy if the diagnosis is malignant, instead of a second anesthesia.

A CAP Q-probe study evaluated 9,164 cases with intraoperative frozen section from 472 institutions for indications (17). Surgeons at the participating institution cooperated in completing questionnaires as to the rationale behind their request for a frozen section consultation. The study found the most common indications were to establish diagnosis to determine type of surgery (51%), confirm adequacy of margins (16%), plan further studies or workup (10%), allow the surgeon to inform the patient of the diagnosis (8%), confirm adequacy of tissue (8%), abate surgeon's curiosity (3%), plan resources (3%), and establish academic protocol (1%). The findings suggest that approximately 10% of frozen sections are done for illegitimate reasons. Another Q probe found that frozen sections were requested in 5.7% of all surgical procedures (18). The frozen section rate was proportional to institutional size, with a 15% rate in hospitals with more than 600 beds. This probably reflects increased complexity of cases at large tertiary centers.

Illegitimate reasons for requesting a frozen section include the following:

1. *Curiosity.* Some frozen sections are requested entirely out of curiosity. The author has personally been requested to perform a frozen section on a "pelvic lesion" specimen, which proved to be seminal vesicle. The surgeon indicated that there was a wager as to whether the pathologist would recognize the normal organ.
2. *Preliminary report to family in the recovery room.* It should be emphasized that because of sampling and technical issues, the diagnosis can only be preliminary, and that any change in diagnosis will be the responsibility of the surgeon to explain.
3. *Surgeon's habit.* Some surgeons perform exactly the same surgery regardless of the outcome of the frozen section.

Obviously there are times when, based on these considerations, a frozen section should be refused, albeit after a conversation with the clinician. Other important considerations that might lead to refusal of a request for frozen section include the following:

1. When the specimen is for primary diagnosis, represents the entire available sample of the lesion, and it is not possible to leave anything nonfrozen for permanent sections. This especially applies to pigmented skin lesions.
2. When the entire specimen appears uniform and grossly benign, for example, a serous cyst, and a frozen section to inspect for subtle microscopic disease would be taken entirely at random.
3. The specimen has a high likelihood of having an infectious agent such as tuberculosis and there are insufficient back-up cryostats to allow one to be decontaminated during the workday.

The Mayo Clinic is perhaps unique in that nearly all operative cases receive a diagnosis rendered entirely by frozen section. In a review of 1 year's experience, Ferreiro et al. reported 24,880 cases with frozen section analysis at the Mayo Clinic (19). By contrast, the percentage of cases undergoing frozen section at most laboratories is nearer to the 5.6% rate reported in a Cap Q-probe study (20). The Mayo Clinic experience includes many intraoperative consultations on cases that would not be considered eligible for frozen section at nearly any other pathology laboratory. For this reason, data regarding frozen section performance and quality assurance from the Mayo clinic cannot be compared to data from other institutions or CAP Q probes (21).

QUALITY ASSURANCE INDICATORS IN FROZEN SECTION

The College of American Pathologists includes standards for the performance of intraoperative frozen sections. The CAP standards are frequently updated. The following discussion is based on the most recent standards (22,23).

General Considerations

Specimens for frozen section are subject to all the CAP standards for specimen identification in the surgical pathology gross room. Particularly when multiple cases for frozen section are handled simultaneously, the risk of switching specimens or introducing cross-contamination is increased. In general, only one frozen section case should occupy each grossing area. Frozen section blocks typically bear no attached accession information while being cut, and a system for identifying the block and slides should be established. One practice is to have a labeled cassette in the cryostat to act as a cradle for the frozen chuck when it is removed from the microtome. Slides should be labeled prior to cutting the sections and if not used, discarded. Unlabeled slides should never be used. In our own laboratory, each frozen section specimen is assigned a unique color for the slide label, cassette, and mounting media during accessioning to reduce the chance of identification errors.

The frozen section slides must be permanently mounted and retained in the archive with the permanent sections from the case. The frozen section block must be processed to a paraffin block and permanent sections produced for correlation with the actual cryostat sections. This is an essential quality assurance tool for the evaluation of discrepancies between frozen and permanent sections. It is also a useful teaching tool for recognizing artifacts and sampling issues in frozen section. Occasionally, the actual frozen section block may be saved frozen for molecular or other studies. This is allowable if there is a policy specifying the types of specimens or situations for which permanent section follow-up may be omitted.

The cryostat must be periodically cleaned and the interior wiped down with 70% alcohol. In most cases this is done once a day, but if the cryostat is used frequently, it is advisable to clean out shavings more frequently to avoid cross-contamination between specimens. Cryostats in daily use should be thawed weekly and decontaminated with a tuberculocidal disinfectant. Less frequently used machines can be decontaminated on a longer cycle. A written procedure and schedule should be followed and documentation of maintenance kept for each cryostat. If a frozen section is performed on tissue from a patient known or suspected to be positive for tuberculosis, hepatitis B or C, human immunodeficiency virus—related disease, or prion disease such as Creutzfeldt-Jakob, the cryostat must be decontaminated before further use.

Several CAP requirements deal with the documentation and transmission of the intraoperative report. Intraoperative consultations must be documented in writing and signed by the pathologist who made the diagnosis. If a verbal report is given, it should correspond to the written documentation and should be given directly to the surgeon, not through an intermediary. Any additional clinical information acquired during the verbal report should be documented on the written report if it influenced the final diagnosis. When a verbal report is given, a routine identification check should be made to confirm that the information is being relayed to the correct surgeon on the correct patient. The intraoperative consultation must be made part of the final surgical pathology report, including the name of the pathologist who rendered the intraoperative diagnosis.

Frozen Section Turnaround Time

The CAP standard for frozen section turnaround time states that 90% of cases should have slides prepared within 15 minutes of receipt of the specimen and the interpretation communicated within 20 minutes of receipt of the specimen. Although CAP requires frozen section turnaround monitoring, it does not specify what percentage of frozen sections must be sampled, or how frequently the sampling should be done. Some pathology computer systems now include a time stamp for receipt and completion of frozen section consultation, which would allow for capture of nearly all cases. However a smaller and less frequent sampling is acceptable if the monitoring procedure is defined, followed, and the results documented, evaluated, and tracked for changes and opportunities for improvement.

The CAP turnaround time standard specifically does not include the transport time prior to receipt of the specimen by the laboratory. Obviously the clinician's impression of the actual timeliness of service may be dependent on transportation factors rather than laboratory performance. The standard also allows exclusion of cases where multiple sequential studies are performed on a single specimen, such as margins. Complex cases requiring additional studies or correlation, for example, examination of radiographs or extensive intradepartmental consultation, can also be excluded from the analysis (24). CAP specifies that if the 90% standard for completion of frozen sections is not met, an analysis of the outliers should be made to ascertain the reason for noncompliance. In practice, our laboratory tracks all frozen sections with a time stamp, and the pathologist of record may indicate if there is a reason for an exclusion from the turnaround time standard. Monthly performance is tracked including percentage of cases with exclusions, number of cases eligible for analysis, and, of those, the percentage, which have met the standard.

Frozen Section Error Rate

CAP requires that frozen sections be compared to the permanent diagnosis and discordance noted and reconciled. This exercise provides the opportunity to track performance over time and identify problem areas and opportunities for improvement (25). The possible sources of discrepancy are as follows:

1. Technical issues
   a. The tissue was difficult to cut; technical problems with mounting or staining, mechanical issues with the cryostat.
2. Sampling error
   a. The lesion is present on permanents of the frozen block, but was not present in the actual cryostat section.
      i. Was the block adequately faced and leveled?
   b. The lesion was not present in the block frozen, but is present in other samples from the submitted specimen.
      i. Was the lesion appropriately sampled?
3. Diagnostic error
   a. Disease process missed, for example, metastasis to a lymph node.
   b. Disease process recognized, but misclassified.
      i. No effect on management.
      ii. Effect on management.
4. Errors in communication of diagnosis

The most recent CAP frozen-section Q probe excluded certain types of discordant cases from analysis (26). These included the following:

1. Discordance in type of carcinoma when it has no effect on management, for example, small cell carcinoma versus non–small cell carcinoma affects operative management, while the diagnosis of squamous cell carcinoma versus adenocarcinoma does not.
2. Discordance in degree of differentiation when it has no effect on management.
3. Discordance in the grade of dysplasia or carcinoma in situ.
4. Discordance in breast biopsy or excision where an area is frozen for calcifications, with no gross lesion.
5. Discordance in well-circumscribed follicular lesions of the thyroid.
6. Frozen sections of breast or other organs undertaken to assess the adequacy of tissue for estrogen and progesterone binding proteins.
7. Discordance in the evaluation of tumor margins when the block is cut en face.

These categories recognize the limitations of frozen section in analyzing certain specimens with a limited sampling and with the artifact inherent in frozen sections. The grading of dysplasia in skin or mucosa section is particularly difficult. The practice of freezing small or mammographically detected breast lesions to confirm diagnostic material for radioimmunoassay of estrogen and progesterone receptors has been supplanted by immunohistochemistry and should be discouraged.

Given limited sampling, frequent paucity of clinical information, and the various artifacts introduced by the freezing process, the frozen section technique is remarkably accurate. A 1991 College of American Pathologist Q-probe study found 4.2% deferral of diagnosis rate and discordance with permanent diagnosis of 1.7%. Major sources of discordance were gross tissue sampling (44.8%), misinterpretation (40%), and sectioning (12.7%). Only 2.5% of discrepancies were felt to have a major impact on patient management. A subsequent Q probe found 1.42% discordance rate, with gross tissue sampling (31.4%), misinterpretation (31.8%), and the presence of diagnostic tissue in the permanents of the frozen block which was not present in the original frozen sections (30%) as major contributors to error (17). Sampling, either of the gross specimen or microscopically by insufficient leveling of the block, accounts for approximately two-thirds of frozen section discrepancy. Diagnostic error at frozen section accounts for less than a third of cases, amounting to a rate of less than 0.5%.

Sources of Discordance in Frozen Sections

The most frequent anatomic sites with discordant frozen section diagnoses in the CAP Q-probe series are skin (17.1%), breast (16%), gynecologic sites (10.2%), lymph nodes for metastases (10%), thyroid (6.1%), lung/mediastinum (5.3%), and gastrointestinal tract (5.2%). The most common source of discordant diagnosis was the false-negative diagnosis of tumor (67.8%) as compared to the 11% false-positive diagnosis rate. Obviously, the actual risk of a discordant diagnosis by anatomic site depends on the volume of cases from that site, and this denominator is not provided in the CAP Q-probe data. The limited sampling done during the frozen section procedure is particularly problematic for large heterogenous tumors such as soft tissue and ovarian tumors. For ovarian mucinous tumors, the predictive value of the frozen section diagnosis is 99% for malignant, 95% for benign, and 65% for borderline lesions (27). Poor technical quality of the prepared slides was cited as a factor in 3% to 5% of cases in Cap Q-probe data. Interestingly, lack of adequate clinical history was cited as a contributing factor in nearly 15% of discrepancies from hospitals with less than 150 beds as opposed to less than 5% of hospitals with more than 450 beds (18).

The frozen section technique played a critical role in the development of diagnostic histopathology in the 19th century and the acceptance of surgical pathology as a specialty in the 20th century. The technique is remarkably accurate when technical and sampling limitations are considered. Frozen section and permanent material should be compared and sources of discordance tracked. The average rate of diagnostic error in published series is less than 0.5%.

REFERENCES

1. Morgagni GB. *The Seats and Causes of Diseases Investigated by Anatomy*. London: A Millar & T Cadell; 1769.
2. Williams HS. *The Story of Nineteenth-Century Science*. New York: Harper and Brothers; 1904.
3. Gal AA. In search of the origins of modern surgical pathology. *Adv Anat Pathol*. 2001;8(1):1–13.
4. Byers JM. Rudolph Virchow-father of cellular pathology. *Am J Clin Pathol*. 1989; 92(suppl):S2–S8.
5. Rather LJ. Rudolph Virchow's views on pathology, pathologic anatomy, and cellular pathology. *Arch Pathol*. 1966;82:197–204.
6. Lin JI. Virchow's pathologic reports on Frederick III's cancer. *N Engl J Med*. 1984; 311(19):1261–1264.
7. Titford M. George Grubler and Karl Hollborn: two founders of the biological stain industry. *J Histotechnology*. 1993;16(2):155–158.
8. Carter D. Surgical pathology at Johns Hopkins. In: Rosai J, ed. *The History of American Surgical Pathology*. Washington, DC: American Registry of Pathology; 1997.
9. Wilson LB. A method for the rapid preparation of fresh tissue for the microscope. *JAMA*. 1905;45:1737.
10. Gal AA, Cagle PT. The 100 year anniversary of the description of the frozen section procedure. *JAMA*. 2005;294(24):3135–3137.
11. Wright JR. The development of the frozen section technique, the evolution of surgical biopsy, and the origins of surgical pathology. *Bull Hist Med*. 1985;59:295–326.
12. Fechner RE. The birth and evolution of American surgical pathology. In: Rosai J, ed. *Guiding the Surgeon's Hand: The History of American Surgical Pathology*. Washington, DC: AFIP; 1997.
13. Bloodgood JC. The relation of surgical pathology to surgical diagnosis. *Detroit Med J*. 1904;3:337–352.
14. Bloodgood JC. When cancer becomes a microscopic disease, there must be tissue diagnosis in the O.R. *JAMA*. 1927;88:1022–1023.

15. Ackerman LV, Ramirez GA. The indications for and limitations of frozen-section diagnosis. *Br J Surg.* 1959;46:336–350.

16. Horn RC. What can be expected of the surgical pathologist from frozen-section examination. *Surg Clin North Am.* 1962;42:443–454.

17. Zarbo RJ et al.; and College of American Pathologists/Centers for Disease Control and Prevention Outcomes Working Group Study. Indications and immediate patient outcomes of pathology intraoperative consultations. *Arch Pathol Lab Med.* 1996;120(1): 19–25.

18. Zarbo RJ, Hoffman GG, Howanitz PJ. Inter-institutional comparison of frozen-section consultation: a College of American Pathologists Q-Probe study of 79,647 consultations in 297 North American institutions. *Arch Pathol Lab Med.* 1991;115:1187–1194.

19. Ferreiro JA, Meyers JL, Bostwick DG. Accuracy of frozen section diagnosis in surgical pathology: review of a 1 year experience with 24,880 cases at Mayo clinic Rochester. *Mayo Clinic Proc.* 1995;70(12):1137–1141.

20. Zarbo RJ, Hoffmann GG, Howanitz PJ. Interinstitutional comparison of frozen-section consultation. A college of American Pathologist Q probe study of 79,647 consultations in 297 North American institutions. *Arch Pathol Lab Med.* 1991;116(12):1187–1194.

21. Page DL, Gray GL. Intraoperative consultations by pathologists at the Mayo Clinic: an unusual experience. *Mayo Clinic Proc.* 1995;70:1222–1223.

22. College of American Pathologists. *Laboratory Accreditation Checklist: Anatomic Pathology.* Northfield, IL: College of American Pathologists; 2007.

23. Rickert RR. Quality assurance goals in surgical pathology. *Arch Pathol Lab Med.* 1990;114:1157–1162.

24. Novis DA, Zarbo RJ. Interinstitutional comparison of frozen section turnaround time. A college of American Pathologists Q probe study of 32868 frozen sections in 700 hospitals. *Arch Pathol.* 1997;121(6):559–567.

25. Raab SS, Tworek JA, Soures R, et al. The value of monitoring frozen section-permanent section correlation data over time. *Arch Pathol.* 2006;130:337–342.

26. Novis DA, Gebhardt GN, Zarbo RJ. College of American Pathologists, Interinstitutional comparisons of frozen section consultation in small hospitals: a College of American Pathologists Q probes study of 18,532 frozen section consultation diagnoses in 233 small hospitals. *Arch Pathol Lab Med.* 1996;120(12):1087–1093.

27. Rose PG, Rubin RB, Nelson BE, et al. Accuracy of frozen section (intraoperative consultation) diagnosis of ovarian tumors. *Am J Obstet Gynecol.* 1994;171(3):823–826.

2

BONE AND SOFT TISSUE

KELLY A. DAKIN HACHÉ AND ANTHONY G. MONTAG

INTRODUCTION

The relative rarity of bone lesions, especially tumors, makes requests for frozen section uncommon. Surgical pathologists may feel uncomfortable in assessing these lesions intraoperatively if major treatment decisions are to be made. It may even occur to pathologists that such requests are unreasonable. However, the recent clinical advances in limb-sparing sarcoma management have created a rationale for intraoperative assessment. The differential diagnosis of bone lesions is considered from clinical, radiological, and pathological perspectives, and a number of cases are provided to illustrate common diagnostic problems and pitfalls.

Most bone lesions have typical clinical presentations and classical radiological features. The pathologist who is able to correlate this information with the morphologic features will avoid making errors in pathological diagnosis by frozen section. If the clinical, radiological, and pathological impressions are concordant, then the pathologist can be reasonably reassured that the diagnosis is correct. However, if any of the three factors is discordant, the diagnosis should be deferred until a permanent section is obtained. It is important to emphasize that the treatment algorithm in the limb salvage era is somewhat backward to what would be ordinarily anticipated:

1. A diagnosis of malignancy made from a frozen section will result in closing of the wound to await permanent sections and confirmation of the diagnosis. After appropriate staging, the definitive limb salvage resection will be preceded by neoadjuvant therapy. If the permanent section and evaluation of nonfrozen tissue reveals a benign diagnosis, the lesion will be reexplored, curetted, and packed with cement or bone chips. The error and possible embarrassment to the pathologist aside, the patient will require a second procedure and the final clinical outcome will be a good one for the patient (1).
2. A benign diagnosis allows the surgeon to curette and pack the lesion directly. If the lesion is in fact benign, then the therapy is complete. If, however, the final interpretation of the frozen and nonfrozen tissue is that the lesion is malignant, then the surgical site has been contaminated and is unsuitable for limb salvage operation. A local recurrence rate of

83% in erroneously diagnosed osteosarcoma treated by limb salvage operation suggests that the patient will require an amputation (2).

Therefore, in conducting intraoperative consultations and analyzing frozen sections for bone lesions, especially tumors, the message for the pathologist is a conservative one. With experience, definitive diagnoses and appropriate treatment can be instituted. However, under any circumstances, if there is a diagnostic question, the interpretation should be deferred for definitive evaluation.

CLINICAL INFORMATION

Most patients with bone lesions present in a characteristic age range of 2 to 3 decades, which can quickly narrow down the clinical differential diagnosis (3) (e-Fig. 2.1). Both chondroblastoma and giant cell tumor occur in younger individuals; but chondroblastoma typically occurs prior to or near the time of epiphyseal closure in the teenage years, while giant cell tumor tends to occur later. Osteosarcoma is the most common malignant bone tumor that occurs in childhood, but it also occurs in older patients.

A history of sickle cell anemia or other potential cause of bone infarct raises the possibility of malignant fibrous histiocytoma of bone. A history of Paget's disease of bone or prior radiation therapy to the region raises the possibility of secondary sarcoma.

A previous history of non-osseous malignancy is particularly helpful. Metastatic lesions to bone are far more common than primary bone lesions: 10% to 15% of patients with metastases of unknown primary tumors present with bone lesions (4) and up to 30% of skeletal metastases constitute the first clinical evidence of a malignancy. As a general rule, any poorly marginated lytic bone lesion in a patient older than 40 years should be suspected to be a metastasis until proven otherwise.

Bone ranks number three (behind lung and liver) as one of the most common sites of clinical metastasis. In autopsy studies, it is the most frequent site of metastasis; up to 60% of patients who die of carcinoma are found to have bone metastases (5). The most common malignancies that metastasize to bone are lung, breast, prostate, kidney, and thyroid malignancies. Although metastases are very uncommon in children, lesions that do metastasize to bone in this population include neuroblastoma, rhabdomyosarcoma, and clear cell sarcoma of the kidney. Metastatic lesions frequently undergo internal fixation, and frozen section confirmation is recommended to avoid the placement of hardware in a primary bone tumor, which results in the loss of the limb in the limb salvage management option.

Fractures may complicate benign or malignant bone tumors, metastases, or may be entirely traumatic in origin but mimic a tumor radiographically. Benign tumors in the small bones of the hand are particularly prone to pathologic fractures (6). Pathologic fractures are uncommon in children, but most frequently occur in association with unicameral bone

TABLE 2.1 Stages of Fracture Maturation	
Days After Fracture	**Feature**
<3 days	Hemorrhage, edema, tissue necrosis
3–7 days	Reactive myofibroblasts, tissue culture appearance
7–10 days	Increasing cellularity, early wisps of osteoid
>10 days	Osteoid and cartilage matrix
2–3 weeks	Osteoblast rimming, broad seams of osteoid

cyst, non-ossifying fibroma, fibrous dysplasia, aneurysmal bone cyst (ABC), osteosarcoma, and Ewing's sarcoma (7–9). In an adult older than 40 years, pathologic fracture should always raise the suspicion of metastasis. Care must be taken not to interpret fracture callus as a malignant neoplasm (10). Fracture callus can present with many of the elements of osteosarcoma including sheets of large osteoblasts, mitotic activity, woven bone, immature cartilage matrix, and cellular fibroblastic proliferation (e-Fig. 2.2A–E). Table 2.1 indicates the morphologic stages of a healing fracture. A comparison of histologic fracture with osteosarcoma is given in e-Figure 2.3. The overall zonal architecture, progressive maturation, broad woven bone trabeculae, and osteoblast rimming are important histologic clues that the lesion is a fracture.

In general, most symptomatic bone lesions present with pain. Cartilaginous tumors of the long bones which present with pain are more likely to be chondrosarcoma, whereas enchondromas are typically asymptomatic. A history of penetrating wound, immunosuppression, sickle cell disease, or previous sepsis raises the possibility of osteomyelitis, which nearly always presents with an elevated sedimentation rate and usually with an elevated C-reactive protein (11). While primary bone tumors are most often solitary, multifocality often indicates a congenital or syndromic condition or metastatic disease (Table 2.2).

TABLE 2.2 Differential Diagnosis of Multifocal Bone Lesions	
Benign	**Malignant**
Vascular lesions	Multiple myeloma
Langerhans cell histiocytosis	Metastases
Fibrous dysplasia	Lymphoma
Enchondromatosis (Ollier and Maffucci)	Hemangioendothelioma/angiosarcoma
Hereditary multiple exostosis	
Paget's disease	

RADIOGRAPHIC IMPRESSION

The radiograph is the gross impression for a bone biopsy, and at the time of frozen section analysis, it is advisable to review the radiograph along with the clinician or at least have the interpretation of a musculoskeletal radiologist available. The radiographic features allow formulation of a differential diagnosis based on the area of the skeleton (extremities, axial, craniofacial), the anatomic location within the bone (epiphyseal, metaphyseal, diaphysial), and the position within the bone (central, eccentric, cortical, juxtacortical) (12). Many of the bone lesions that occur in the extremities have a predilection for characteristics sites (Table 2.3); for example, giant cell tumors occur mostly around the knee, enchondromas are common in the bones of the hands and feet, and adamantinoma nearly always occurs in the tibia.

In general, a slow-growing bone lesion will display an abrupt margin of transition with the surrounding bone, usually with a rim of sclerotic

TABLE 2.3 Extremity Bone Lesions by Location		
Epiphysis	**Metaphysis**	**Diaphysis**
Chondroblastoma	**Eccentric/cortical**	**Cortical**
Giant cell tumor	Non-ossifying fibroma	Osteofibrous dysplasia
Clear cell chondrosarcoma	Chondromyxoid fibroma	Adamantinoma
	Central	Osteoid osteoma
	Nearly anything	Metastatic renal cell carcinoma
		Central
		Fibrous dysplasia
		Non-ossifying fibroma
		Epithelioid hemangioma
		Chondrosarcoma
		Osteosarcoma
		Angiosarcoma
		Medullary/permeative
		Ewing's sarcoma
		Lymphoma
		Langerhans cell histiocytosis
		Myeloma
		Metastasis
		Infection

host bone. Malignant lesions are more likely to have an indistinct transition and a "moth-eaten" appearance, while lacking a rim of sclerosis.

Cortical destruction and periosteal extension are characteristic of malignant tumors. The infiltration of the periosteal tissues is associated with thickening and elevation of the periosteum and, when associated with mineralization, appears as Codman triangle. Expansile tumors such as giant cell tumor and ABC may markedly distort the cortex, but usually retain a thin shell. Soft-tissue extension is frequently difficult to see on a standard radiograph, but is more easily seen on CT or MRI scans.

The pattern of mineralization also gives clues for tumor diagnosis. Benign bone-forming tumors tend to have a uniform distribution of osteoid matrix, while osteosarcoma tends to be less homogenous. Fibrous dysplasia has a "ground-glass" appearance on radiographs because of the numerous and fairly evenly spaced bone spicules. Enchondromas tend to have ossification and calcification at the edge of lobules, and they usually present a pattern of interlacing arcs of matrix on radiographs.

During definitive excision, the marrow at the bony margin is frozen or subjected to imprint preparations so as to assess the presence of tumor. The marrow in long bones is usually fatty; however, use of colony-stimulating factors during chemotherapy may result in a disconcertingly hypercellular marrow. The MRI is extremely accurate and helpful in evaluating the extent of marrow involvement (13), and in practice, at our institution we have not seen a positive marrow margin on frozen section for more than a decade.

IMPORTANT DIFFERENTIALS THROUGH CASE STUDIES

Epiphyseal Lesions

A 16-year-old adolescent boy presented with knee pain 6 weeks after an athletic injury. Imaging showed a well-delineated, lytic, and partially cystic lesion with variable calcification involving the epiphysis of the distal femur (Fig. 2.1). An imprint of a curetted specimen demonstrated polygonal, mononuclear cells, mildly atypical in appearance with nuclear folds (Fig. 2.2). The frozen section showed a "chicken-wire" pattern of calcification of the matrix (Fig. 2.3) and mononuclear stromal cells with scattered osteoclastlike giant cells (Fig. 2.4). These features are diagnostic of chondroblastoma and are consistent with the clinical and radiographic features. The differential diagnosis of an epiphyseal lesion includes chondroblastoma, giant cell tumor, and clear cell chondrosarcoma. Chondroblastoma occurs in a younger age group, typically before the closure of the epiphysis, and has a characteristic matrix. The giant cell tumor typically has a diffuse distribution of giant cells (e-Fig. 2.4), but this feature can also be seen in areas of chondroblastoma. The nucleus of the

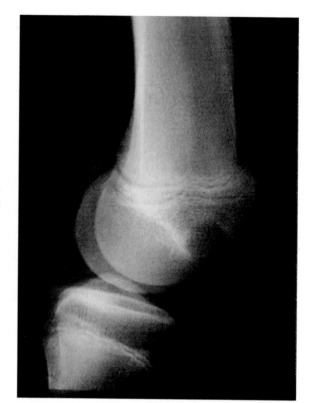

FIGURE 2.1 Radiograph displays an epiphyseal lesion with mineralization.

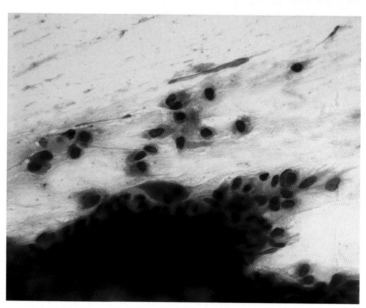

FIGURE 2.2 Touch preparation revealing hyperchromatic folded nuclei and osteoclastlike giant cells.

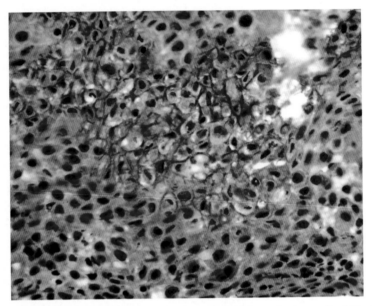

FIGURE 2.3 Chondroblastoma frequently displays a chicken-wire type of calcification of the fine chondroid matrix produced by the tumor.

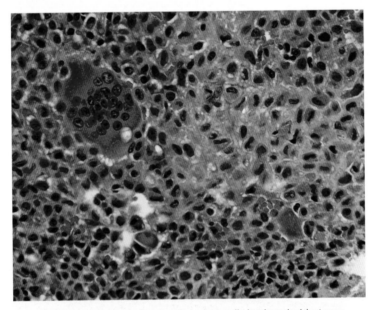

FIGURE 2.4 Chondroblasts and osteoclastlike giant cells in chondroblastoma.

TABLE 2.4	Features of Epiphyseal Lesions		
	Chondroblastoma	Giant Cell Tumor	Clear Cell Chondrosarcoma
Radiology	Epiphyseal, central, usually not expanding the contour of the bone	Epiphyseal, often with metaphyseal involvement, expansile, lytic	Epiphyseal, central, not expansile, but may extend from epiphysis to articular cartilage
Age	10–20 y	20–40 y	20–40 y
Cells	Polygonal	Oval to plump, spindled stromal cells	Abundant clear cytoplasm
Nucleus	Smudgy, notched, atypical looking, but uniform	Oval and similar to giant cell nuclei	Uniform, large, clear blown out chromatin, large nucleoli
Matrix	Cartilage, chicken-wire calcified matrix, pink osteoidlike matrix	Reactive bone at edges or secondary to fracture; no matrix	Loose cartilage matrix with calcification; well-formed spicules of lamellar bone
Giant cells	Scattered to numerous	Usually diffuse and numerous	Scattered

mononuclear stromal cell of chondroblastoma is folded, hyperchromatic, and somewhat atypical in appearance, while the nucleus in the stromal cell of giant cell tumor is similar to that of the giant cells. Well-formed spicules of lamellar bone are characteristic of clear cell chondrosarcoma (e-Fig. 2.5), and the nucleus is large and vesicular. Neither giant cell tumor nor clear cell chondrosarcoma exhibit the characteristic "chicken-wire" pattern of matrix calcification seen in chondroblastoma. The features of the epiphyseal tumors are summarized in Table 2.4.

Expansile Cystic Lesions

A 12-year-old boy presented with a foot drop and a slowly enlarging leg mass, seen radiographically as a solitary lytic, expansile lesion of the proximal fibula without soft-tissue extension (Fig. 2.5). The MRI revealed fluid-fluid levels in the cystic spaces. A frozen section of this lesion demonstrated cystic, blood-filled spaces lacking an endothelial lining with septae composed of fibroblasts, mononuclear cells, hemosiderin, and multinucleated giant cells (Figs. 2.6, 2.7). These are the classic features of an ABC. An ABC may be a primary lesion or may result as secondary degeneration

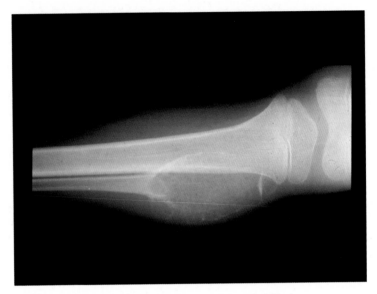

FIGURE 2.5   Radiograph of expansile cystic lesion of proximal fibula.

of another bone tumor, including chondroblastoma, giant cell tumor, and non-ossifying fibroma among others. The most important differential diagnosis of an ABC is illustrated by another 12-year-old boy presenting with knee pain, radiographically represented by a mixed sclerotic and lytic diaphyseal lesion with soft-tissue extension (Fig. 2.8). The frozen section

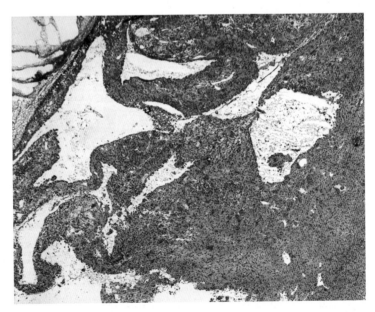

FIGURE 2.6   Low-power examination reveals numerous spaces separated by fibrous webs.

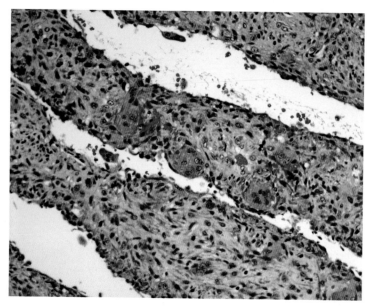

FIGURE 2.7 High power shows mixed fibroblastic and mononuclear population with osteoclastlike giant cells. No atypia is present.

FIGURE 2.8 Radiograph of expansile bone lesion with mineralization and periosteal reaction.

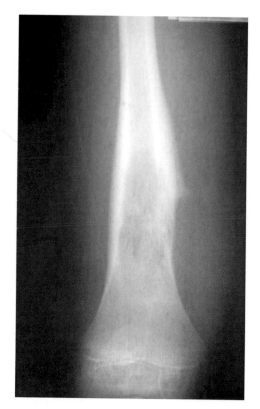

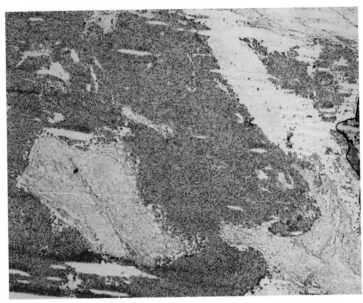

FIGURE 2.9 Low power reveals cystic spaces and cellular septae, consistent with telangiectatic osteosarcoma.

showed blood-filled, cystic spaces associated with dense cellularity and osteoclastlike giant cells, similar to an ABC, but in areas there are obviously malignant stromal cells (Figs. 2.9, 2.10) indicative of telangiectatic osteosarcoma (Table 2.5). The presence of necrosis in the absence of fracture in a cystic lesion of bone is an ominous sign and is highly suggestive of telangiectatic osteosarcoma. Telangiectatic osteosarcoma typically produces little or no osteoid in the aneurysmal areas. An ABC may have associated osteoid production, but it is similar to fracture repair with broad seams and osteoblast rimming. A more conventional osteosarcoma is depicted in e-Fig. 2.5 as an ill-defined medullary lesion with periosteal elevation and mineralization. Morphologically, osteoblastic cells with pleomorphic nuclei are arrayed in a matrix of fine woven neoplastic osteoid (e-Fig. 2.6). The osteoblastic or chondroblastic osteosarcoma must be differentiated from fracture callus, which is shown in e-Figure 2.3.

Marrow Processes

An 18-month-old male child presented with decreased use of his left arm over a period of 1 week. There were no constitutional symptoms. The left forearm and elbow were tender, but there was no swelling, erythema, or increased warmth. The white blood count, C-reactive protein, and erythrocyte sedimentation rate were slightly elevated. The radiograph (Fig. 2.11) showed a destructive proximal ulnar marrow lesion with periosteal reaction. The frozen section (Fig. 2.12) demonstrated a mixed inflammatory infiltrate including eosinophils and mononuclear histiocytic cells. On

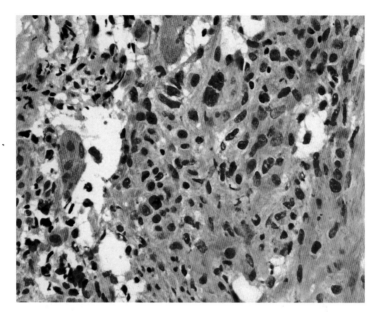

FIGURE 2.10 High power reveals nuclear atypia. Telangiectatic osteosarcoma typically produces little osteoid.

TABLE 2.5 Features Differentiating Aneurysmal Bone Cyst From Telangiectatic Osteosarcoma

	Aneurysmal Bone Cyst	Telangiectatic Osteosarcoma
Radiology	Expansile, lytic, cystic fluid-fluid levels	Expansile, lytic, cystic fluid-fluid levels
Peak age	10–20 y	10–20 y
Low power	Cystic spaces, webs, filled with blood	Cystic spaces, webs, filled with blood
Cells	Short spindled stromal cells, fibroblasts	Spindled to polygonal stromal cells, pleomorphic giant cells
Nucleus	Sometimes reactive but uniform	Pleomorphic, variable size
Mitoses	Occasional, but normal	Atypical
Giant cells	Osteoclastlike, frequently at edges of cyst wall	Osteoclastlike and pleomorphic
Matrix	Reactive woven and lamellar bone may be present	Rare fine network of osteoid
Necrosis	Hemorrhage, but not tumor necrosis	Tumor necrosis is highly suggestive of telangiectatic osteosarcoma

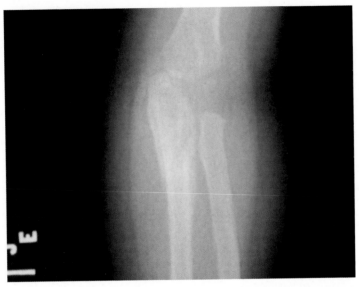

FIGURE 2.11 Radiograph of medullary lesion of the proximal ulna, with periosteal reaction.

permanent section study, this lesion was shown to be Langerhans cell histiocytosis. The differential diagnosis of a radiographic "marrow process" lesion includes chronic osteomyelitis, Langerhans cell histiocytosis, Ewing's sarcoma, lymphoma, and metastasis. Although chronic osteomyelitis may occur at any age, osteomyelitis from hematogenous seeding is most common in children and immunocompromised adults. Both Langerhans cell histiocytosis and Ewing's sarcoma are most common in those younger than 30 years, and metastases are more common in adults older than 40 years. Histologically, the differential diagnosis is divided into blue cell lesions, mixed inflammatory lesions, and metastases. The blue cell tumors require triage for further cytogenetic and molecular workup. Both chronic osteomyelitis and Langerhans cell histiocytosis have a mixed cell population of histiocytes and other inflammatory cells. The folded nucleus of the Langerhans cell and the bilobed nucleus of the eosinophils characterize Langerhans cell histiocytosis, although the inflammatory infiltrate may have a predominance of neutrophils or lymphocytes. Fragmented devitalized bone with empty lacunae, a blue dusty discoloration at the edge of the bone fragment, and a neutrophilic infiltrate are highly suggestive of osteomyelitis. In practice, cultures should be sent whenever the differential diagnosis is Langerhans cell histiocytosis versus osteomyelitis. A comparison case is that of a 12-year-old male child with right hand swelling of several weeks' duration without constitutional symptoms or fever. Radiographically, a destructive, marrow-based lesion of the fourth metacarpal

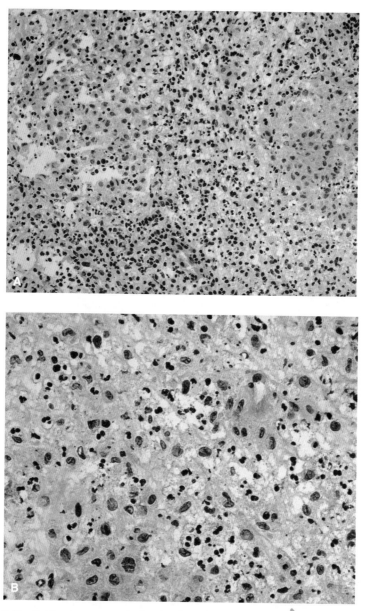

FIGURE 2.12   **A.** Low power reveals sheets of mononuclear histiocytic cells and inflammatory cells. Poor staining of the eosinophils fails to reveal their granules, but the bilobed nuclei are characteristic. **B.** High power reveals grooved nuclei characteristic of Langerhans cell histiocytosis.

TABLE 2.6 Features Differentiating Langerhans Cell Histiocytosis From Chronic Osteomyelitis

	Langerhans Cell Histiocytosis	Chronic Osteomyelitis
Radiology	Intramedullary ill-defined lytic diaphyseal lesion; frequently craniofacial bones	Intramedullary ill-defined lytic diaphyseal lesion; rarely effects craniofacial bones
Peak age	<30 y	Hematogenous spread is more common in children
Low power	Mixed infiltrate of inflammatory and mononuclear cells	Mixed infiltrate of inflammatory and mononuclear cells; devitalized bone
Cells	Langerhans cells, eosinophils, but sometimes neutrophils or plasma cells predominate	Neutrophils, lymphocytes, and plasma cells; sometimes prominent histiocytic infiltrate or granulomas
Nucleus	Grooved Langerhans nuclei, bilobed eosinophils	Reniform macrophages
Mitoses	Not prominent	Not prominent
Giant cells	May have giant cells composed of Langerhans cells, with similar nuclei	Osteoclasts, or foreign body giant cells if chronic (fungal) or Langerhans cells if TB
Matrix	No matrix unless fracture or reactive border	Devitalized bone and remodeling may be present

was found (e-Fig. 2.7). Frozen section also showed a mixed inflammatory infiltrate with numerous epithelioid histiocytes and acute inflammatory cells, with rare budding yeast forms, consistent with granulomatous osteomyelitis (e-Fig. 2.8), which was subsequently found to be caused by North American blastomycosis. A more typical osteomyelitis is shown in e-Figure 2.9, with a fragment of dead bone and inflamed reactive fibrous marrow. A comparison of the features of Langerhans cell histiocytosis and chronic osteomyelitis is presented in Table 2.6.

In adults, the differential of a lytic medullary process includes lymphoma, osteomyelitis, and most importantly, metastasis. e-Figure 2.10 shows a radiograph from a 45-year-old man who presented with a 6-month history of right proximal thigh pain. The review of systems was otherwise negative. Touch preparation (e-Fig. 2.11) revealed clusters of epithelial cells, but the frozen section showed that it was primarily reactive bone consistent with fracture repair. Rare groups of epithelial cells were present (e-Fig. 2.12). The patient was subsequently found to have a renal cell carcinoma. Metastases frequently present with a component of fracture, and secondary repair changes often complicate the histologic picture. The first specimen submitted for frozen section evaluation is frequently periosteum with fracture callus or procallus. Further sampling and touch preparations may be required to identify the underlying lesion. The majority of carcinomas are easily differentiated from a primary bone tumor because of specific features of epithelial differentiation (gland formation, cellular cohesion, intercellular bridges, keratin formation, or mucin production). However, poorly differentiated carcinomas must be distinguished from lymphoma, melanoma, or sarcoma. A sarcomatoid carcinoma should also be considered in the differential diagnosis of primary bone tumors with spindle cell morphology; sarcomatoid differentiation occurs in 10% of renal cell carcinomas. Primary bone lesions may also mimic epithelial tumors, particularly in the case of epithelioid hemangioendothelioma or epithelioid angiosarcoma.

Cartilaginous Lesions

A 52-year-old woman presented with recent onset of pain in the right distal thigh. The radiograph showed an ill-circumscribed medullary lesion with erosion of the cortex (Fig. 2.13). The frozen section revealed mildly cellular cartilage (Fig. 2.14) with trapping of preexisting lamellar bone (Fig. 2.15), consistent with the infiltrating margin of a chondrosarcoma.

Differentiation of chondrosarcoma from enchondroma on frozen section should be approached with full knowledge of clinical history,

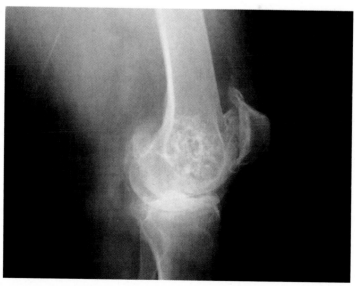

FIGURE 2.13 Central lytic lesion with indistinct mineralization and cortical erosion.

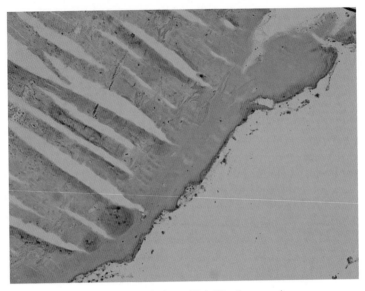

FIGURE 2.14   Low cellularity cartilage lesion with infiltrative margin.

symptoms, radiology, site, and surgical intraoperative impression. There are several rules regarding cartilaginous lesions that should be heeded:

1. Asymptomatic lesions are usually benign.
2. Lesions of the hand and feet (although they may be cellular and atypical enough to warrant a diagnosis of grade II chondrosarcoma in other sites) are benign until proven otherwise.

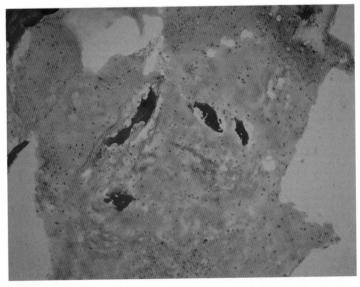

FIGURE 2.15   Trapping of native lamellar bone is a reliable feature of chondrosarcoma.

3. Small lesions and lesions in patients younger than 30 years of age are almost always benign.
4. Lesions with myxoid stroma are more likely malignant (e-Fig. 2.13).
5. The presence of necrotic cartilage (in the absence of a fracture) usually indicates that the lesion is malignant.
6. Infiltrative growth with trapping of lamellar bone is diagnostic of chondrosarcoma.
7. Expansile growth with no trapping of lamellar bone is more indicative of enchondroma.
8. A rim of lamellar bone at the edge of the cartilage lobule is more indicative of a benign process (e-Fig. 2.14).

A comparison of the features of enchondroma and chondrosarcoma is presented in Table 2.7.

TABLE 2.7	Features of Enchondroma and Low-Grade Chondrosarcoma	
	Enchondroma	Low-Grade Chondrosarcoma
Age group	Teenagers to elderly persons	Mostly in those older than 50 y
Symptoms	Usually asymptomatic, incidentally discovered; if painful, usually associated with fracture	Progressive pain, night pain, mass
Distribution	Hands and feet, femur, humerus, tibia	Pelvis, femur, humerus, ribs, scapula
Location	Diaphysis, metaphysis, uncommon epiphyseal lesion	Same
Size	Usually 6 cm or less	Larger
Low power	Islands of cartilage with ossification to lamellar bone at rim, no trapped lamellar bone	Infiltrative pattern, trapped native lamellar bone, infiltration of Haversian canal, lobules separated by fibrous bands
Cellularity	Low cellularity; fewer than 25 cells per hpf (400×), likely benign	Variable, but if greater than 100 cells per hpf (400×) then likely malignant
Mitoses	<1/50 hpf	More than 2/50 hpf
Radiology	Sharply defined radiolucency with cloudlike calcification; without erosion of cortex and without periosteal extension	Less well-defined, may expand the contour of the bone, scallop the cortex and show periosteal reaction
Matrix	Hyaline, not myxoid	May be myxoid
Cytology	Small nuclei	Atypia, prominent nucleoli

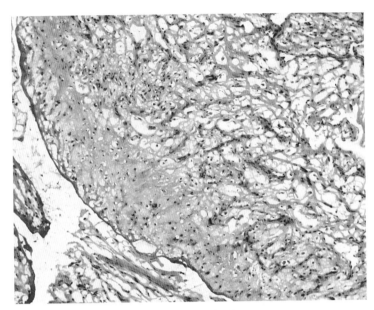

FIGURE 2.16   Fibrous membrane from joint prosthesis.

Previous Joint Replacement and Evaluation for Infection

A 62-year-old man with a knee replacement surgery 8 years earlier presented with loosening of the prosthesis and resorption of the bone surrounding the stem. The surgeon submitted several specimens of fibrous tissue from around the prosthesis asking for a "poly count."

Intraoperative neutrophil counts are a frequent source of frozen section requests when the surgeon is replacing a prosthetic joint that has loosened or shows radiologic evidence of resorption of bone. Collections of neutrophils in the prosthetic pseudocapsule increase the likelihood of infection, and, if present, will prompt the surgeon to remove the hardware and treat for infection before inserting a new joint. The most commonly used criterion is five neutrophils or more in each of five high-power fields (14). Fibrin and surface inflammatory exudates are excluded, as are marginating neutrophils in capillaries (Figs. 2.16–2.18). Patients with active rheumatoid arthritis cannot be accurately evaluated. Macrophages and lymphocytes are not counted, and the differentiation of macrophages from neutrophils is the most difficult aspect of the procedure. Definite constriction between nuclear lobes, as opposed to a twisted nucleus, is the most reliable diagnostic feature.

A recent study found that, as compared with cultures, the specificity of a positive intraoperative neutrophil count was 95% but the sensitivity was low (at 29%). The predictive value of a negative count was 92%, which indicates that intraoperative neutrophil counts are a valuable test when infection is suspected in a prosthetic joint (15). Other studies have

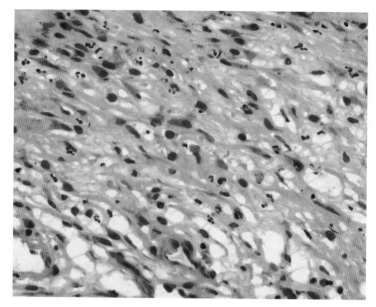

FIGURE 2.17   Neutrophilic infiltration of fibrous prosthetic joint capsule.

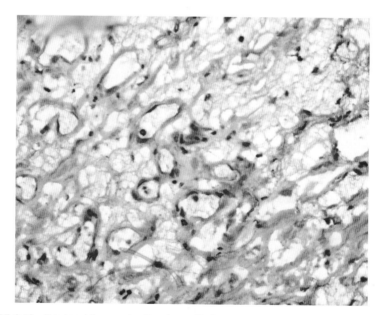

FIGURE 2.18   Neutrophils marginating in capillaries may result from manipulation during surgery and should not be counted in neutrophil counts.

found better sensitivity by setting the criteria at an average of 1 or more neutrophils per high power field in a set of 10 fields (16).

SUMMARY

Errors in the diagnosis of bone lesions by frozen section can be avoided by correlating clinical and radiologic impression with morphologic features. A complete understanding of the surgeon's algorithm for intraoperative decision making is also vital. The diagnosis should be deferred if there is any doubt about the nature of the lesion, which could jeopardize definitive management of the lesion, or if there is any discordance among the clinical, radiological, or pathological impressions.

REFERENCES

1. Simon MA. Current concepts review: limb salvage for osteosarcoma. *J Bone Joint Surg Am.* 1988;70-A:307–310.
2. Bui MM, Smith P, Agresta SV, et al. Practical issues of intraoperative frozen section diagnosis of bone and soft tissue lesions. *Cancer Control.* 2008;15:7–12.
3. Unni KK. *Dahlin's Bone Tumors: General Aspects and Data on 11,087 Cases.* 5th Ed. Philadelphia: Lippincott-Raven, 1996.
4. Rougraff BT, Kneisl JS, Simon MA. Skeletal metastases of unknown origin: a prospective study of a diagnostic strategy. *J Bone Joint Surg Am.* 1993;75:1276–1281.
5. Peabody T, ed. The rodded metastasis is a sarcoma: strategies to prevent inadvertent surgical procedures on primary bone malignancies. *Instr Course Lect.* 2004;53:657–661.
6. Shenoy R, Pillai A, Reid R. Tumours of the hand presenting as pathological fractures. *Acta Orthop Belg.* 2007;73:192–195.
7. Ortiz EJ, Isler MH, Navia JE, et al. Pathologic fractures in children. *Clin Orthop Relat Res.* 2005;432:116–126.
8. Wagner LM, Neel MD, Pappo AS, et al. Fractures in pediatric Ewing sarcoma. *J Pediatr Hematol Oncol.* 2001;23:568–571.
9. Papagelopoulos PJ, Mavrogenis AF, Savvidou OD, et al. Pathologic fractures in primary bone sarcomas. *Injury.* 2008;39:395–403.
10. Mirra JM. Teaching case: stress fracture versus osteosarcoma. In: Mirra JM, ed. *Bone tumors: Clinical, Radiologic, and Pathological Parameters.* Philadelphia: Lea & Febiger, 1989:172–173.
11. Gutierrez K. Bone and joint infections in children. *Pediatr Clin North Am.* 2005;52: 779–794.
12. Letson D, Falcone R, Muro-Cacho CA. Pathologic and radiologic features of primary bone tumors. *Cancer Control.* 1999;6:283–293.
13. Meyer MS, Spanier SS, Moser M, et al. Evaluating marrow margins for resection of osteosarcoma: a modern approach. *Clin Orthop Relat Res.* 1999;363:170–175.
14. Mirra JM, Marder RA, Amstutz HC. The pathology of failed joint arthroplasty. *Clin Orthop Relat Res.* 1982;170:175–183.
15. Kanner WA, Saleh KJ, Frierson HF. Reassessment of the usefulness of frozen section analysis for hip and knee revisions. *Am J Clin Pathol.* 2008;130:363–368.
16. Pandey R, Drakoulakis E, Athanasou NA. An assessment of the histological criteria used to diagnose infection in hip revision arthroplasty tissues. *J Clin Pathol.* 1999;52: 118–123.

3

INTRAOPERATIVE CONSULTATION IN GYNECOLOGIC PATHOLOGY

ANTHONY G. MONTAG

Specimens from the gynecologic organs are among the most common in surgical pathology. The major sources of intraoperative consultations are ovarian masses, hysterectomy specimens, and vulvectomy specimens for margins (1). In both the ovarian and uterine specimens, the frozen section diagnosis may direct the surgeon to perform lymph node dissection and other staging procedures, with the accompanying risk of increased morbidity and potential loss of fertility. It is therefore particularly important to know the clinical history, age, gravidity and parity of the patient, and the decision algorithm that the surgeon will employ based on the intraoperative diagnosis. The evaluation of margins from vulvectomy specimens is similar to that of other skin specimens, an area covered in the chapter on frozen sections of skin lesions.

OVARIAN MASSES

Ovarian masses are rarely removed with a previous study confirming malignancy; a solid and cystic ultrasound appearance on ultrasound suggests malignancy but is correct only 25% of the time, and only a quarter of stage I ovarian tumors have elevated serum markers. Apparently localized lesions are found to have other sites of involvement on staging in a quarter of cases (2). Underdiagnosis at frozen section may lead to understaging, while overdiagnosis of malignancy may result in inappropriate loss of fertility. As in all intraoperative consultations, the pathologist should know the surgeon's treatment algorithm based on the diagnosis rendered.

A careful documentation of the intactness of the ovarian capsule and examination for surface involvement should precede opening the specimen. The extent of solid and cystic components and the nature of cyst contents should be noted. A fairly reliable test for mucinous versus serous content is whether the material flows easily through the fenestrated plate that covers most gross room sink drains. Unilocular cysts may be follicular or epithelial in origin, and rarely a cystic granulosa cell tumor may present as a unilocular cyst. The latter is not a diagnosis that is comfortably made on frozen section. Unilocular cysts with a smooth lining lacking solid areas or excrescences can be given a gross diagnosis of "simple cyst" without frozen section, as sampling would be completely at random and the chance of finding an occult lesion small. A unilocular mucinous cyst with a solid fibroma component is usually a Brenner tumor, which can be confirmed on frozen section.

Sebaceous contents, hair, or other features of a cystic teratoma directs attention to the Rokitansky tubercle, the site of the solid component. If no soft fleshy component is present, the lesion can be given a diagnosis of benign cystic teratoma on gross examination, otherwise the area is frozen. When evaluating for immature elements, most commonly neuroepithelium, the possibility of mature teratomatous mimics such as retina and cerebellar granular layer should be considered. As most of teratomas occur in women of reproductive age and the vast majority is benign, one should be hesitant to make a diagnosis of immature teratoma based on frozen section.

A unilocular "chocolate-cyst" appearance is indicative of endometriosis, and in the absence of a solid component or other clinical indication of malignancy, a presumptive diagnosis can be made without performing a frozen section. Solid elements are most commonly normal structures trapped in fibrosis, but clear cell and endometrioid carcinomas may be encountered.

Serous borderline tumors frequently present as unilocular serous cysts with a papillary lining that resembles a shag carpet (e-Fig. 3.1). In the absence of solid mural areas, a representative frozen to confirm borderline histology is sufficient (e-Fig. 3.2). Surgeons frequently stage patients with serous borderline tumors. Serous carcinoma typically presents as a solid or solid and cystic tumor and displays obvious cytological atypia on frozen section. If a malignant serous tumor presents with primarily surface ovarian involvement, the fallopian tube should be entirely sampled for permanent sections to evaluate for occult fallopian tube carcinoma.

Mucinous Tumors

Mucinous ovarian tumors present two clinical problems: are they benign, borderline, or malignant; and are they primary or metastatic? The evaluation of mucinous tumors is the largest source of discrepancy in intraoperative examination of gynecologic specimens (3–5). Lesions with one or few smooth-walled dominant cysts and no solid areas on gross examination prove to be benign more than 95% of the time, (6) and do not require frozen section examination. Multiloculated and solid and cystic mucinous lesions require frozen section, however in the absence of a solid component gross inspection rarely indicates where to find the focal area of borderline or malignant histology. Figure 3.1 shows a multiloculated mucinous tumor, which was found to have focal borderline histology on frozen section (Fig. 3.2). On permanent section, areas of invasive mucinous carcinoma were found. Although adequate sampling for permanent sections requires one section per centimeter of the largest diameter of the tumor, it is impractical to do more than one or two frozen sections. The predictive

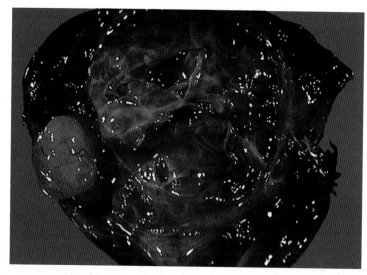

FIGURE 3.1 Gross specimen of multiloculated mucinous tumor.

value of the frozen section diagnosis is 95% for benign, 99% for malignant, and 65% for borderline mucinous tumors (7). Approximately a fourth of frozen section diagnoses of borderline tumor will have carcinoma in the final pathologic sections. For this reason, a diagnosis of "at least borderline" is sometimes warranted. In practice, most surgeons stage mucinous borderline tumors.

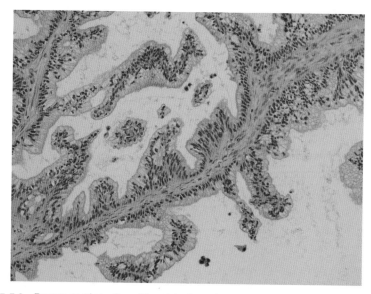

FIGURE 3.2 Frozen section of multiloculated mucinous tumor, displaying borderline features including stratification and epithelial tufting.

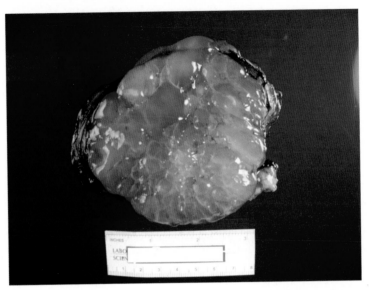

FIGURE 3.3 Gross specimen of a metastatic mucinous tumor to the ovary from a pancreatic primary.

Figure 3.3 illustrates a multicystic mucinous tumor without solid areas. The frozen section, shown in Figure 3.4, displays a single layer of columnar cells with minimal atypia. In this case, both ovaries were involved by mucinous carcinoma, and a pancreatic primary was found on abdominal exploration. Metastases to the ovary may originate from all parts

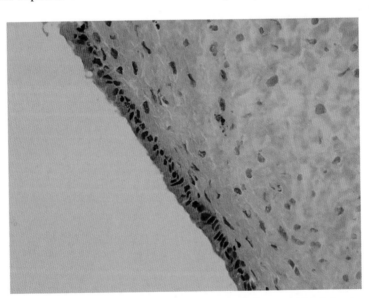

FIGURE 3.4 Microscopic of specimen from Figure 3.3. Although the lining is a simple columnar epithelium, there is mild cytologic atypia. Metastatic mucinous tumors may have areas indistinguishable from primary mucinous cystadenoma.

TABLE 3.1	Features of Primary and Metastatic Mucinous Tumors		
	Primary	Metastatic	*p* Value
Laterality	Unilateral 95%	Bilateral 60%–75%	<.0001
Microscopic surface involvement	Absent	79%	<.0001
Nodular growth pattern	Absent	42%	<.0003
Infiltrative invasive pattern	16%	91%	<.0001
Small glands/tubules	12%	94%	<.0001
Expansile invasive pattern	88%	18%	<.0001
Complex papillae	60%	8%	.0004
Benign-appearing areas	76%	36%	.008
Borderline with atypia	57%	31%	.035

of the gastrointestinal tract, as recently reviewed by Young (8). The gross appearance varies from a solid lesion to multiloculated to even occasionally unilocular. Krukenberg tumors (e-Fig. 3.3) classically present as bilateral large fibrous ovarian tumors, which weep mucin on the cut surface. Histologically, the classic Krukenberg tumor has a dense reactive stroma with infiltrating glands and single cells (e-Fig. 3.4). Metastatic mucinous carcinoma in the ovary may resemble primary mucinous carcinoma, borderline tumors, or endometrioid ovarian primaries; e-Figures 3.5 and 3.6 display an endometrial carcinoma metastatic to the ovary. The presence of dirty necrosis on both the touch preparation and the cryostat section suggests metastatic disease. Useful clinical and histologic features have been analyzed recently by Lee and Young (9) and are partially summarized in Table 3.1. The features most predictive for metastatic disease and useful on frozen section are bilaterality, microscopic surface involvement, macroscopic nodular growth pattern, infiltrative invasive growth pattern, and infiltration of stroma by small glands or individual cells. Interestingly many features had no discriminatory value: gross necrosis; cribriform, villous, or solid growth pattern; goblet cells or colonic carcinoma-like appearance, and low-grade histology. Although histologically benign-appearing areas favored a primary ovarian mucinous tumor, 36% of metastatic tumors had benign-appearing areas. Any time an ovarian mucinous tumor is found on frozen section, the surgeon should be immediately queried as to the status of the other ovary and any previous history of gastrointestinal carcinoma. All patients with bilateral tumors or suspicious histology should have the gastrointestinal tract evaluated during laparotomy. Many surgeons routinely remove the appendix when a mucinous tumor of the ovary is found, as this is a frequent occult source for metastases. Any patient with an ovarian mucinous tumor associated with pseudomyxoma peritonei should be suspected to have appendiceal carcinoma (10).

TABLE 3.2 Features of Granulosa Cell Tumor vs Undifferentiated Carcinoma		
	Granulosa Cell Tumor	Undifferentiated Carcinoma
Age	Peak 45–55	Peak 55–60
Stage	90% stage I	90% stage III or greater
Bilaterality	5%	50%
Gross	Predominantly solid	Predominantly solid
Low power	Solid sheets, cords, usually no necrosis if no torsion	Solid sheets, poorly formed papillae or glands, necrosis
High power	Usually uniform nuclei, smaller, scant cytoplasm, grooves better seen on touch preparations	Pleomorphic, large nuclei scant cytoplasm
Mitoses	Occasional, rarely atypical	Frequent and atypical

Ovarian Small Blue Cell Tumor

Several ovarian tumors may present as a sheet of blue cells on frozen section. Ovarian lymphoma and desmoplastic round cell tumor are rare, and the more typical differential is granulosa cell tumor versus undifferentiated carcinoma (Table 3.2). Granulosa cell tumors are typically unilateral, and although they may occur in all ages, they are more common in adults. The tumors may be large, and occasionally present as an acute abdomen because of ovarian torsion, rupture, or hemoperitoneum. Ninety percent of cases present as stage I lesions; standard management is to do unilateral oophorectomy and inspect peritoneal surfaces for implants. Particularly for women in the reproductive years, the misdiagnosis of granulosa cell tumor as an undifferentiated carcinoma can lead to inappropriate surgery. Histologically, granulosa cell tumors typically present as sheets of monotonous cells with relatively uniform nuclear size and shape, occasionally with cord-like arrangements, which can mimic abortive gland formation, and, particularly in poorly executed frozen sections, lead to consideration of a poorly differentiated carcinoma (Fig. 3.5). Touch preparations can be particularly helpful in evaluating a granulosa cell tumor, as nuclear grooves and other cytologic features are much more readily seen in a touch preparation than on frozen section (Fig. 3.6).

Undifferentiated carcinoma of the ovary includes tumors with little or no differentiation toward the traditional histologic subtypes. Patients tend to be older, with average age in the mid-fifties. Approximately 50% of patients have bilateral ovarian involvement, and the majority present at an advanced stage. Microscopically, undifferentiated carcinoma may present sheets of cells with scant cytoplasm and deceptively uniform hyperchromatic nuclei,

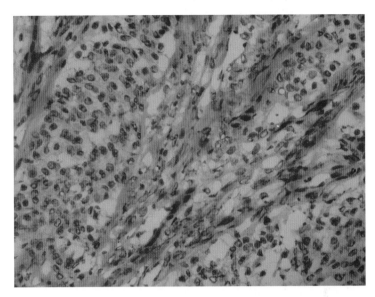

FIGURE 3.5 Frozen section of solid ovarian mass, revealing sheets of blue tumor cells.

superficially resembling a granulosa cell tumor (Figs. 3.7, 3.8). Abortive gland formation may be mistaken for sex cords or Cal-Exner bodies. Pleomorphism, increased mitotic activity atypical mitoses, and tumor necrosis not associated with torsion all suggest undifferentiated carcinoma as opposed to granulosa cell tumor. Cytologic examination is particularly useful to

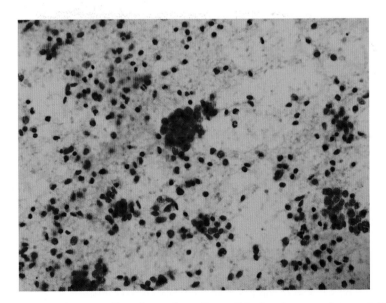

FIGURE 3.6 Touch preparation of case from Figure 3.5, showing monotonous cells with scant cytoplasm and occasionally grooved nuclei, consistent with granulosa cells.

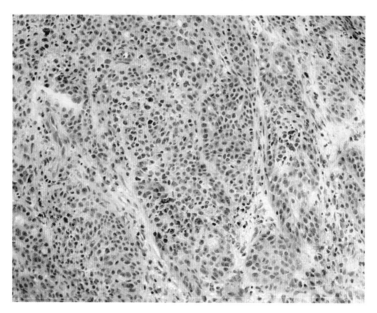

FIGURE 3.7 Solid sheets of undifferentiated cells with cytologic atypia. A vague nesting arrangement is present.

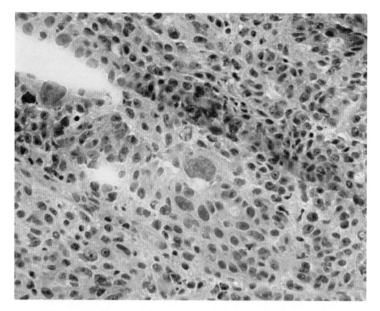

FIGURE 3.8 Higher magnification of Figure 3.7. The cytologic atypia is atypical for granu-losa cell tumor, and is more consistent with undifferentiated carcinoma.

compare nuclear detail. The clinical history will generally separate granulosa cell tumor from undifferentiated carcinoma.

Ovarian Tumors in Pregnancy

Ovarian lesions presenting in pregnancy reflect the tumors characteristic of the age group and the special functional tumor-like lesions that arise during pregnancy. The incidence of adnexal masses during pregnancy is variable, dependent on the use of imaging and the inclusion in studies of functional lesions that involute without being biopsied. Retrospective studies have found adnexal masses in 1 per 632 pregnancies (11) and 1 per 1,000 pregnancies (12). The majority of benign lesions are mature cystic teratomas (27%–50%), cystadenomas (20%–34%), and functional lesions (13%–18%). Malignant or borderline tumors make up around 6% of tumors, (13) including germ cell tumors (30%–45%), borderline tumors (30%–35%), cystadenocarcinomas (5%–10%), and sex cord stromal tumors (10%–20%). Torsion with and without rupture is a common presentation of adnexal tumors during pregnancy. In general, any ovary which has undergone torsion has an underlying mass, which should be carefully documented. Although the risk of malignancy in ovarian torsion associated with pregnancy is small, torsion in the postmenopausal patient is associated with malignancy in about a quarter of cases (14).

Figure 3.9 illustrates a 29-year-old G3P2 presenting for cesarean section in whom an incidental 8-cm ruptured ovarian mass was discovered during the procedure. The tumor cells have abundant pink cytoplasm and

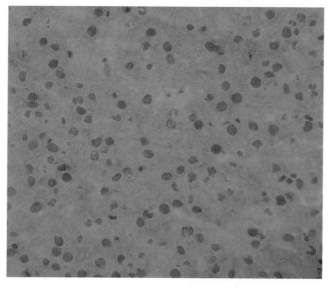

FIGURE 3.9 Solid sheets of cells with abundant pink cytoplasm and monotonous nuclei, suggesting luteinized cells.

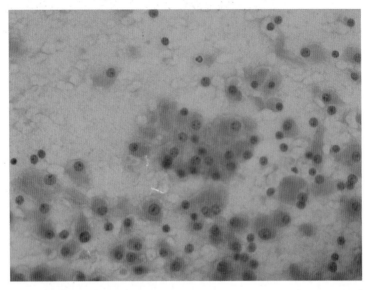

FIGURE 3.10 Touch preparation revealing abundant pink cytoplasm and small distinct nucleoli characteristic of luteinized cells.

on touch preparation have distinct nucleoli, indicating a steroid-producing cell (Fig. 3.10). The differential of a solid eosinophilic cell lesion presenting in pregnancy includes luteoma of pregnancy, corpus luteum of pregnancy, stromal hyperthecosis, stromal hyperplasia, steroid (lipid) cell tumor, Leydig cell tumor, luteinized granulosa cell tumor, oxyphilic variant of clear cell carcinoma, and metastatic carcinoma with marked stromal luteinization (Table 3.3). Clear cell carcinoma is rare before the age of 40, and has cystic and papillary structures. Metastatic carcinoma typically has stromal reaction and epithelial islands in addition to the luteinized stoma cells. In terms of intraoperative management, the separation of functional lesions from tumor is most important. Functional lesions such as luteoma and luteal cysts require no surgery beyond wedge excision, and will involute after pregnancy.

INTRAOPERATIVE EVALUATION OF ENDOMETRIAL CARCINOMA

The diagnosis of endometrial carcinoma is typically made on biopsy or curetting prior to surgery. Intraoperative evaluation of hysterectomy specimens is done to document the extent of disease and tumor grade so that a decision regarding pelvic lymph node dissection may be made. Features indicating a high risk of metastasis are shown in Table 3.4. If no risk factors are present, there is 2.8% risk of pelvic and <1% risk of paraaortic node involvement (15–17). If the preoperative biopsy shows a high-grade endometrioid tumor or unfavorable histology (clear cell or

TABLE 3.3 Differential of Ovarian Tumors in Pregnancy			
	Luteoma	Steroid Cell Tumor	Granulosa Cell Tumor
Age	Twenties to thirties	Forties to fifties	Twenties to seventies
Race	80% in African Americans	No tendency	No tendency
Laterality	Multifocal or bilateral	Unilateral	Unilateral
Symptoms	No symptoms or torsion	Most are virilizing	Hyperestrogenic
Histology	Uniformly pink cells, rarely lipid vacuoles	Pink and clear cells, lipid	Solid, cords, trabeculae, may have vacuoles
Cytology	Uniform nuclei, small nucleoli	Variable nuclei, small nucleoli	Nucleoli, but frequently grooves

serous carcinoma), then no intraoperative evaluation is necessary; a lymph node dissection has already been directed by the biopsy results. Failure to document significant prognostic factors during the intraoperative examination leads to the omission of pelvic node dissection, resulting in re-operation to perform the node dissection or, more commonly pelvic radiation therapy. Overdiagnosis of adverse prognostic factors leads to unnecessary pelvic node dissection and increased potential for morbidity (up to 15%).

The serosa and adnexa of the hysterectomy specimen are inspected grossly for extrauterine involvement, which is rarely seen. The corpus is bivalved at 3- and 9-o'clock positions and the lining inspected. Full thickness cuts from mucosa to serosa at 5-mm intervals and are then made to identify areas of possible myometrial invasion (Fig. 3.11). The deepest

TABLE 3.4 Prognostically Significant Features for Endometrial Carcinoma	
Feature	Relative Risk Increase of Lymph Node Metastasis
Serous or clear cell histology	3×
Grade 3 histology	3×
Outer half myometrial involvement	5×
Cervical involvement	4×
Adnexal involvement	4×

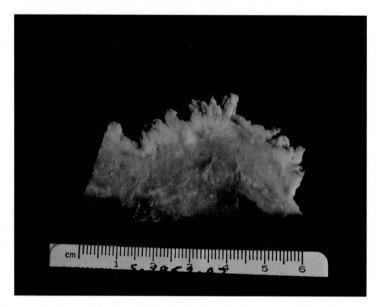

FIGURE 3.11 Gross examination of uterus for depth of invasion. The uterus has been bi-valve and bread-loafed. This section shows superficial invasion of the myometrium.

apparent focus is then frozen, ideally as a full thickness, or in a manner to preserve the overall depth and total thickness measurements (Fig. 3.12). Any mucosal abnormality in the lower uterine segment and endocervical canal should also be frozen (e-Fig. 3.7).

Accuracy of intraoperative assessment of grade is between 80% and 96%, with undergrading the common problem (2,18), and usually due to sampling error. Gross assessment of myometrial invasion alone is difficult, particularly with high-grade tumors, and is overall probably no better than 70% accuracy (19). Most discrepancies in depth involve superficial lesions. Generally management of intraendometrial and superficial (<50%) lesions is similar, and a recent review of prognostic factors in endometrial staging suggests that the outcome is not significantly different (20).

ENDOMETRIAL BIOPSY FOR PRODUCTS OF CONCEPTION

Evaluation of endometrial biopsy material for evidence of an intrauterine pregnancy is done to rule out the possibility of ectopic pregnancy. Simultaneous intrauterine and ectopic conceptuses occur in approximately 1 of 10,000 pregnancies, and even more frequently in patients conceiving with in vitro fertilization. The practice of freezing products of conception is less common today because ultrasound examination of the Fallopian tubes, particularly transvaginal ultrasound, is highly accurate in detecting ectopic pregnancy (21). Sensitivity of transvaginal ultrasound is 91% and

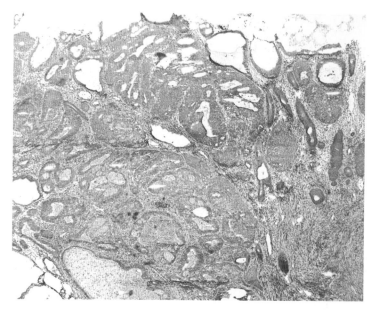

FIGURE 3.12 Frozen section confirms superficial infiltration of a grade 1 endometrioid carcinoma.

specificity is >99%. By comparison the sensitivity of frozen section is 76% and the specificity 98% (22). If the material is copious it can be floated in saline and presumptive villi sampled based on the apparent branched villous architecture. Because of the large amount of fluid in villi freezing should be rapid to avoid ice crystal artifact. Because of the low sensitivity, a negative frozen result does not rule out the presence of an intrauterine pregnancy.

CONCLUSION

Intraoperative consultation in gynecologic pathology is usually performed to assess diagnosis, local prognostic factors, and to determine necessity of further surgical staging. With the exception of ovarian mucinous tumors, frozen section diagnosis is highly accurate.

REFERENCES

1. Coffey D, Kaplan AL, Ramzy I. Intraoperative consultation in gynecologic pathology. *Arch Pathol.* 2005;129:1544–1557.
2. Acs G. Intraoperative consultation in gynecologic pathology. *Semin Diagn Pathol.* 2002;19:237–254.
3. Boriboonhirunsarn D, Sermboon A. Accuracy of frozen section in the diagnosis of malignant ovarian tumor. *J Obstet Gynaecol Res.* 2004;30:394–399.
4. Twaalfhoven FC, Peters AA, Trimbos JB, et al. The accuracy of frozen section diagnosis of ovarian tumors. *Gynecol Oncol.* 1991;41:189–192.

5. Tempfer CB, Polterauer S, Bentz EK, et al. Accuracy of intraoperative frozen section analysis in borderline tumors of the ovary: a retrospective analysis of 96 cases and a review of the literature. *Gynecol Oncol.* 2007;107:248–252.

6. Lim FK, Yeoh CL, Chong SM, et al. Pre and intraoperative diagnosis of ovarian tumours: how accurate are we? *Aust N Z J Obstet Gynaecol.* 1997;37:223–227.

7. Rose PG, Nelson RR, Hunter RE, et al. Accuracy of frozen section (intraoperative consultation) diagnosis of ovarian tumors. *Am J Obstet Gynecol.* 1994;171(3):823–826.

8. Young RH. From Krukenberg to today: the ever present problems posed by metastatic tumors of the ovary. Part II. *Adv Anat Pathol.* 2007;14:149–177.

9. Lee KR, Young RH. The distinction between primary and metastatic mucinous carcinomas of the ovary. *Am J Surg Pathol.* 2003;27:281–292.

10. Young RH. From Krukenberg to today: the ever present problems posed by metastatic tumors to the ovary: part 1. Historical perspective, general principles, mucinous tumors including the Krukenberg tumor. *Adv Anat Pathol.* 2006;13:205–227.

11. Sherard GB, Hodson CA, Williams HJ, et al. Adnexal masses and pregnancy: a 12 year experience. *Am J Obstet Gynecol.* 2003;189:358–362.

12. Hermans RH, Fischer DC, vander Putten HW, et al. Adnexal masses in pregnancy. *Oncology.* 2003;26:167–172.

13. Whitecar MP, Turner S, Higby MK. Adnexal masses in pregnancy: a review of 130 cases undergoing surgical management. *Am J Obstet Gynecol.* 1999;181:19–24.

14. Eitan R, Galoyan N, Zuckerman B, et al. The risk of malignancy in post-menopausal women presenting with adnexal torsion. *Gynecol Oncol.* 2007;106:211–214.

15. Mikuta JJ. Preoperative evaluation and staging of endometrial cancer. *Cancer.* 1995; 76:2041–2043.

16. Fanning J, Tsukada Y, Piver MS. Intraoperative frozen section diagnosis of depth of myometrial invasion in endometrial adenocarcinoma. *Gynecol Oncol.* 1990;37:47–50.

17. Creasman WT, Morrow CP, Bundy BN, et al. Surgical pathologic spread patterns of endometrial cancer. A Gynecologic Oncology Group Study. *Cancer Control.* 1987;60; 8(suppl):2035–2041.

18. Quinlivan JA, Petersen RW, Nicklin JL. Accuracy of frozen section for the operative management of endometrial cancer. *BJOG.* 2001;108:798–803.

19. Goff BA, Rice LW. Assessment of depth of myometrial invasion in endometrial adenocarcinoma. *Gynecol Oncol.* 1990;38:46–48.

20. Zaino RJ. FIGO staging of endometrial adenocarcinoma: a critical review and proposal. *Int J Gyn Pathol.* 2009;28:1–9.

21. Condous CG, Okaro E, Khalis A, et al. The accuracy of transvaginal ultrasonography for the diagnosis of ectopic pregnancy prior to surgery. *Hum Reprod.* 2005;20:1404–1409.

22. Barak S, Oettinger M, Perri A, et al. Frozen section examination of endometrial curettings in the diagnosis of ectopic pregnancy. *Acta Obstet Gynecol Scand.* 2005;84:43–47.

4

LUNG, MEDIASTINUM, AND PLEURA

ILYSSA O. GORDON, KIMIKO SUZUE, AND ALIYA N. HUSAIN

INTRODUCTION: LUNG FROZEN SECTION

Frozen sections of pulmonary specimens are used to assess nodules or to determine the presence of an infectious process in immunocompromised hosts. Rarely, intraoperative evaluation in the transplant setting of a small nodule or an enlarged lymph node found in a donor lung may be requested. In general, frozen sections on tissue with suspected interstitial lung disease are not useful because of the typically small tissue sample obtained and the freezing artifact distortion. Rare exceptions may include acute exacerbations of undiagnosed interstitial lung disease in patients who are in the intensive care unit and for whom an urgent diagnosis is needed to direct clinical decision-making. In these cases, consultation with the clinical team, and consideration of a 4- to 6-hour rapid processing, if available, may be preferable.

Solitary lung nodules, which are the most common lung specimen submitted for intraoperative evaluation, are typically preceded by preoperative radiologic evaluation, a key component in the diagnostic pathway. With the goal of obtaining a tissue diagnosis prior to definitive surgery, radiologic evidence of a nodule larger than 2 cm would lead to a preoperative transbronchial biopsy by flexible bronchoscopy or a CT-guided transthoracic needle core biopsy. Tissue obtained from these procedures is submitted for permanent sections as well as for more immediate cytologic evaluation. Frozen section does not typically have a role in this setting. A nodule smaller than 2 cm or a surgically inaccessible nodule would lead to an intraoperative endobronchial biopsy by rigid bronchoscopy or to a wedge biopsy, most often by video-assisted thoracoscopy. Frozen section evaluation of these tissues would aid in the determination of whether definitive surgery, namely lobectomy and lymph node dissection, should be undertaken during the same operation. When completion lobectomies are performed, frozen section determination of bronchial margin involvement is also common. Central lung nodules are considered surgically unresectable when they involve the carina, as seen radiologically, and therefore frozen section diagnosis is not necessary; however, tissue may be examined to determine if it is adequate for diagnosis. Radiologically suspicious lymph nodes are also an important component of the staging workup and are discussed further in the mediastinum section.

The Lung Frozen Section: Major Intraoperative Questions

The intraoperative evaluation of a lung wedge biopsy needs to be accompanied by important clinical history, including suspicion of tuberculosis or lymphoma, and the appropriate precautions taken. The specimen should be measured and inked. The staple line should be removed with minimal disruption of the underlying tissue, and the resection margin should then be inked a different color than used before. In some cases, freezing a portion of the nodule with a portion of adjacent lung parenchyma may reveal an adjacent in situ component, which would indicate a primary lung lesion. It is important to note that sections of the nodule at its closest approach to the pleura should not be frozen, as pleural involvement by carcinoma is important for surgical staging of tumors smaller than 3 cm. These sections should always be submitted for permanent paraffin sections for adequate assessment of pleural involvement.

The major clinical question for malignant peripheral lung nodules, which are surgically resectable, is whether it is a small cell or a non-small cell carcinoma (Figs. 4.1, 4.2, e-Fig. 4.1). Small cell lung carcinoma is not typically resected, except for the small minority that present in stage I disease, while non-small cell carcinoma is surgically resected when possible. The distinction between small cell carcinoma and non-small cell carcinoma

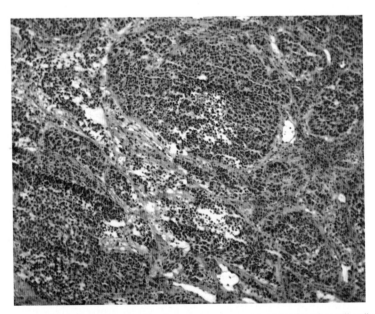

FIGURE 4.1 Small cell carcinoma. The tumor is composed of nests of small cells within which some pseudorosettes can be identified.

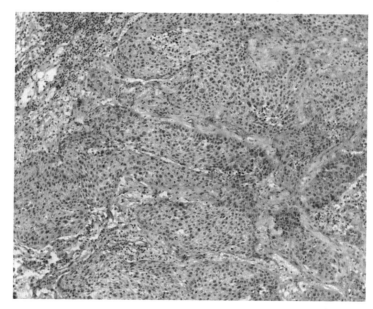

FIGURE 4.2 Non–small cell carcinoma. There are nests of large cells with abundant cytoplasm.

is therefore very important in determining whether or not to continue to definitive lobectomy and lymph node dissection. If the distinction cannot be made on frozen section, documentation that diagnostic tissue has been obtained is helpful, and the actual diagnosis can be deferred, with further surgical management as necessary.

Once a malignant diagnosis is rendered on frozen section, another clinical question may be whether the lesion represents primary or metastatic disease. A round, well-circumscribed nodule lacking a central scar favors a metastasis (Fig. 4.3). Metastatic adenocarcinoma may have more complex architecture (Figs. 4.4, 4.5), dirty necrosis (e-Fig. 4.2), or bland cytology, and metastatic squamous cell carcinoma may be more differentiated with keratinization and minimal atypia compared to primary tumors (1). This may be a difficult distinction, especially by frozen section, even with previous documentation of a non–lung primary carcinoma. The expertise of the pathologist, deferral to paraffin sections, and immunohistologic workup are all factors to be considered. In equivocal cases, it is best to document that a non–small cell carcinoma is present, and that the primary site cannot be determined.

Subpleural scars (Fig. 4.6), which are linear and parallel to the pleural surface, are a common finding in adults, and may be either subclinical incidental findings or identified on CT scan. The presence of a subpleural scar on gross inspection should not distract from the search for a distinct peripheral nodule, which is more likely to be the lesion in question.

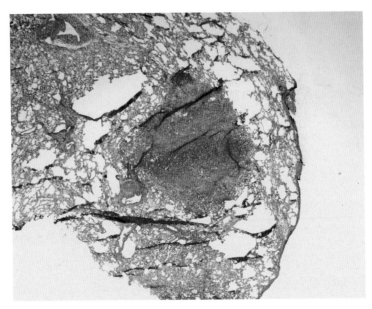

FIGURE 4.3 Metastatic carcinoma. Subpleural location and rounded well-defined nodule without central scar favors metastasis.

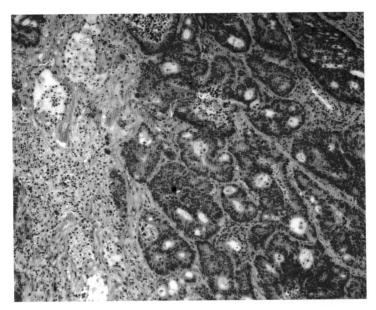

FIGURE 4.4 Complex cribriforming architecture is seen in this case of metastatic colon carcinoma.

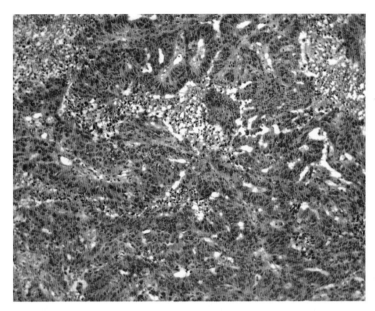

FIGURE 4.5 Adenocarcinoma. Left upper lobe nodule with cribriforming glands and dirty necrosis. It may be difficult to differentiate a primary versus a metastatic adenocarcinoma. In this case, the circumscribed nature of this lesion and the "dirty" appearance is consistent with colonic primary.

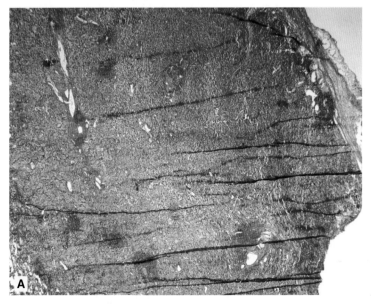

FIGURE 4.6 Subpleural scar. Low power (**A**) shows a mass lesion which on high power (**B**) has only fibrosis and no evidence of malignancy. (*continued*)

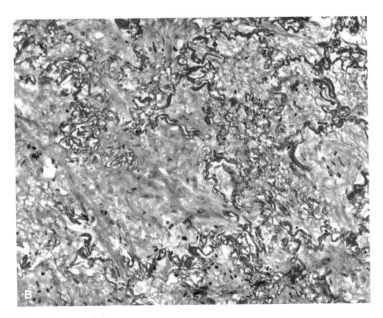

FIGURE 4.6 (*Continued*)

Reviewing the CT scan may be helpful in these cases. Upon thorough gross inspection of any lung wedge biopsy, incidental nodules less than 5 mm should not be frozen. These small nodules are not usually clinically worrisome and most often represent benign lesions or atypical adenomatous hyperplasia, which is best evaluated on nonfrozen sections. For cases in which it is necessary to freeze a small pulmonary nodule, it may be useful to inflate the lung with a 2:3 dilution of embedding medium in saline (2). Regardless, at least a portion of each distinct nodule larger than 5 mm should be frozen in any lung wedge biopsy sent for intraoperative consultation, as there may be more than one process present, such as a malignant tumor and organizing pneumonia (Fig. 4.7).

Another common clinical question pertains to involvement of bronchial resection margins for lobectomy specimens. Surgical resection margins should be inked, and careful gross examination can reveal margin involvement. Areas of questionable involvement of a margin should be frozen to permit a thorough intraoperative assessment (e-Fig. 4.3). A study at the University of North Carolina (3) found that 5.4% of bronchial margins were positive for either in situ or invasive carcinoma, and that lymphoma, adenoid cystic/mucoepidermoid carcinoma (e-Fig. 4.4), and small cell carcinoma had a higher frequency of positive margins than non–small cell tumors. It should be noted that the presence of preinvasive bronchial squamous lesions (dysplasia or in situ carcinoma) in frozen margins may not have clinical significance (4), but should always be reported.

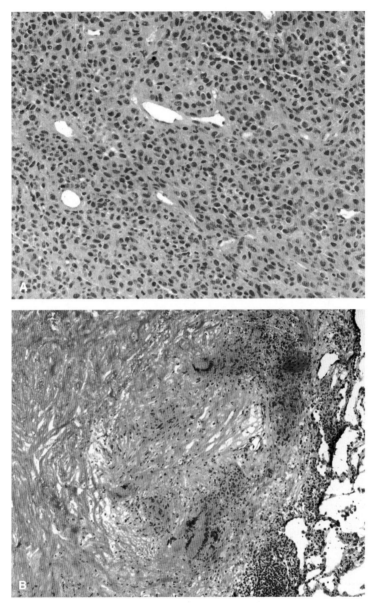

FIGURE 4.7   Two distinct nodules were present in this wedge biopsy. **A**. Metastatic malignant melanoma. **B**. Partially hyalinized granuloma.

At the University of Chicago, between 2005 and 2007, there were 226 cases of lung wedge biopsies with an intraoperative frozen section. Of these 92 (41%) were benign and 134 (59%) were malignant. Benign lesions included granulomas, intrapulmonary lymph nodes, and pulmonary hamartomas (Fig. 4.8), among others. Of the malignant lesions, 113 (84%)

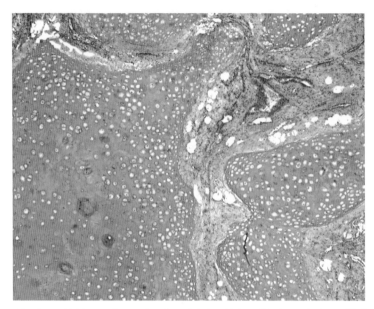

FIGURE 4.8 Bronchial hamartoma. Small endobronchial cartilaginous lesion with bronchial epithelium and fat.

were non–small cell carcinomas, and the remaining were small cell carcinomas, carcinoid tumors, sarcomas, lymphomas, and melanomas. In eight of the malignant cases, the specific diagnosis was deferred for permanent sections, two of which were sarcomas, and one of which was lymphoma. There were a total of eight cases in which the final diagnosis differed from the frozen section diagnosis, the most common reason being incorrect specific diagnosis (Table 4.1).

The Lung Frozen Section and Its Interpretation

There are several important factors to consider when evaluating a frozen section of a lung nodule. It is easier to interpret sections cut at a thickness of 5 μm. In thinner cuts, the architectural features are less apparent, making the diagnosis of carcinoma more difficult. Standard hematoxylin and eosin staining is adequate for most cases, and care should be taken to ensure adequate hematoxylin staining to best visualize nuclear features.

Fortunately, the majority of malignant lung nodules can be readily diagnosed as small cell carcinoma or non–small cell carcinoma on a well-cut and stained frozen section. Features that favor small cell over non–small cell include lack of prominent nucleoli, presence of salt and pepper chromatin, high mitotic activity, necrosis, and cellular crowding (Figs. 4.9, 4.10). A potential pitfall is that resected small cell carcinoma on frozen section may exhibit a moderate amount of cytoplasm and frequently lacks the crush artifact commonly seen on nonfrozen tissue (Fig. 4.11). Imprints

TABLE 4.1 Reasons for Incorrect Diagnosis (n = 8) on Frozen Section of Lung Wedge Biopsies (n = 226) at the University of Chicago Hospitals between 2005 and 2007	
Sampling error	
Findings insufficient to diagnose malignancy (one case, Fig. 4.15)	
Multiple nodules in specimen, diagnostic nodule not frozen (one case)	
Carcinoma not on levels cut for frozen section (one case, Fig. 4.16)	
Major discrepancy	
Carcinoma at edge of necrotic nodule (one case, Fig. 4.13)	
Incorrect diagnosis affecting operative course[a] (one case)	
Frozen section diagnosis	*Final diagnosis*
Non–small cell carcinoma	Carcinoid tumor
Minor discrepancy	
Incorrect specific diagnosis, not affecting operative course[b] (four cases)	
Frozen section diagnosis	*Final diagnosis*
Case 1 Hodgkin lymphoma	Follicular lymphoma
Case 2 Pulmonary hamartoma	Inflammatory myofibroblastic tumor
Case 3 Neuroendocrine tumor, favor carcinoid	Metastatic myoepithelial carcinoma

[a]An intraoperative diagnosis of non–small cell carcinoma typically leads to completion lobectomy, whereas carcinoid tumor does not usually require lobectomy.

[b]In most instances, a broad intraoperative diagnosis, such as "lymphoma" (case 1), "benign neoplasm" (case 2), "carcinoid tumor," "non–small cell carcinoma," or "small cell carcinoma" will be sufficient. In case 3, the operative management is the same (wedge resection).

may be helpful in distinguishing small cell carcinoma from non–small cell carcinoma.

Lung carcinoma is frequently surrounded by an inflammatory reaction or an obstructive/organizing pneumonia (Fig. 4.12), or the lesion may be partially necrotic (Fig. 4.13), which may lead to consideration of necrotizing granuloma (Fig. 4.14). Therefore, if initial sections of a suspected lung carcinoma do not reveal definitive carcinoma, deeper sections of the frozen tissue or sampling another block, ideally through the center of the lesion, should be obtained before finalizing an intraoperative diagnosis. Deeper sections of the frozen tissue should also be cut if there are only a few atypical cells present on the initial sections (Fig. 4.15), and if a nodule is suspected clinically, but not seen on initial sections (Fig. 4.16).

A diagnostic conundrum is distinguishing a well-differentiated adenocarcinoma, including bronchioloalveolar carcinoma, from bronchial metaplasia on frozen section (Fig. 4.17, e-Fig. 4.5). Both well-differentiated adenocarcinoma and bronchial metaplasia have fibrosis, but a higher ratio

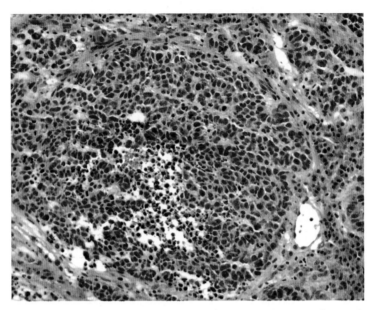

FIGURE 4.9 Small cell carcinoma frozen section showing nuclear crowding and necrosis. These features favor small cell carcinoma over non–small cell carcinoma.

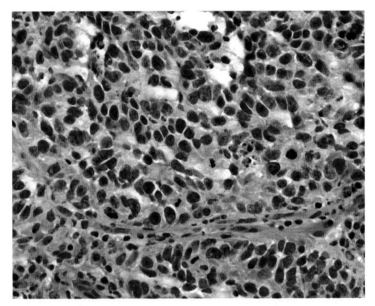

FIGURE 4.10 Higher power of tumor in Figure 4.9 shows small cells that lack prominent nucleoli, and have salt and pepper chromatin and high mitotic activity, features that favor small cell carcinoma.

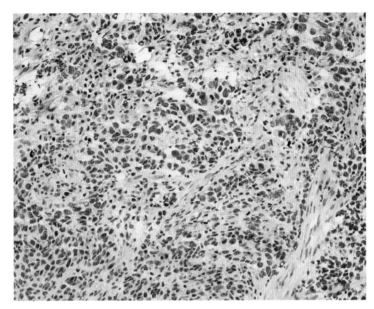

FIGURE 4.11 As opposed to bronchoscopic biopsies, frozen sections of small cell carcinoma often are well-preserved, have moderate cytoplasm, and lack crush artifact.

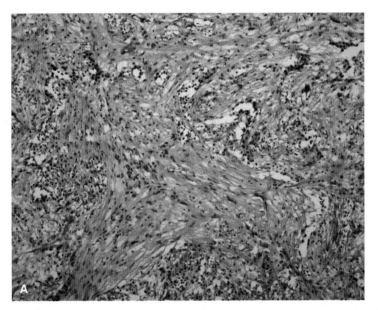

FIGURE 4.12 **A.** Organizing pneumonia only was seen in the first section submitted from this 0.9-cm nodule. **B.** Additional block was submitted from the center of the nodule, which showed squamous cell carcinoma. (*continued*)

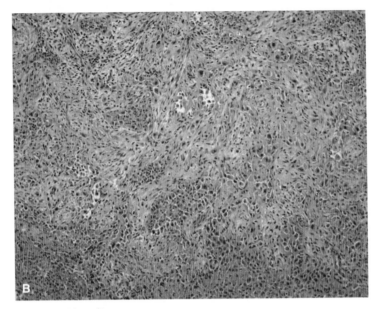

FIGURE 4.12 (*Continued*)

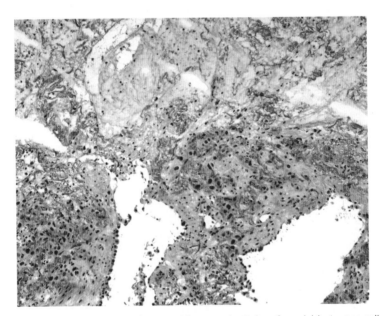

FIGURE 4.13 Non–small cell carcinoma with necrosis. Only a few viable tumor cells were present in this case, which led to the misdiagnosis of benign lesions on frozen section.

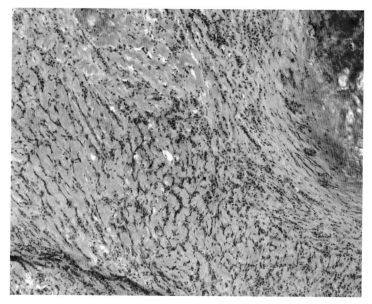

FIGURE 4.14   Necrotizing granuloma. The periphery is cellular and can mimic malignancy.

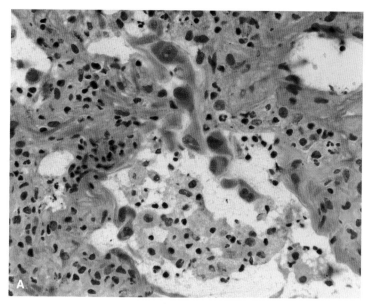

FIGURE 4.15   **A.** Frozen section of nodule shows only a few atypical cells. **B.** Permanent section did show non–small cell carcinoma. (*continued*)

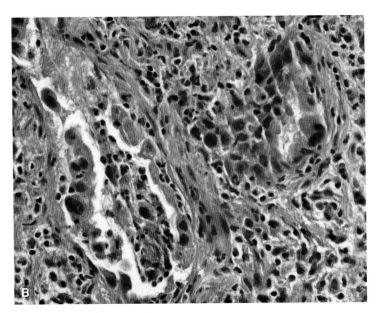

FIGURE 4.15 *(Continued)*

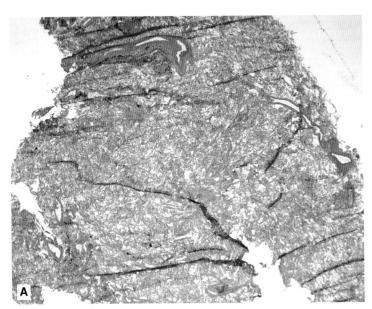

FIGURE 4.16 **A.** Frozen section of nodule showed only benign lung parenchyma. **B.** Deeper section cut from the same block after paraffin embedding shows adenocarcinoma. *(continued)*

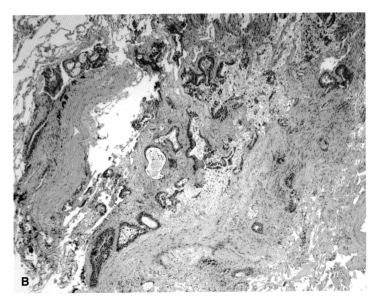

FIGURE 4.16 (*Continued*)

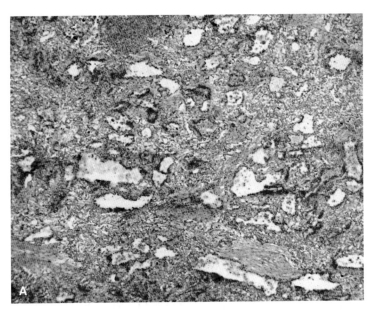

FIGURE 4.17 Well-differentiated adenocarcinoma that was called bronchial metaplasia on frozen section. Clues to malignancy are crowding of glands and variation in nuclear size. **A.** Low power. **B.** High power. (*continued*)

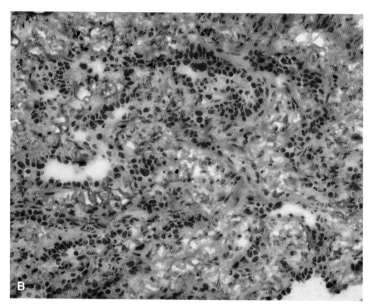

FIGURE 4.17   (*Continued*)

of glands to fibrotic tissue, as well as crowding of the glands, in the presence of minimal inflammation is strongly suggestive of carcinoma (1). The nuclear features of metaplasia are more uniform in contrast to uneven atypia and hobnailing of nuclei suggestive of carcinoma. A prospective single-institution study by Gupta et al. (5) determined that the presence of macronucleoli, anisocytosis, atypical mitoses, multiple growth patterns, and more than 75% atypia are features strongly in favor of well-differentiated adenocarcinoma. Granulomas strongly suggest reactive atypia. Probably the most important factor to consider in these cases is that generally metaplasia does not present as a mass. Therefore, with a high clinical suspicion of malignancy, a frozen section of a lung nodule with well-differentiated glandular features is more likely adenocarcinoma. While the tendency is more often to call the lesion benign on intraoperative evaluation, any doubt should prompt the pathologist to defer the diagnosis. The permanent sections could certainly reveal a true malignancy. In any case, additional surgery can be performed later if the lesion proves to be malignant, inconvenience notwithstanding.

In the assessment of bronchial resection margins, microscopic features that can mimic carcinoma include squamous metaplasia (Fig. 4.18, e-Fig. 4.6), radiation changes, submucosal glands, and clusters of peribronchial lymphocytes (3). While tumor in a frozen resection margin specimen may be most conspicuous on the mucosal surface, the systematic assessment of the extramucosal tissue for microscopic peribronchial spread as well as intravascular and lymphatic invasion should not be ignored (3,6).

The use of imprints in the intraoperative evaluation of lung nodules is a valuable adjunct, but often dependent on the preference of the

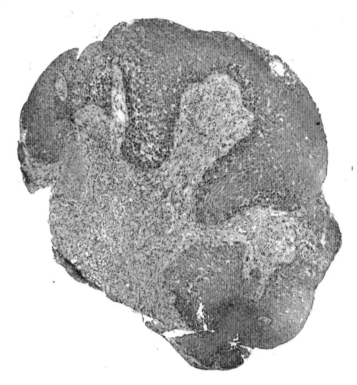

FIGURE 4.18 Squamous metaplasia. Extensive metaplasia can mimic carcinoma as seen in this low-power photomicrograph of bronchial mucosa from a person who smokes heavily.

pathologist. The architectural features of a lesion are often diagnostically helpful, a feature lacking in imprints (Fig. 4.19). Also, atypia of type II pneumocytes may be misinterpreted as malignancy on imprints. Imprints may be useful for appreciating the nuclear features of carcinoid tumors (Fig. 4.20) or for identifying pigment in a metastatic melanoma (Fig. 4.21). Paucicellular imprints may be due to fibrosis, desmoplasia, or the presence of a central scar in the lesion.

There are several other considerations when evaluating a frozen section of a lung nodule. Previous therapy may induce atypia and/or hyperplasia of type II pneumocytes, which can be mistaken for malignancy. Carcinoid tumors should be considered in the differential of a small cell carcinoma, because wedge resection or partial lobectomy is typically sufficient surgical therapy for a carcinoid tumor (Fig. 4.22). The morphologic similarities between carcinoid tumors and small cell carcinomas include small nuclei, salt and pepper chromatin, and indistinct nucleoli. Lack of mitotic figures and necrosis favors carcinoid tumor. Although frozen section evaluation is not typically requested in cases with multiple nodules suspected of being metastatic, the possibility of multiple pulmonary carcinoid tumorlets may be a consideration (7). Other malignancies, such as sarcoma or hematologic malignancies, rarely present initially as lung nodules, but may be encountered.

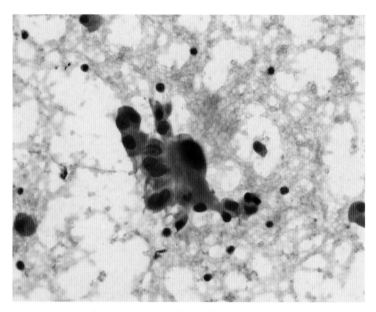

FIGURE 4.19 Intraoperative touch preparation of adenocarcinoma shows cellular features of malignancy.

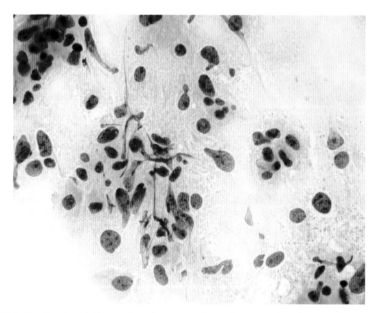

FIGURE 4.20 Carcinoid tumor. Touch preparation (Giemsa stain) shows salt and pepper chromatin and small nucleoli.

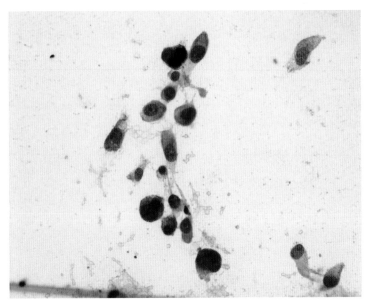

FIGURE 4.21 Malignant melanoma metastatic to lung. On touch preparation (Giemsa stain), melanin pigment is easily identified in the tumor cells.

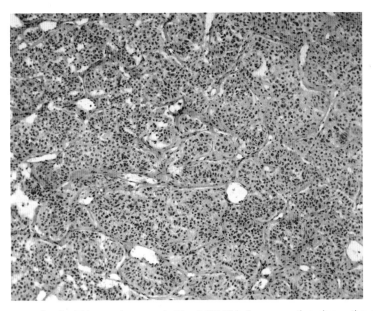

FIGURE 4.22 Carcinoid tumor (same as in Fig. 4.20). This frozen section shows the characteristic organoid pattern of uniform cells without necrosis.

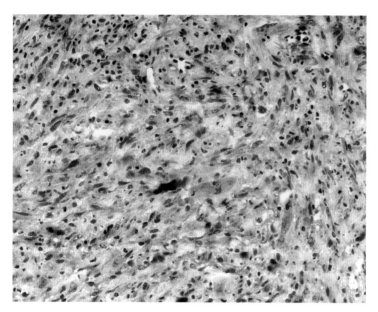

FIGURE 4.23 Spindle cell lesions. **A.** High-grade pleomorphic sarcoma. **B.** Neurofibroma.
C. Organizing pneumonia. (*continued*)

Lesions with a spindle cell component may be difficult to interpret on frozen section, and may represent malignant or benign neoplasms or non-neoplastic entities (Fig. 4.23, e-Fig. 4.7). Pulmonary inflammatory myofi-broblastic tumor (Fig. 4.24), which may be misinterpreted as pulmonary sarcoma (8), and pulmonary sclerosing hemangioma (9) are examples of rare benign neoplasms with spindle cell components. Pulmonary sclerosing hemangioma is best identified by the presence of more than one of the typical histologic growth patterns, as well as circumscription of the tumor nodule and bland cytology on imprints (10,11). The presence of chronic lung disease in the background of a malignant lesion is usually not a major intraoperative concern and can be better evaluated on permanent sections.

Finally, there are several nonneoplastic conditions that may present as a solitary lung nodule, including the metaplasia associated with an in-farct, granulomatous diseases (e-Figs. 4.8, 4.9), and organizing pneumo-nia. Squamous metaplasia involving the bronchial, bronchiolar, and alve-olar epithelia, may be mistaken for squamous cell carcinoma. Similarly, mucinous metaplasia of the airway or bronchiolar metaplasia of the alve-olar epithelium can be mistaken for adenocarcinoma. Finding hyaline membranes should prompt consideration of diffuse alveolar damage (Fig. 4.25), and finding intraalveolar fibroblastic nodules (Masson bodies) should prompt consideration of organizing pneumonia (Fig. 4.26). An ex-cellent review by Sienko et al. (1) presents a thorough discussion of the differential diagnoses for various histologic patterns encountered on lung nodule frozen sections.

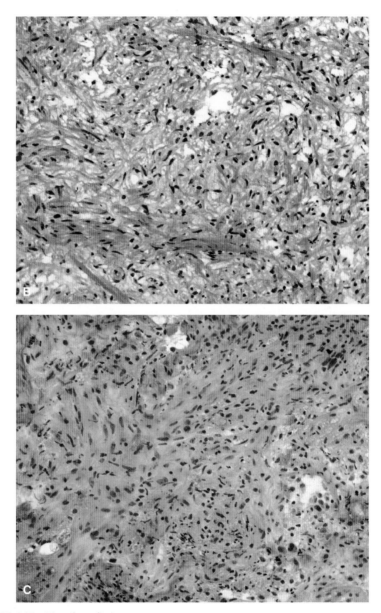

FIGURE 4.23 (*Continued*)

The immunocompromised host presents a special patient population in whom fungal pneumonias are in the differential diagnosis of a lung nodule. Fungal hyphae and large budding yeasts of blastomycosis are easily recognized on frozen section. To aid in identifying fungus, Giemsa and Diff-Quick stains may be used, or the section may be left 30 seconds longer than usual in hematoxylin. Invasive fungal hyphae are often found

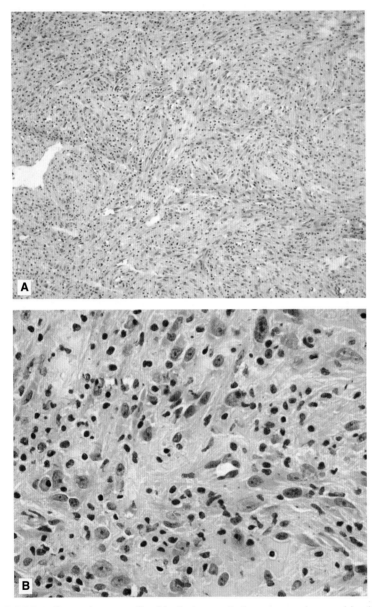

FIGURE 4.24 Inflammatory myofibroblastic tumor. **A.** Low power shows a bland spindle cell tumor. **B.** High power shows spindle cells admixed with lymphocytes and plasma cells.

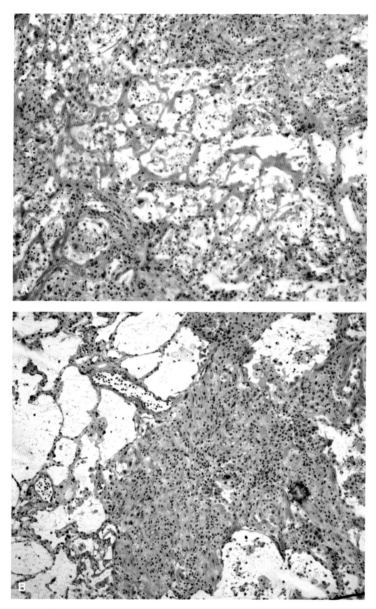

FIGURE 4.25 Diffuse alveolar damage. **A.** Striking hyaline membranes lining the alveolar septae with intraalveolar foamy macrophages. **B.** Focal areas of organizing diffuse alveolar damage are also present. **C.** Higher power shows random large reactive type II pneumocytes. (*continued*)

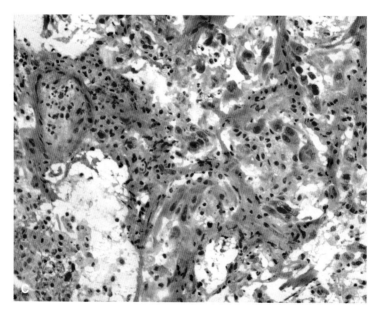

FIGURE 4.25 (*Continued*)

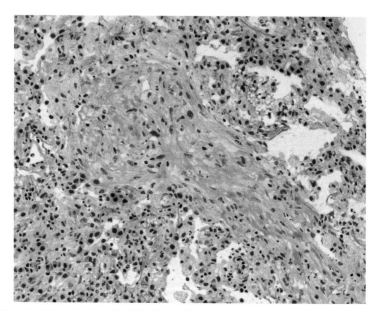

FIGURE 4.26 Intraalveolar fibroblastic proliferation (Masson body) streaming from one alveolus to the next with normal background lung architecture is characteristic for organizing pneumonia.

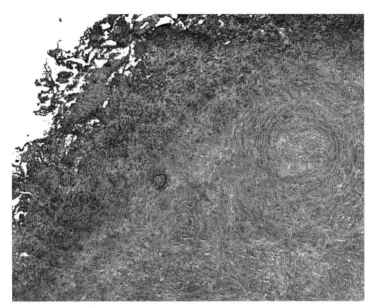

FIGURE 4.27 Granulomatous inflammation with necrosis. There was concern for malignancy in this immunocompromised patient with lung nodules seen on imaging. Frozen section showed necrotic granulomas with no evidence of tumor. Silver stains later highlighted the presence of *Pneumocystis jiroveci.*

in the wall of an abscess, and focusing up and down helps in their identification. *Pneumocystis jiroveci* infection (Fig. 4.27) rarely presents as a mass, although it may be associated with an infarction, which may be surgically removed. Infection by cytomegalovirus is usually already clinically known through the use of sensitive PCR serologic methods, but cytomegalovirus may still be present incidentally on a frozen lung section and should be reported. Overall, multiple organisms should be kept in mind when evaluating the frozen section lung biopsy of immunocompromised hosts. Other diagnostic considerations in immunocompromised patients include recurrent leukemia or lymphoma after bone marrow transplant and posttransplant lymphoproliferative disorder after solid organ transplant.

INTRODUCTION: MEDIASTINAL LYMPH NODE FROZEN SECTION

Over the past several years, it has become standard practice to evaluate metastatic disease prior to definitive resection in patients with a lung nodule suspicious for carcinoma. A common metastatic site of primary lung cancer is the regional lymph nodes, which are divided into N1, N2, and N3 nodes. The treatment principle for mediastinal lymph node evaluation in cases of suspected lung cancer is that N1 node status does not alter the decision to resect the tumor. However, if an N2 node is positive, the patient will have stage IIIA disease, and neoadjuvant therapies will be undertaken prior to surgical management. N3 disease renders the tumor unresectable.

Surgical excision and intraoperative evaluation of mediastinal lymph nodes are not analogous to a sentinel lymph node biopsy: there is no dye or radioactive tracer used to find these nodes intraoperatively. In patients with a known lung nodule, the clinical evaluation will often include a PET scan for any suspicious mediastinal lymph nodes seen on CT. If the PET scan is negative, then the workup of the lung nodule can proceed as described earlier in the chapter. However, if suspicion remains, or if the mediastinal lymph node is positive on PET scan, a transbronchial fine needle aspiration or Wang needle biopsy of the lymph node may be obtained prior to surgery. In the surgical setting, clinically suspicious and PET-positive mediastinal lymph nodes are excised for intraoperative frozen section diagnosis to determine metastatic disease prior to resection of the target lung nodule. The biopsy may be obtained by mediastinoscopy or in an open procedure, with the intent to halt surgical intervention if a lymph node metastasis is found on frozen section.

Mediastinal Lymph Node Frozen Section: Major Intraoperative Questions

The major question for frozen section evaluation of mediastinal lymph nodes in a suspected lung cancer patient is whether metastatic disease is present. If the frozen section reveals metastatic disease in N2 nodes, surgical intervention will typically be interrupted in favor of multimodality therapy. If the lymph node is negative, either additional suspicious lymph nodes will be sent for intraoperative evaluation, or the surgeon will proceed with wedge biopsy of the lung nodule.

Lymph nodes obtained by mediastinoscopy may be fragmented, but all tissue is frozen regardless of whether the nodes are intact or fragmented. Confirmation of a grossly positive node may be accomplished by freezing a portion of the tissue, with the caveat that the remaining tissue should be frozen if the first portion is not positive. For lung cancer staging, although the number of positive lymph nodes is not a key consideration, the station is important (12), and care should be taken to transcribe this information exactly as written by the surgeon on the specimen container and requisition.

Mediastinal Lymph Node Frozen Section and Its Interpretation

In a mediastinal lymph node, microscopically identifiable epithelial cells constitute metastatic disease. The presence of any extracapsular extension should also be reported (12). Crushed normal lymphoid tissue should not be misinterpreted as a small cell carcinoma (13). The use of imprints in cases of suspected metastatic carcinoma is at the discretion of the pathologist; however, imprints should always be evaluated prior to freezing lymph nodes in cases where lymphoma is a diagnostic consideration. Lymphoma may be suspected clinically or upon gross inspection of the node. Mediastinal lymph nodes rarely harbor metastases from primary tumors other than from the lung. The Mayo Clinic has reported that in patients with extrathoracic primary carcinomas, up to 28% of mediastinal lymph nodes can harbor secondary metastases from the lung metastases (13).

Mediastinal Mass Frozen Section and Its Interpretation

Mediastinal masses other than those associated with a suspected lung carcinoma are occasionally sent for intraoperative evaluation. The diagnostic considerations include lymphoma (Fig. 4.28, e-Fig. 4.10), thymoma (Fig. 4.29), and germ cell tumor (Fig. 4.30). In our experience, it may be difficult to distinguish thymoma from lymphoma on frozen section. Clues to thymoma include presence of epithelioid cells and lack of lymphocyte atypia. Consideration of the patient's age when faced with a small blue cell tumor of the mediastinum may also be helpful since patients in the second to fourth decade are more likely to have germ cell tumors or lymphomas, while older patients are more likely to have carcinoma and thymoma. If thymoma can be definitively diagnosed by frozen section, this may help avoid a second surgery. In cases of suspected lymphoma, document that adequate tissue has been obtained for workup and diagnosis. Mediastinal tuberculosis and infectious pseudotumor can be mistaken for tumor necrosis and lymphoma (14). Thymic tissue (Fig. 4.31) may be confused

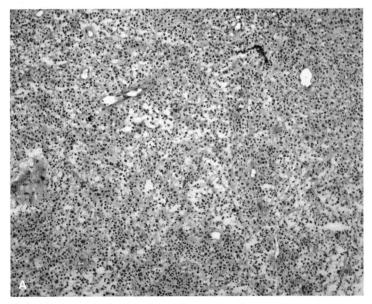

FIGURE 4.28 Large B-cell lymphoma. **A.** A lymphoid infiltrate partially obliterating the lung architecture is seen on low power, the differential diagnosis for which includes inflammation. **B.** On higher power, large atypical dyscohesive lymphoid cells, some with prominent nucleoli, are seen. (*continued*)

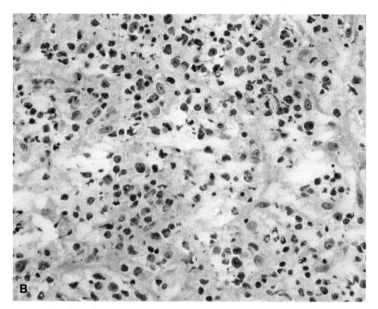

FIGURE 4.28 (*Continued*)

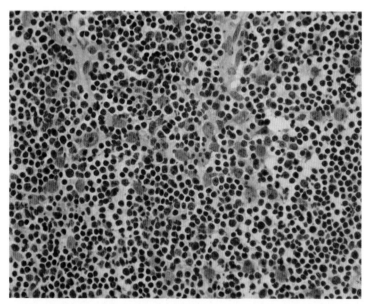

FIGURE 4.29 Thymoma. Single large epithelioid cells are seen within a small lymphoid cell background, which was reported as "lymphoma versus thymic neoplasm." Final diagnosis was WHO type B2 thymoma.

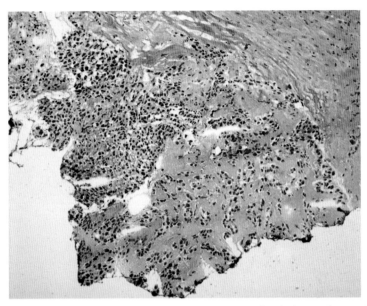

FIGURE 4.30   Yolk sac tumor. On frozen section of this mediastinal mass from a 27-year-old, a cellular myxoid lesion is seen which was reported as "malignant tumor, defer to permanent sections."

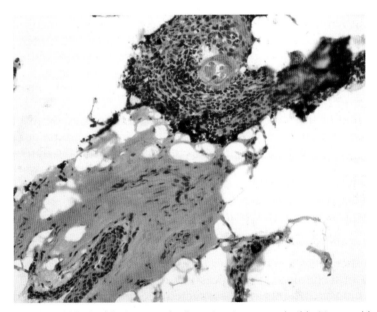

FIGURE 4.31   Atrophic thymic tissue and adjacent cyst are seen in this 61-year-old patient with mediastinal mass.

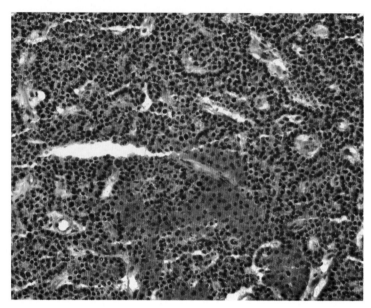

FIGURE 4.32 Ectopic hypercellular parathyroid tissue is seen in this frozen section from the mediastinum.

for lymphoid tissue with metastatic tumor, especially if specimen designation/site is lacking because of uncertainty of the surgeon. Ectopic thyroid and parathyroid tissues (Fig. 4.32) may also be seen in the mediastinum.

At the University of Chicago, between 2000 and 2007, there were a total of 91 mediastinal specimens for frozen section in 67 different patients, excluding cases of lymph nodes for lung cancer staging. Of these, 23 (25%) were mediastinal lymph nodes, 54 (59%) were mediastinal masses, and 14 (16%) were other diagnoses, including ectopic mediastinal parathyroid or thyroid glands. Of the mediastinal masses, 34 (63%) were malignant and 20 (37%) were benign. Malignancies were predominantly lymphomas and benign diagnoses were mostly nonspecific fibrous tissue or scar. Fourteen (41%) of the malignant mediastinal masses were called malignant on frozen section, but deferred to permanent sections for specific typing. There was only one case that was misdiagnosed as a malignancy on frozen section that proved to be benign on permanent sections.

Pleural Frozen Section and Its Interpretation

Pleural specimens are no longer commonly evaluated by frozen section because of technological advances including the video-assisted thoracoscopic biopsy. Patients with suspected pleural lesions will undergo a video-assisted thoracoscopy procedure, with the biopsy specimen submitted only for permanent paraffin sections. In rare cases where a frozen section of a pleural biopsy is requested, the main clinical questions are

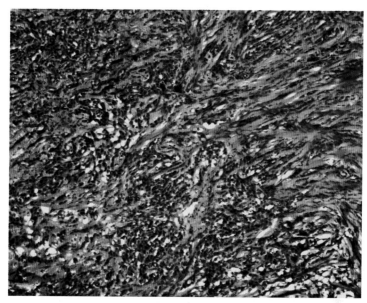

FIGURE 4.33 Malignant mesothelioma. A malignant infiltrate was seen on frozen section but it is difficult to determine whether this is an adenocarcinoma or mesothelioma; however, it does represent diagnostic tissue.

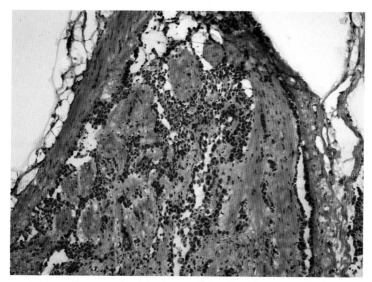

FIGURE 4.34 Malignant mesothelioma. The frozen section of this pleural biopsy displays mesothelial proliferation with areas suspicious for infiltration into adipose tissue. This was read as "most consistent with mesothelioma."

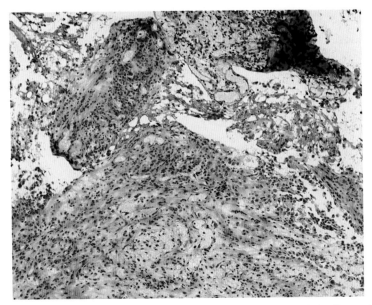

FIGURE 4.35 Reactive mesothelial proliferation. Fibrin with mesothelial cells overlying fibrosis creates a layering effect, suggestive of a benign mesothelial process.

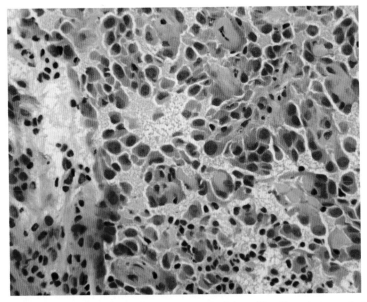

FIGURE 4.36 High power of this reactive mesothelial proliferation shows cells indistinguishable from those seen in malignant mesothelioma.

whether there is adequate tissue for definitive diagnosis, whether the diagnosis is mesothelioma (Fig. 4.33) or metastatic carcinoma, and whether mesothelioma can be distinguished from benign reactive mesothelial proliferations. Clues to the diagnosis of mesothelioma are definitive invasion into fat or muscle (Fig. 4.34), complex architecture, necrosis, and the absence of a layering effect. A layering or zone effect consisting of a layer of fibrin with mesothelial cells and a layer of granulation tissue with fibrosis is suggestive of reactive hyperplasia (Fig. 4.35). The presence of atypical mesothelial cells is not diagnostic of malignancy, as these are commonly seen in reactive conditions (Fig. 4.36).

REFERENCES

1. Sienko A, Allen T, Zander D, Cagle P. Frozen section of lung specimens. *Arch Pathol Lab Med*. 2005;129(12):1602–1609.
2. Myung J, Choe G, Chung D, et al. A simple inflation method for frozen section diagnosis of minute precancerous lesions of the lung. *Lung Cancer*. 2008;59(2):198–202.
3. Maygarden S, Detterbeck F, Funkhouser W. Bronchial margins in lung cancer resection specimens: utility of frozen section and gross evaluation. *Mod Pathol*. 2004;17(9): 1080–1086.
4. Kutlu C, Urer N, Olgac G. Carcinoma in situ from the view of complete resection. *Lung Cancer*. 2004;46(3):383–385.
5. Gupta R, McKenna R, Marchevsky A. Lessons learned from mistakes and deferrals in the frozen section diagnosis of bronchioloalveolar carcinoma and well-differentiated pulmonary adenocarcinoma: an evidence-based pathology approach. *Am J Clin Pathol*. 2008;130(1):11–20.
6. Thunnissen F, den Bakker M. Implications of frozen section analyses from bronchial resection margins in NSCLC. *Histopathology*. 2005;47(6):638–640.
7. Darvishian F, Ginsberg M, Klimstra D, et al. Carcinoid tumorlets simulate pulmonary metastases in women with breast cancer. *Hum Pathol*. 2006;37(7):839–844.
8. Takeda S, Onishi Y, Kawamura T, et al. Clinical spectrum of pulmonary inflammatory myofibroblastic tumor. *Interact Cardiovasc Thorac Surg* 2008;7(4):629–633.
9. van Wyk Q, Suvarna S. Frozen section diagnosis of fibrotic sclerosing pneumocytoma with psammomatous calcification. *Histopathology*. 2003;43(5):504–505.
10. Chan A, Chan J. Can pulmonary sclerosing haemangioma be accurately diagnosed by intra-operative frozen section? *Histopathology*. 2002;41(5):392–403.
11. Majak B, Bock G. Pulmonary sclerosing haemangioma diagnosed by frozen section. *Histopathology*. 2003;42(6):621–622.
12. Lardinois D, De Leyn P, Van Schil P, et al. ESTS guidelines for intraoperative lymph node staging in non-small cell lung cancer. *Eur J Cardiothorac Surg*. 2006;30(5): 787–792.
13. Ercan S, Nichols F, Trastek V, et al. Prognostic significance of lymph node metastasis found during pulmonary metastasectomy for extrapulmonary carcinoma. *Ann Thorac Surg*. 2004;77(5):1786–1791.
14. de Montpreville V, Dulmet E, Nashashibi N. Frozen section diagnosis and surgical biopsy of lymph nodes, tumors and pseudotumors of the mediastinum. *Eur J Cardiothorac Surg*. 1998;13(2):190–195.

5

PEDIATRIC FROZEN SECTION

AJIT PAINTAL AND ALIYA N. HUSAIN

At the University of Chicago Hospitals and Medical Center, the most frequent indications for intraoperative consultation in children are bone tumors and brain tumors which are discussed in their respective chapters. Approximately 9% of our pediatric intraoperative consultations are performed for the evaluation of Hirschsprung's disease and the vast majority of the remaining consultations are done for tumors. Evaluation of an immunocompromised child is a rare indication for frozen section and is discussed elsewhere in this volume. Our overall frozen section concordance rate (95%) and deferral rate (11%) are roughly comparable to what has been reported in the literature at other institutions (1,2).

INTRODUCTION: PEDIATRIC SOLID TUMORS

Relative to adults, malignancies in children are uncommon, accounting for approximately 7,000 cases per year in the United States. Hematopoietic neoplasms are the largest single group of cancers leaving solid tumors to account for approximately 60% of all cases. The spectrum of malignancy in infants and children differs markedly from that seen in the adult population and most of these patients receive treatment at specialized tertiary centers. Because of these factors, most nonpediatric pathologists do not accrue substantial amounts of experience with these diseases.

Over the past several decades, outcomes in pediatric cancer have improved dramatically as a result of improved accuracy in diagnosis, recognition of biologically significant prognostic features, and tailored therapy using multiple modalities. Successful treatment of these diseases hinges on the correct initial classification of the malignancy and recognition of significant morphologic (e.g., anaplasia in Wilms tumors) and genetic (e.g., N-*myc* amplification in neuroblastoma) prognostic factors.

Pediatric Solid Tumors: Major Intraoperative Questions

Because of the important role that molecular and genetic testing play in the diagnosis of pediatric tumors, a request for a specific primary diagnosis is generally inappropriate and often not possible intraoperatively. Definitive surgery and therapy are properly based only upon thorough histologic examination of fixed tissues and interpretation of ancillary data. The frozen section in this setting may address the basic question of the benign versus malignant nature of a tumor so that a catheter may be placed for future chemotherapy. A malignant diagnosis may also initiate staging bone marrow biopsies which can be performed while the patient is under anesthesia.

A second use for frozen section in pediatric tumors is in the assessment of margin status and extent of disease. Margins are critically important in most pediatric tumors, and in the case of hepatoblastoma, complete resection is essential for disease cure (3). In most cases, 1- to 2-mL margins are sufficient, particularly when operating in the head and neck regions (4).

Last, frozen section may facilitate triage and assessment of adequacy of a biopsy. In this scenario, requesting an intraoperative consultation serves to bring the specimen to the pathologist's attention allowing the viability of the tissue to be assessed and tissue to be apportioned for cytogenetics, electron microscopy, and molecular studies (5). Additionally, cytologic preparations (imprints) can be made at this time which are often a valuable adjunct in arriving at the final diagnosis (6).

Pediatric Solid Tumors and Frozen Section Interpretation

As in other settings, the nature of the question being posed usually determines how the intraoperative consultation is performed. In the case of determining adequacy or whether a lesion is benign or malignant, intraoperative cytology often proves invaluable, especially if material is limited. In a single series, intraoperative cytology to evaluate masses in pediatric patients with knowledge of the clinical and radiographic data had an accuracy rate ranging from 93% to 98% among three observers and was shown to be particularly effective in the case of small round blue cell tumors allowing general classification as such in more than 95% of cases. Interestingly, performing a concurrent frozen section and intraoperative evaluation of histology only increased the accuracy rates by 0% to 3%, depending on the observer (7). If material is limited, intraoperative cytology alone is almost always sufficient to determine if diagnostic tissue is present and to classify a lesion as benign or malignant.

A major potential pitfall in interpreting frozen sections in pediatric neoplasms lies in misreading inflammatory atypia as a malignant process, particularly in spindle cell lesions. Florid inflammatory processes may display marked atypia and hypercellularity rendering them treacherous in the setting of a frozen section. The importance of correlating intraoperative histology and cytology with clinical and radiographic data before rendering a diagnosis cannot be overemphasized. A lack of correlation between morphology and the clinical picture should make one strongly consider deferring any evaluation to permanent sections and a more thorough examination of the material. In a series of soft-tissue lesions of unknown etiology in adults, a specific or general (benign vs malignant) diagnosis could only be obtained intraoperatively in 84% of cases (9).

In regard to the amount of viable material required for an appropriate workup including histology and ancillary studies, we find that 2 cm^3 of tissue is adequate. This tissue should be obtained via "cold knife" rather than cautery and be sent to pathology for triage immediately after it is obtained in a fresh, unfixed state (5). In any case, the top priority is always to fix an adequate amount of tissue in formalin for diagnostic examination by light microscopy and immunohistochemical stains. The second priority is to snap-freeze at least 100 mg of viable tissue for molecular studies, often crucial in evaluating pediatric tumors. If material is limited, tissue that has been frozen intraoperatively may be maintained in its frozen state. Unstained touch preparations made at the time of tissue triage are useful in that they may be used for FISH studies. Cytogenetics is another potentially useful diagnostic modality and generally requires a piece of viable tissue measuring 0.5 cm × 0.5 cm × 0.2 cm (10–12). A small portion of tissue may additionally be submitted in glutaraldehyde for electron microscopy. If there is any suspicion that a case is infectious in nature, material should be sent for culture from the operating room rather than from pathology to minimize the risk of contamination. When evaluating margins intraoperatively, once the specimen is inked appropriately, we advocate examining perpendicular margins as opposed to "shave" margins. Particularly when the margins are likely to be close, perpendicular margins provide a better evaluation of whether the inked margin is involved, and if not, an actual distance of tumor to the resected edge can be reported as opposed to simply "positive" or "negative."

INTRODUCTION: INTRAOPERATIVE PEDIATRIC LYMPH NODE EVALUATION

Lymphadenopathy is extremely common in the pediatric population. Almost half of all children younger than 5 years who present for routine well-child visits will exhibit some form of lymphadenopathy if carefully examined (13). In most cases, lymphadenopathy in children is reactive. In a single series, even when clinical and laboratory findings were suspicious enough to warrant excisional biopsy, only 13% of cases of lymphadenopathy were found to be the result of lymphoma (14).

Lymphomas are broadly categorized as Hodgkin and non-Hodgkin lymphomas. Hodgkin lymphoma is rare in children younger than 5 years and its incidence gradually increases throughout childhood. Overall, in children younger than 15 years, non-Hodgkin lymphomas are somewhat more common than Hodgkin lymphomas. In the 15- to 19-year age group, the reverse is true with Hodgkin lymphomas outnumbering non-Hodgkin lymphomas by a ratio of approximately 2:1.

Among pediatric Hodgkin lymphomas, the most frequent subtypes are nodular sclerosing (70% of cases) and mixed cellularity (16% of cases)

(15). The most frequent forms of non-Hodgkin lymphomas in children are Burkitt lymphoma, lymphoblastic lymphoma, and large cell lymphoma respectively. Together, these three entities account for 85% of all pediatric non-Hodgkin lymphomas (16). It is worth noting that unlike their adult counterparts, pediatric non-Hodgkin lymphomas are high-grade malignancies that frequently present with extranodal disease. Indolent low-grade B-cell lymphomas that make up the majority of adult cases of non-Hodgkin lymphoma are extremely rare.

Pediatric Lymph Nodes: Major Intraoperative Questions

Similar to nonhematopoietic pediatric solid tumors, the final diagnosis in pediatric lymphomas rests heavily upon ancillary techniques which include flow cytometry, cytogenetics, and molecular studies. The accuracy of the evaluation of lymph nodes in adult patients by imprint cytology as would be used in intraoperative diagnosis has been reviewed and found to be relatively poor with a mean diagnostic accuracy of 78% in regard to classifying lymph nodes as reactive lymph nodes, Hodgkin and non-Hodgkin lymphomas, or nonhematopoietic malignancy (17). Given that most non-Hodgkin lymphomas in children are high-grade diffuse processes, one would expect more accuracy in the pediatric population.

Because induction chemotherapeutic regimens differ for different forms of lymphoma, definitive treatment should not be based solely upon an intraoperative assessment of morphology. Rather, the appropriate intraoperative question that should be posed to the pathologist is whether diagnostic tissue has been obtained. If tissue is limited, the pathologist can then use the initial morphologic impression to triage tissue in a way that best utilizes the specimen in light of the suspected diagnosis (18).

Intraoperative Interpretation of Pediatric Lymph Nodes

Specimens obtained for the workup of a potential lymphoma should be received fresh and as sterile as possible to ensure the viability of cells for ancillary studies. Lymph nodes are initially dissected with a sterile scalpel blade and forceps from a sterile surgical suture kit to prevent contamination. The lymph nodes are then sectioned and the cut surface is examined.

The gross examination of a lymph node often provides a valuable initial impression. Reactive lymph nodes are tan gray and rubbery while lymphomas are often pale with a firm "fish-flesh" consistency. The gross appearance of nodular sclerosing Hodgkin lymphoma is particularly characteristic and may show multiple matted lymph nodes with a firm nodular cut surface. Granulocytic sarcomas, although rare, may display a green tinge.

Frozen section evaluation of potential lymphomas is discouraged in that it consumes diagnostic material and does not provide the detailed cellular morphology required to make a definitive diagnosis (5). Imprint cytology is useful in this setting in that it allows a rapid assessment of morphology and fine cytologic detail (e-Figs. 5.1, 5.2). Unstained imprints prepared at the time of intraoperative evaluation can also be saved for FISH studies and cytochemical stains. Cytologic imprints additionally provide a valuable adjunct once permanent histologic sections are available.

In general, the presence of a mixed lymphocytic population is suggestive of a benign reactive process. In this setting, a spectrum of cells ranging from small lymphocytes to large reactive centroblasts and immunoblasts is generally seen. Scattered "tingible-body" histiocytes are also usually abundant. Even though this pattern is generally reassuring, a similar milieu may also be seen in malignant conditions including nasopharyngeal carcinoma, Hodgkin lymphoma, and anaplastic large cell lymphoma (ALCL). Necrotic debris is also often seen in reactive lymphadenopathies and should prompt a workup for an infectious etiology, including special stains and culture if the quantity of tissue permits. Although common in benign conditions, necrosis is also seen in malignancy and may be extensive in Hodgkin lymphomas as well as high-grade non-Hodgkin lymphomas (19).

The diagnostic accuracy of imprint cytology for Hodgkin lymphoma has been reported to range from 69% to 85%. Even if this diagnosis cannot definitively be made on the basis of an imprint alone, a cytologic preparation can suggest it in up to 95% of cases (20). When using imprints alone, familiarity with the stain (H&E or Diff-Quick) is essential, as the tinctorial properties of the Reed-Sternberg cells will show minor variations. Recognizing Hodgkin lymphoma requires the identification of two components: (i) a reactive background and (ii) Reed-Sternberg cells (19). The background in Hodgkin lymphoma is generally heterogeneous and contains a spectrum of reactive lymphocytes, often with admixed eosinophils, plasma cells, neutrophils, and necrosis (21). Granulomatous inflammation may occasionally be the dominant cytologic feature (22). Diagnostic Reed-Sternberg cells, while often rare and difficult to locate, should at least focally have the classic morphology (Figs. 5.1, 5.2, e-Figs. 5.3, 5.4). In addition to being large and multinucleated, the chromatin is coarse and often marginates against the nuclear envelope. Each nucleus should contain a single dark inclusion which is at least the size of an erythrocyte and is surrounded by a pale halo. Several disease processes may contain cells which closely mimic Reed-Sternberg cells, and for this reason, one should consider other possible diagnoses if the cytologic features of the Reed-Sternberg cells are not classic or if the typical reactive background is lacking.

ALCL occasionally involves lymph nodes focally and may resemble Hodgkin lymphoma on imprint cytology. Helpful features to distinguish between the two include the presence of more neoplastic cells (usually >30% of all cells) in ALCL and a tendency by the neoplastic cells to cluster. In addition, although some of the neoplastic cells may resemble Reed-Sternberg cells, a spectrum of morphology is usually seen and other forms

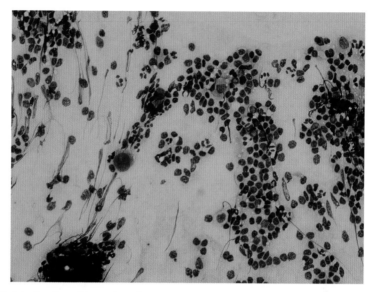

FIGURE 5.1 Scattered large lymphocytes are present in a background of reactive small lymphocytes and neutrophils in a case of Hodgkin lymphoma (imprint, Diff-Quick stain, 200×). This should prompt a search for Reed-Sternberg cells, which were present in other fields.

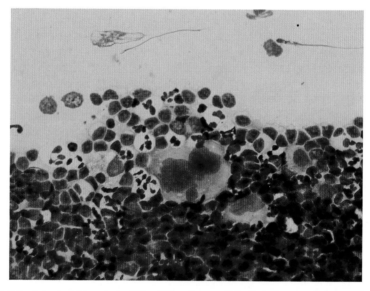

FIGURE 5.2 A typical binucleated Reed-Sternberg cell in the characteristic reactive background. Note the prominent inclusion-like nucleoli (imprint, Diff-Quick stain, 400×).

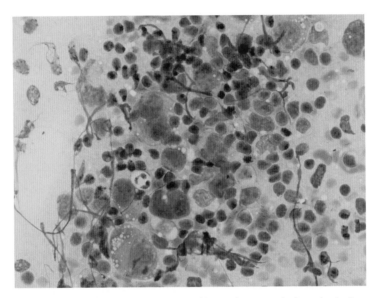

FIGURE 5.3 Numerous large lymphocytes with varying morphology including a Reed-Sternberg-like cell are present in a reactive inflammatory background in this case of anaplastic large cell lymphoma (imprint, Diff-Quick stain, 600×). The morphologic spectrum and abundance of large cells speak against this being Hodgkin lymphoma.

with more characteristic "hallmark" or multinucleated "wreath" morphology are often present (23) (Figs. 5.3, 5.4, e-Figs. 5.5, 5.6). Another potential mimic of Hodgkin lymphoma in the pediatric age group is "lymphoepithelioma" or undifferentiated nasopharyngeal carcinoma. Although the reactive background in this disease may be identical to that seen in Hodgkin lymphoma and the malignant epithelial cells may closely resemble Reed-Sternberg cells, aggregates of neoplastic basaloid cells suggest the correct diagnosis. In addition, even though there are macronucleoli in the large epithelial cells, it has been reported that they are often poorly demarcated from the rest of the nucleus and usually lack the characteristic halos seen in Reed-Sternberg cells (24). A final entity that may be confused with Hodgkin lymphoma is infectious mononucleosis. Although the background in this condition is reactive and binucleated immunoblasts reminiscent of Reed-Sternberg cells may be present, a continuum of morphology from reactive to enlarged atypical lymphocytes is usually seen rather than the biphasic picture of Reed-Sternberg cells in sharp contrast to the reactive background that characterizes Hodgkin lymphoma (25).

Burkitt lymphoma classically presents a distinct clinical picture and appearance in cytologic preparations. In the United States, the most common presentation is in the form of an abdominal mass. The cells are monotonous, typically somewhat larger than small lymphocytes (intermediate in size), and have a scant to intermediate quantity of deeply azurophilic cytoplasm. Multiple cytoplasmic vacuoles are present, and the

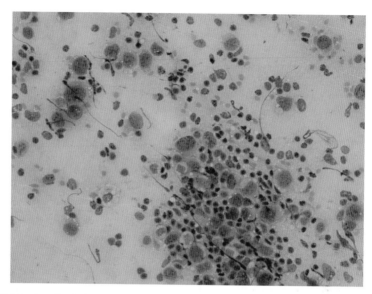

FIGURE 5.4   Anaplastic large cell lymphoma. Note that the proportion of large cells is much greater than would be expected in a case of Hodgkin lymphoma (imprint, Diff-Quick stain, 400×).

nuclei are round with multiple nucleoli and a granular chromatin texture (Figs. 5.5, 5.6, e-Figs. 5.2, 5.7). Tingible body macrophages and mitotic figures are often abundant. The diagnosis of Burkitt-like lymphoma is applied when cases deviate from the classic morphology but otherwise show the characteristic genetic lesion (*myc* rearrangement) and immunophenotype (26). These cases have more variation in cell size relative to typical Burkitt lymphoma, but frequently contain the same characteristic blue vacuolated cytoplasm. Burkitt and Burkitt-like lymphomas are not thought to differ clinically (27).

Lymphoblastic lymphoma and diffuse large B-cell lymphoma are also usually considerations when entertaining a diagnosis of Burkitt or Burkitt-like lymphoma. The cells in diffuse large B-cell lymphoma are usually larger and more pleomorphic with irregular nuclear membranes (Fig. 5.7). Because the diagnosis of Burkitt lymphoma hinges upon the demonstration of a genetic lesion involving *myc*, a definitive distinction between these entities should not be made on morphology alone (Fig. 5.8, e-Fig. 5.8). Rather the identification of the characteristic morphology should prompt triage of tissue for the appropriate molecular and genetic testing.

Acute lymphoblastic leukemia may present as a mass (lymphoblastic lymphoma), classically in adolescent males in the mediastinum. In these cases, the cells often display a T-cell phenotype. Cytologically, the cells are dyscohesive and monotonous with a high nuclear to cytoplasmic ratio. The nuclei are commonly round with evenly distributed chromatin and

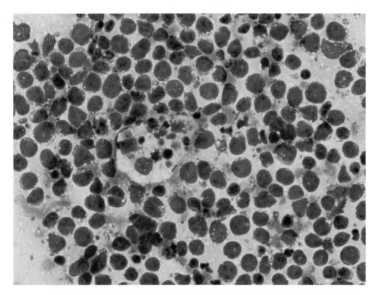

FIGURE 5.5   Classic case of Burkitt lymphoma with a somewhat monotonous population of intermediate-size lymphocytes containing azurophilic vacuolated cytoplasm. Note the tingible body macrophage (imprint, Diff-Quick stain, 400×). Genetic testing subsequently identified a *myc* translocation.

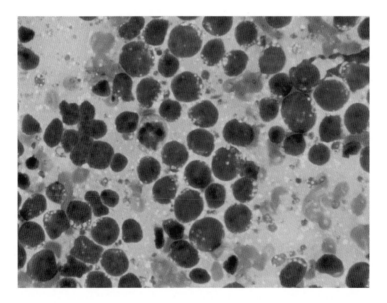

FIGURE 5.6   This case of Burkitt lymphoma is notable for the mitotic figure in this field. Mitotic figures should be easy to find in a case of Burkitt lymphoma given the high proliferative index that is characteristic of this disease. Note the abundant lymphoglandular bodies in the background (imprint, Diff-Quick stain, 600×).

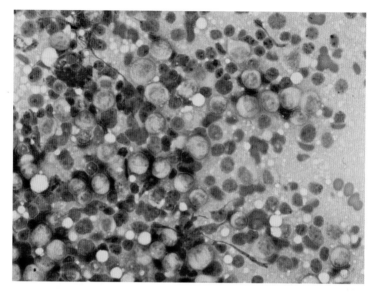

FIGURE 5.7 This case of diffuse large B-cell lymphoma contains a population of intermediate to large cells with some variation in size and somewhat irregular nuclei (imprint, Diff-Quick stain, 400×).

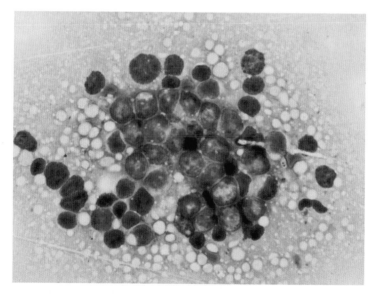

FIGURE 5.8 Many of the cells in this case of diffuse large B-cell lymphoma are intermediate in size with cytoplasmic vacuoles (imprint, Diff-Quick stain, 600×). Genetic studies failed to uncover evidence of a *myc* translocation precluding a diagnosis of Burkitt lymphoma.

inconspicuous nucleoli. Flow cytometry can confirm the impression of an acute leukemic process and allows rapid treatment (18) in an emergent situation.

Other pediatric small round blue cell tumors frequently enter into the cytologic differential diagnosis when considering lymphoblastic lymphoma or other forms of non-Hodgkin lymphoma. Helpful features in distinguishing a lymphoid process generally include dyscohesion and a somewhat monotonous growth pattern. This is in contrast to Wilms tumor, which often shows tubular structures and a triphasic growth pattern and PNET/Ewing sarcoma, which characteristically has a biphasic cell populations on cytologic examination (28). Other useful features in nonlymphoid tumors include a fibrillary background and rosette formation in neuroblastoma and spindled cells in rhabdomyosarcoma.

Lymphoglandular bodies are perhaps the most important diagnostic feature in distinguishing lymphoma from other tumors in cytologic preparations (29). Lymphoglandular bodies are round basophilic cytoplasmic fragments between 2 and 7 μm in size (Fig. 5.6). Although they are more common in FNA specimens, they are generally abundant in imprints of both benign and neoplastic lymphoid tissue. In a single study, abundant lymphoglandular bodies were seen in 93% of non-Hodgkin lymphoma and only 4.8% of non-lymphoid round cell tumors (30). An important caveat is that imprints of lymph nodes containing metastatic nonlymphoid tumors may also contain abundant lymphoglandular bodies proportional to the amount of residual lymphoid tissue.

Although conveying a tentative initial impression to the clinical service may be useful in some circumstances, distinguishing Hodgkin lymphoma, non-Hodgkin lymphoma, and nonlymphoid tumors is most important to determine how tissue will be allocated if the specimen is limited. Assuming that the sample size is adequate, we submit tissue for formalin fixation, B5 fixation, cytogenetics, flow cytometry, and snap-freeze a small piece (at least 100 mg) for molecular studies. Regardless of the scenario, the top priority is that tissue be submitted for formalin fixation, since H&E–stained formalin-fixed sections allow for standard morphologic evaluation and immunohistochemical stains. In addition, most molecular studies can be performed on paraffin-embedded tissue. Fixing a portion of the specimen in B5 provides superior nuclear morphology; however, molecular studies are not as reliable when performed on B5 fixed tissue. Cytogenetics is especially critical in Burkitt lymphoma, ALCL, and lymphoblastic lymphoma, where the demonstration of various cytogenetic abnormalities has both diagnostic and prognostic weight. A sterile piece of viable tissue measuring 0.5 cm $\times$ 0.5 cm $\times$ 0.2 cm contains a sufficient number of cells for cytogenetic studies. Flow cytometry is also useful in these neoplasms and allows rapid discrimination of a mature versus immature and B-cell versus T-cell phenotype. A piece of tissue measuring 0.3 cm $\times$ 0.3 cm $\times$ 0.3 cm is sufficient for a comprehensive lymphoma panel. Flow cytometry and cytogenetics do not provide any meaningful information in Hodgkin lymphoma, and depending on the clinical and initial morphologic impression tissue may be triaged accordingly if material is limited.

INTRODUCTION: HIRSCHSPRUNG'S DISEASE

Hirschsprung's disease is a relatively common congenital disorder (incidence of 1 in 5,000 live births) characterized by abnormal innervation of a variable length of the distal colon (8). The disease clinically announces itself by delayed passage of meconium in the first few days of life. Radiographically, it is characterized on contrast barium enema by a dilated properly innervated proximal colon, an aganglionic contracted distal colon, and an intervening funnel-shaped transition zone, which normally develops after the first 1 to 2 weeks of life (31). The length of the affected portion of distal colon is variable and the extent of disease can be classified as short-segment, long-segment, or total colonic aganglionosis.

The definitive therapy for Hirschsprung's disease is surgical, and the particular surgical approach determines to some extent the material submitted for frozen section. The traditional surgical strategy involves two separate operations. The first operation, performed in the neonatal period, involves laparotomy, identification of normal ganglionated bowel via seromuscular biopsy and intraoperative frozen section, and creation of a diverting colostomy. A definitive procedure is then performed several months later and involves either removal of the aganglionic portion of bowel and creation of a colorectal anastomosis (Swenson procedure) or creation of a neorectum with an anterior portion composed of the aganglionic rectal stump and a posterior portion composed of ganglionated normal colon (Duhamel procedure) (4).

The two-stage surgical treatment of Hirschsprung's disease has largely been superseded by the use of a one-stage transanal endorectal pull through. This is generally performed within the first few weeks of life and involves a transperineal approach, mucosal stripping of the aganglionic distal bowel, and pull-through of the normal ganglionated bowel. In this procedure, the role of the frozen section is central, as identification of normally ganglionated colon determines the level of bowel excision (32). Generally, two to five separate biopsies are provided for evaluation and these may either take the form of full-thickness or seromuscular biopsy. While waiting for the intraoperative biopsy results, the surgeon may perform further dissection and preparation but in general is likely to delay further action until receiving the pathologist's report.

Hirschsprung's Disease: Major Intraoperative Questions

At its root, the question is, "Are ganglion cells present or not?" Despite the apparent simplicity of this question, evaluation of frozen sections for

Hirschsprung's disease can be an intimidating task even for experienced pediatric pathologists. Several recent series have reported a discordance rate between frozen and permanent sections of 3% to 10% (33,34). An erroneous diagnosis of the absence of ganglion cells (false positive) will result in unnecessary resection of a portion of bowel while an erroneous diagnosis of the presence of ganglion cells (false negative) results in significant postoperative morbidity and may necessitate reoperation and resection of an additional length of colon.

The Frozen Section

In the assessment and management of patients with Hirschsprung's disease, there are several possible specimen sources. The initial diagnostic specimen is generally a superficial mucosal suction biopsy containing mucosa and submucosa, presumably with Meissner plexus. Evaluation of this specimen via intraoperative frozen section is strongly discouraged, as the concordance rate between permanent and frozen sections in this setting has been found to be particularly poor (67%) (33). This initial diagnostic suction rectal biopsy should be submitted entirely for permanent sections and routine H&E evaluation.

The specimen received for intraoperative evaluation should be a seromuscular or full-thickness biopsy from the distal colon. This should be taken from more than 2 cm above the anorectal junction as the distal 2 cm of the rectum is normally devoid of or sparsely populated by ganglion cells. Additional biopsy specimens are then generally obtained proximal to the contracted aganglionic distal colon and funnel-shaped transition zone as the surgeon attempts to determine the most distal level of normally innervated bowel for anastomoses.

Upon receiving a specimen for intraoperative evaluation, the first task is to determine adequacy. Biopsy specimens should be seromuscular or preferably full thickness and measure at least 0.5 cm in length (we have found 1.0 cm to be ideal) or be at least hemicircumferential to ensure that a sufficient number of nerves are present for evaluation (35) (Fig. 5.9).

The specimen is embedded so that the full thickness of the entire circumference of the specimen is examined on each histologic section. Cutting somewhat thicker sections (6 μm) and over staining in hematoxylin (90 seconds) may facilitate visualization of the cytologic detail of the ganglion cells. Our practice is to initially cut and stain two frozen section slides and subsequently cut and stain two more if our initial set of slides is equivocal or negative for ganglion cells. If the first four sections are negative for ganglion cells, additional levels from the same piece of tissue are unlikely to be rewarding and we report the absence of ganglion cells.

On initial histologic examination of a full-thickness biopsy, the submucosal and myenteric neuronal plexus should be identified. The submucosal plexus is present throughout the submucosa and the myenteric

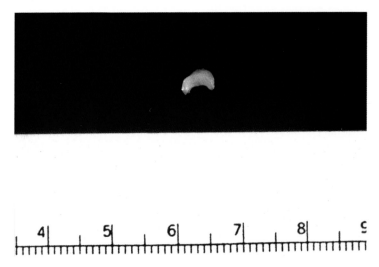

FIGURE 5.9 This is an adequate full-thickness biopsy for the purpose of evaluating the presence of ganglion cells. The specimen curls in the direction of the mucosal surface (gross photograph). This feature allows for proper orientation of the specimen.

plexus courses through the muscularis propria but is best evaluated in the area between the longitudinal and circumferential muscle layers. The ganglion cells are more easily recognized and abundant in the myenteric plexus (36,37), and therefore attention should primarily be directed toward identifying nerves in this region. Due in part to increased tortuosity, nerve density is increased in segments of bowel involved by Hirschsprung's disease (38). It should also be noted that the level of termination of ganglion cells in Hirschsprung's patients is the same in both neuronal plexuses so that the finding of ganglion cells in either the myenteric or submucosal plexus implies their presence in both (39).

The identification of ganglion cells is best facilitated by first locating "neural units" as described by Yunis et al. in the seminal 1976 publication (40). These neural units are vaguely organoid structures consisting of a horseshoe-shaped array of two to ten nuclei surrounding a central core of pale, "bubbly" neural tissue. Within the submucosal plexus, the ganglion cells are most easily identified and commonly located at the periphery of these neural units (Figs. 5.10, 5.11, e-Fig. 5.9). These neural units are less well characterized in the myenteric plexus and the cells at the periphery of the neural units in this location are often more heterogeneous and contain more prominent Schwann cells with rounded nuclei which are admixed with immature and mature ganglion cells.

The appearance of the mature ganglion cell has been well characterized. The typical ganglion cell is intermediate to large in size with an eccentric nucleus. The cytoplasm is moderately to deeply amphophilic (appreciation of this feature is facilitated by over staining and cutting a thick

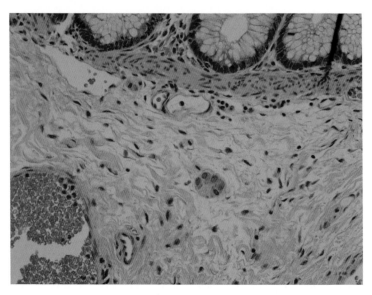

FIGURE 5.10 A well-formed neural unit in the submucosal plexus. Note the horseshoe-shaped arrangement of the ganglion cells around a core of "bubbly" neural material (permanent section, 200×).

section as previously detailed) with sharply defined cell borders (Fig. 5.12, e-Figs. 5.10A–C). The nucleus is round, large, and vesicular, with one or more prominent nucleoli. In an appropriately innervated section of bowel, multiple ganglion cells should be present throughout the circumference. Given the potential morbidity of a false-negative diagnosis and

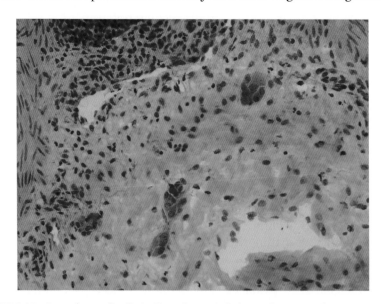

FIGURE 5.11 Several neural units in the submucosal plexus (frozen section 200×).

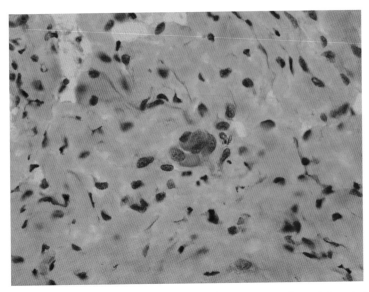

FIGURE 5.12 Several ganglion cells with visible nucleoli, eccentric nuclei, and abundant amphophilic cytoplasm (frozen section, 400×).

inappropriate anastomoses, we do not report the presence of ganglion cells unless the location, size, cytoplasmic character, and nuclear detail of the prospective cells are typical (Figs. 5.13, 5.14, e-Figs. 5.11–5.13). Additionally, one should not report the presence of appropriate innervation

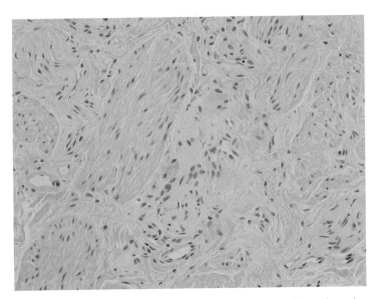

FIGURE 5.13 Several of the cells within this nerve contain somewhat enlarged nuclei and appear to contain a quantity of amphophilic cytoplasm. The cytologic features are not well developed enough to be confidently diagnosed as ganglion cells (frozen section, 200×).

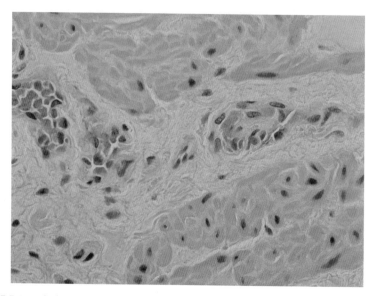

FIGURE 5.14 Similar to Figure 5.13. Activated endothelial cells add to the confusion in this case (frozen section, 400×).

based on solitary or few ganglion cells present in only a small portion of the circumference of the tissue section.

In a newborn patient, many of the ganglion cells may have a more immature phenotype and may not display the classic morphologic features. Immature ganglion cells are smaller, contain scant cytoplasm, and have hyperchromatic nuclei that may not display prominent nucleoli (Fig. 5.15). As definitive surgical intervention is now being performed at an increasingly early age, this becomes a critical issue. Despite the overall immaturity of the ganglion cells in a neonatal patient, mature ganglion cells with the classic morphology should still be present and identifiable even in preterm infants (36). The maturation of ganglion cells in the submucosal plexus trails those in the myenteric plexus by several weeks (41) and this reinforces the point that the myenteric plexus is superior to the submucosal plexus for the purpose of identifying ganglion cells.

Several potential mimics exist for ganglion cells in the setting of the frozen section. Awareness of these pitfalls and adherence to the strict morphologic criteria detailed earlier are thus critical. Blood vessels normally run with the neural units in the bowel wall, and activated endothelial cells may vaguely resemble ganglion cells if strict criteria are not used (Figs. 5.16, 5.17, e-Fig. 5.14, 5.15). While the presence of an adjacent vascular space with erythrocytes is useful to avoid this mistake in permanent section, red blood cells are lysed during frozen section preparation and cannot be relied upon in this setting. A heavy inflammatory infiltrate may obscure the neural unit and should generally preclude any attempt to identify ganglion cells in a given area (Fig. 5.18, e-Fig. 5.16). Adjacent

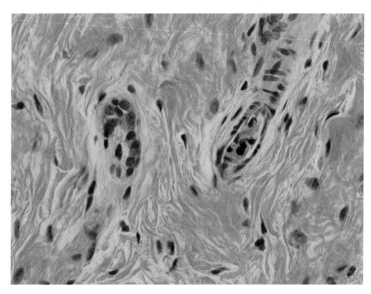

FIGURE 5.15 A neural unit with immature ganglion cells from a preterm patient. The cytologic features are not well developed. One should be wary of reporting the presence of ganglion cells based on this cluster of cells alone (frozen section, 400×).

smooth muscle cells are another possible mimic, which can be avoided by paying attention to the more eosinophilic character of the cytoplasm. A misinterpretation of fibroblasts and histiocytes can also be avoided by paying close attention to cytoplasmic and nuclear detail.

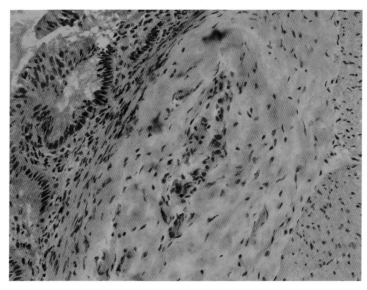

FIGURE 5.16 The activated endothelial cells lining this blood vessel are a potential mimic of ganglion cells (frozen section, 200×).

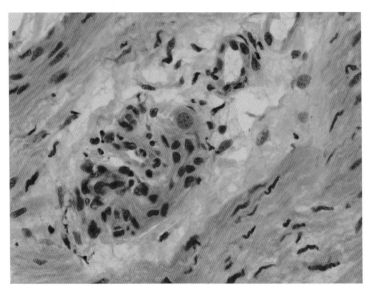

FIGURE 5.17 Nerves where ganglion cells may be identified are often located adjacent to blood vessels in the myenteric plexus (frozen section, 400×).

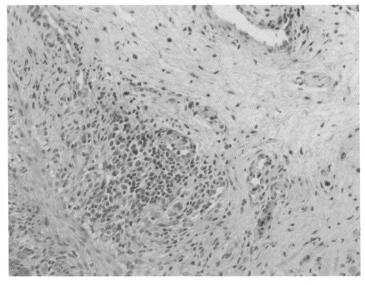

FIGURE 5.18 Inflammation obscures the neural units in this case and makes the assessment of ganglion cells impossible. In addition, large plasma cells, activated lymphocytes, and activated endothelial cells may be mistaken for ganglion cells in this setting (frozen section, 200×).

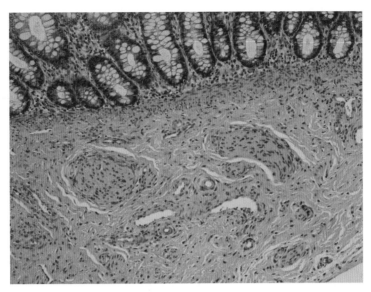

FIGURE 5.19   Hypertrophic nerves in the submucosa (permanent section, 200×).

Although the evaluation of a portion of bowel for involvement by Hirschsprung's disease rests on the presence or absence of ganglion cells, assessment of submucosal nerve diameter constitutes an objective ancillary finding that is strongly correlated with the presence or absence of ganglion cells (38) (Fig. 5.19). Nerve trunk hypertrophy is associated with Hirschsprung's disease and in a single study, 90% of aganglionic portions of bowel examined contained hypertrophic submucosal nerve trunks measuring more than 40 μm. In contrast, the vast majority of submucosal nerve trunks in normal portions of bowel measured between 10 and 20 μm and no nerve trunks more than 40 μm were identified. The investigators also reported that hypertrophic nerve trunks were only infrequently found in total colonic aganglionosis where nerve trunks may actually be hypoplastic or absent, making this finding inapplicable in that setting. Although nerve trunk hypertrophy is also seen in the myenteric plexus in the setting of Hirschsprung's disease, it must be reiterated that the findings of this study apply only to the submucosal plexus.

In addition to nerve trunk hypertrophy, aganglionic portions of bowel often show hypertrophy of the muscularis propria. Despite this, assessment of muscularis propria thickness does not constitute a useful ancillary finding in determining the absence or presence of ganglion cells. Muscularis propria hypertrophy is a nonspecific finding that can be seen as a consequence of constipation of any etiology.

Even when ganglion cells are focally present in a level of bowel, this does not absolutely indicate normal innervation. As alluded to earlier, in the setting of Hirschsprung's disease, the aganglionic and normally inner-vated portions of bowel are separated by an intervening transition zone that can measure up to 2.4 cm in length (42). Surgical anastomosis of this transition zone to the rectal stump can cause significant morbidity in the form of constipation, enterocolitis, and incontinence often necessitating surgical revision (43,44). Concordance between the radiographic and his-tologic transition zones is poor, particularly in long-segment disease (45); thus, awareness of the morphologic features of the transition zone is es-sential. Ganglion cells are absent or very rare, and the spacing of the nerve bundles is wider than normal in the transition zone. As in aganglionic por-tions of bowel, submucosal nerve trunks may be hypertrophic measuring 40 μm or more. The junction between normally innervated and agan-glionic bowel is not symmetric around the circumference of the bowel wall and so a "leading edge" of normal innervation with an appropriate num-ber of ganglion cells is found in a portion of the circumference of the bowel wall (42). Hypertrophic submucosal nerves and aganglionic neural units are often not found in the immediate area of normal innervation in the leading edge and so small point biopsies from this location can appear completely normal. This fact underlines the need for at least hemicircum-ferential specimens for intraoperative evaluation. Even if properly gan-glionated areas are present in a circumferential tissue section, if ganglion cells are only seen focally and/or hypertrophic nerves bundles are seen, the impression of transition zone histology should be conveyed to the sur-geon.

In summary, the main recommendations are (i) isolated ganglion cells are insufficient, (ii) neural units should be identified, (iii) the pres-ence of rare ganglion cells with or without hypertrophic nerve trunks sug-gests transition zone histology, and (iv) normal clusters of ganglion cells and neural units should be present for placement of colostomy or level of resection.

REFERENCES

1. Coffin CM, Spilker K, Zhou H, et al. Frozen section diagnosis in pediatric surgical pathology: a decade's experience in a children's hospital. *Arch Pathol Lab Med.* 2005; 129:1619–1625.
2. Preston HS, Bale PM. Rapid frozen section in pediatric pathology. *Am J Surg Pathol.* 1985;9:570–576.
3. Dicken BJ, Bigam DL, Lees GM. Association between surgical margins and long-term outcome in advanced hepatoblastoma. *J Pediatr Surg.* 2004;39:721–725.
4. Warner B. Pediatric surgery. In: Townsend CM, ed. *Sabiston Textbook of Surgery.* 17th ed. Philadelphia, PA: Saunders; 2004.
5. Fisher JE, Burger PC, Perlman EJ, et al. The frozen section yesterday and today: pediatric solid tumors–crucial issues. *Pediatr Dev Pathol.* 2001;4:252–266.
6. Berkley C, Stanley MW, Wolpert J, et al. Adult Wilms' tumor. Intraoperative cytology and ancillary studies performed in a case as an adjunct to the histologic diagnosis. *Acta Cytol.* 1990;34:79–83.
7. Wakely PE, Frable WJ, Kornstein MJ. Role of intraoperative cytopathology in pediatric surgical pathology. *Hum Pathol.* 1993;24:311–315.

8. Dahms BB. The gastrointestinal tract. In: Stocker TJ, Dehner LP, eds. *Pediatr Pathol.* 2nd ed. Philadelphia, PA: Lippincott Williams and Wilkins; 2001.

9. Golouh R, Bracko M. Accuracy of frozen section diagnosis in soft tissue tumors. *Mod Pathol.* 1990;3:729–733.

10. Qualman SJ, Bowen J, Fitzgibbons PL, et al.; College of American Pathologists. Protocol for the examination of specimens from patients with neuroblastoma and related neuroblastic tumors. *Arch Pathol Lab Med.* 2005;129:874–883.

11. Qualman SJ, Bowen J, Amin MB, et al.; College of American Pathologists. Protocol for the examination of specimens from patients with Wilms tumor (nephroblastoma) or other renal tumors of childhood. *Arch Pathol Lab Med.* 2003;127:1280–1289.

12. Qualman SJ, Bowen J, Parham DM, et al. Protocol for the examination of specimens from patients (children and young adults) with rhabdomyosarcoma. *Arch Pathol Lab Med.* 2003;127:1290–1297.

13. Herzog LW. Prevalence of lymphadenopathy of the head and neck in infants and children. *Clin Pediatr (Phila).* 1983;22:485–487.

14. Knight PJ, Mulne SF, Vassy LE. When is lymph node biopsy indicated in children with enlarged peripheral nodes? *Pediatrics.* 1982;69:391–396.

15. United States National Cancer Institute. *Survival Epidemiology and End Result Data.* http://seer.cancer.gov. Accessed September 2008.

16. Wright D, McKeever P, Carter R. Childhood non-Hodgkin lymphomas in the United Kingdom: findings from the UK Children's Cancer Study Group. *J Clin Pathol.* 1997;50: 128–134.

17. Molyneux AJ, Attanoos RL, Coghill SB. The value of lymph node imprint cytodiagnosis: an assessment of interobserver agreement and diagnostic accuracy. *Cytopathology.* 1997;8:256–264.

18. Mann G, Attarbaschi A, Steiner M, et al. Early and reliable diagnosis of non-Hodgkin lymphoma in childhood and adolescence: contribution of cytomorphology and flow cytometric immunophenotyping. *Pediatr Hematol Oncol.* 2006;23:167–176.

19. DeMay RM. *The Art and Science of Cytopathology.* Chicago, IL: American Society of Clinical Pathology; 1996.

20. Funamoto Y, Nagai M, Haba R, et al. Diagnostic accuracy of imprint cytology in the assessment of Hodgkin's disease in Japan. *Diagn Cytopathol.* 2005;33:20–25.

21. Kardos TF, Vinson JH, Behm FG, et al. Hodgkin's disease: diagnosis by fine-needle aspiration biopsy. Analysis of cytologic criteria from a selected series. *Am J Clin Pathol.* 1986;86:286–291.

22. Khurana KK, Stanley MW, Powers CN, et al. Aspiration cytology of malignant neoplasms associated with granulomas and granuloma-like features: diagnostic dilemmas. *Cancer.* 1998;84:84–91.

23. Mourad WA, al Nazer M, Tulbah A. Cytomorphologic differentiation of Hodgkin's lymphoma and Ki-1+ anaplastic large cell lymphoma in fine needle aspirates. *Acta Cytol.* 2003;47:744–748.

24. Kollur SM, El Hag IA. Fine-needle aspiration cytology of metastatic nasopharyngeal carcinoma in cervical lymph nodes: comparison with metastatic squamous-cell carcinoma, and Hodgkin's and non-Hodgkin's lymphoma. *Diagn Cytopathol.* 2003;28:18–22.

25. Kardos TF, Kornstein MJ, Frable WJ. Cytology and immunocytology of infectious mononucleosis in fine needle aspirates of lymph nodes. *Acta Cytol.* 1988;32:722–726.

26. Harris NL, Horning SJ. Burkitt's lymphoma–the message from microarrays. *N Engl J Med.* 2006;354:2495–2498.

27. Kelly DR, Nathwani BN, Griffith RC, et al. A morphologic study of childhood lymphoma of the undifferentiated type. The Pediatric Oncology Group experience. *Cancer.* 1987; 59:1132–1137.

28. Silverman JF, Joshi VV. FNA biopsy of small round cell tumors of childhood: cytomorphologic features and the role of ancillary studies. *Diagn Cytopathol.* 1994;10:245–255.

29. Thunnissen FB, Kroese AH, Ambergen AW, et al. Which cytological criteria are the most discriminative to distinguish carcinoma, lymphoma, and soft-tissue sarcoma? A probabilistic approach. *Diagn Cytopathol.* 1997;17:333–338.

30. Francis IM, Das DK, al-Rubah NA, et al. Lymphoglandular bodies in lymphoid lesions and non-lymphoid round cell tumours: a quantitative assessment. *Diagn Cytopathol.* 1994;11:23–27.

31. Wyllie R. Stomach and intestines: normal development, structure and function. In: Behrman RE, ed. *Nelson Textbook of Pediatrics.* 17th ed. Philadelphia, PA: Saunders; 2004.

32. Wilcox DT, Bruce J, Bowen J, et al. One-stage neonatal pull-through to treat Hirschsprung's disease. *J Pediatr Surg.* 1997;32:243–245.

33. Maia DM. The reliability of frozen-section diagnosis in the pathologic evaluation of Hirschsprung's disease. *Am J Surg Pathol.* 2000;24:1675–1677.

34. Shayan K, Smith C, Langer JC. Reliability of intraoperative frozen sections in the management of Hirschsprung's disease. *J Pediatr Surg.* 2004;39:1345–1348.

35. Berrebi D, Fouquet V, de Lagausie P, et al. Duhamel operation vs neonatal transanal endorectal pull-through procedure for Hirschsprung disease: which are the changes for pathologists? *J Pediatr Surg.* 2007;42:688–691.

36. Smith B. Pre- and postnatal development of the ganglion cells of the rectum and its surgical implications. *J Pediatr Surg.* 1968;3:386–391.

37. Swenson O, Fisher JH, McMahon HE. Rectal biopsy as an aid in the diagnosis of Hirschsprung's disease. *N Engl J Med.* 1955;253:632–635.

38. Monforte-Muñoz H, Gonzalez-Gomez I, Rowland JM, et al. Increased submucosal nerve trunk caliber in aganglionosis: a "positive" and objective finding in suction biopsies and segmental resections in Hirschsprung's disease. *Arch Pathol Lab Med.* 1998;122: 721–725.

39. Gherardi GH. Pathology of the ganglionic-aganglionic junction in congenital megacolon. *Arch Pathol.* 1960;69:520–523.

40. Yunis EJ, Dibbins AW, Sherman FE. Rectal suction biopsy in the diagnosis of Hirschsprung disease in infants. *Arch Pathol Lab Med.* 1976;100:329–333.

41. Junqueira LC, Tafuri WL, Tafuri CP. Quantitative and cytochemical studies on the intestinal plexuses of the guinea pig. *Exp Cell Res.* 1958;14:568–572.

42. White FV, Langer JC. Circumferential distribution of ganglion cells in the transition zone of children with Hirschsprung disease. *Pediatr Dev Pathol.* 2000;3:216–222.

43. Farrugia MK, Alexander N, Clarke S, et al. Does transitional zone pull-through in Hirschsprung's disease imply a poor prognosis? *J Pediatr Surg.* 2003;38:1766–1769.

44. Ghose SI, Squire BR, Stringer MD, et al. Hirschsprung's disease: problems with transition-zone pull-through. *J Pediatr Surg.* 2000;35:1805–1809.

45. Jamieson DH, Dundas SE, Belushi SA, et al. Does the transition zone reliably delineate aganglionic bowel in Hirschsprung's disease? *Pediatr Radiol.* 2004;34:811–815.

6

BREAST AND SENTINEL NODE

JEROME B. TAXY

INTRODUCTION: BREAST FROZEN SECTION

The historical importance of the breast frozen section in the evolution of surgical pathology practice is the basis for including this topic. The paradigm for clinically relevant immediate decision making in surgical pathology is the breast frozen section. Indeed, the practical history of the frozen section as a diagnostic modality could be traced by its implementation related to breast cancer. In the current era, a decline in the number of frozen section diagnoses in the management of breast cancer is a reflection of the significant changes in the clinical detection and therapy of this disease over the last approximately 40 years.

In the premammography era, breast tumors were discovered by palpation, usually by the patient herself or her spouse, partner, or physician. The definitive diagnosis was made by open biopsy, incisional or excisional. While the patient was still anesthetized, a fresh tissue sample, even if grossly benign, was sent to the surgical pathology laboratory for immediate analysis by frozen section. If the frozen section showed carcinoma in any form, in situ or invasive, a mastectomy was immediately done. Since mastectomy was the only therapeutic option, the objective of this sequence was to provide definitive therapy without a second anesthesia. In the later years in which this practice was common, fresh samples of invasive tumors, 0.5 to 1.0 g, were required for estrogen receptor determination, which was done by competitive binding assay. Because tumors were relatively large and biopsy samples were of generous size, there was typically ample tumor to spare.

The advent of screening mammography in the 1970s and subsequent generations of refined imaging techniques have been major factors in changing both the histologic evaluation and therapeutic approach to breast cancer by detecting tumors of small size. The size of the tumors is perhaps best summarized by a premammography era tabulation of 1,355 cases seen at the Memorial Hospital in New York from 1935 to 1942, where more than half the tumors were between 2 and 4 cm and almost 20% were larger than 5 cm (1). In the current era, most tumors are smaller than 2.0 cm and many are not palpable at all. Diminished tumor size is encountered in both community hospitals as well as referral

TABLE 6.1 Size of Invasive Breast Cancer in Community and University Setting		
Tumor Size	LGH[a]	U of C[b]
T1mic	40	8
T1a	51	55
T1b	173	113
T1c	284	258
T2	233	281
T3	29	75

[a]Advocate Lutheran General Hospital, 1999 to 2001 ($n = 830$).
[b]University of Chicago, 2000 to 2006 ($n = 891$).
Source: Cancer Registries at Advocate Lutheran General Hospital and University of Chicago.

settings. Table 6.1 illustrates the comparable sizes of invasive breast cancers as encountered at the time of diagnosis over several recent years at the Advocate Lutheran General Hospital, a large community hospital in the Chicago suburbs, and the University of Chicago (data supplied by the Cancer Registries in the respective institutions). The decrease in size of the tumors is largely due to screening mammography, which has concomitantly solidified the concept of breast conservation surgery. The combination of the accepted efficacy of conservation procedures coincident with the radiographic discovery of smaller tumors has changed the treatment algorithm for this disease.

Small size is a major disadvantage for frozen section diagnosis in this context. There would be a risk of having to freeze the entire sample and then having to deal potentially with frozen artifact on both the frozen and the paraffin-embedded material. Consequently, the number of breast frozen sections has markedly diminished. At the University of Chicago for the last several years, the numbers are in single digits. Currently, the diagnosis of breast carcinoma is established by core needle biopsy or aspiration cytology. Immediate definitive surgery is not typical; the patient herself is likely to be consulted about the therapeutic options after the diagnosis is established on permanent paraffin-embedded material.

The Breast Frozen Section: Major Intraoperative Questions

Current published studies on breast frozen sections are uncommon (2–5). It is perhaps of some relief to pathologists that legal actions related to breast cancer are relatively few for frozen section (6), with the legal burden, in general, having been shifted to the radiologists (7). While the prior habit of freezing all breast specimens is no longer advocated (8), in the context of individualizing therapy, there is an occasional request for a frozen section of a breast mass. The major question has not changed, i.e., to definitively and immediately identify and treat a malignant tumor. The treatment decision remains a major one; however, these circumstances are exceptional. In addition, the price that has been paid for decreased frequency is that the pathologist is less experienced and perhaps not as confident as in the past. In an attempt to minimize error, therefore, interpreting a breast frozen section may negatively influence the therapeutic goal by resulting in a deferred diagnosis or a descriptive nondiagnostic response.

Occasionally, a request may be received for a frozen section on a definitive lumpectomy specimen, either for a primary diagnosis or an assessment of margins. The potential immediate consequences of such evaluations would be either a wider excision or possibly a mastectomy. However, given the fat composition of such specimens and the probable small size of the tumor, a frozen section is ill advised not to mention difficult to interpret. The optimal evaluation for such resection specimens under intraoperative conditions requires a good gross assessment; actual frozen sections should be used judiciously (2,3). Definitive microscopic examination should be done on inked, well-fixed, and processed tissue.

The Breast Frozen Section and Its Interpretation

The most important parameter in the analysis of a breast frozen section is the gross examination. This is negated if the sample is a core needle biopsy, necessitating freezing the entire sample. This may be clinically suboptimal. In an excisional biopsy, the specimen should be inked according to departmental practice and all sectioned surfaces should be inspected to minimize sampling error (Fig. 6.1, e-Fig. 6.1). To minimize potential artifacts, the freezing of fatty areas should be avoided; the need for sharp

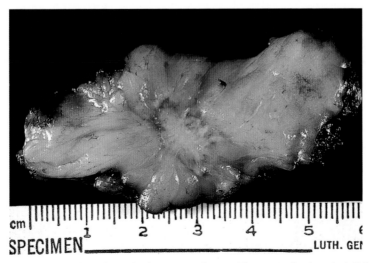

FIGURE 6.1 Cross section of an inked gross specimen with a centrally placed, stellate, gray-white tumor grossly typical for infiltrating carcinoma. The size of the tumor is approximately 1.0 cm. The margins are free of tumor.

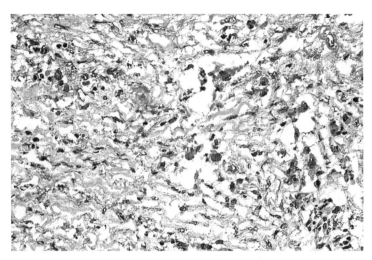

FIGURE 6.2   Infiltrating ductal carcinoma. Dense fibrous tissue investing poorly oriented cords of large, pleomorphic malignant cells. No normal breast tissue is present.

blades and cryostats, for which the temperature is properly monitored and maintained, cannot be overstated. The histologic examination of the actual frozen section requires no special skill or secret maneuver other than attention to traditional morphologic detail: Recognition of the standard alterations in growth pattern, under low-power observation, just as would be appreciated on routine paraffin-embedded sections (Fig. 6.2). Employing imprint preparations along with the actual frozen section facilitates the

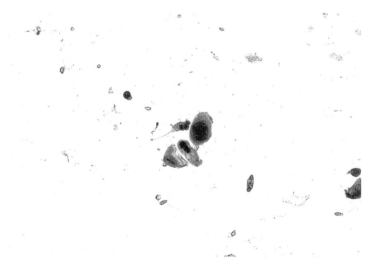

FIGURE 6.3   H&E imprint of the tumor in Figure 6.2. A group of pleomorphic cells with pyknotic nuclei and variable amounts of dense cytoplasm, similar to the cells in the tissue section. The single layer preparation allows for increased appreciation of nuclear detail.

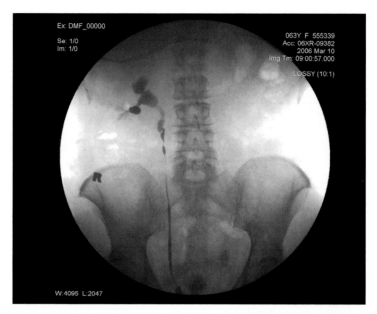

FIGURE 6.4 A retrograde pyelogram of a 63-year-old woman with a remote history of in-filtrating breast cancer who presented with flank pain. Note the kinking of the right ureter (*arrow*) with proximal hydronephrosis due to a poorly defined retroperitoneal mass. A surgical ureterolysis was undertaken to ease the external obstruction to the urinary tract.

appreciation of cytologic detail (Fig. 6.3, e-Figs. 6.2–6.4). The ability to discriminate infiltrating cancer from a radial scar lesion, inflammatory in-filtrates, fat necrosis, sclerosing adenosis, and involutional changes in a papilloma relies on adequate sampling and basic morphology. It is not good practice, not to mention potentially dangerous, for the pathologist to ignore these fundamental morphologic and technical principles.

In part because of early diagnosis and effective treatment, breast cancer has now become a chronic disease. Patients may present years after their primary diagnosis with metastatic lesions. The diagnostic context depends heavily on the history and a consideration of breast cancer by the pathologist (Figs. 6.4–6.7). The most important point to remember is that if the frozen section is not absolutely diagnostic of cancer defer the diagnosis (Figs. 6.8, 6.9, e-Figs. 6.5–6.7).

INTRODUCTION: THE SENTINEL NODE FROZEN SECTION

The staging and prognostic parameters used to evaluate each new case of infiltrating breast cancer are many. However, the two most important factors remain the size of the primary tumor and the status of the regional lymph nodes. While it is a principle of clinical management that smaller invasive tumors are less likely to have regional node metastases, 10% to 30% of tumors smaller than 1.0 cm have axillary metastases. It is widely

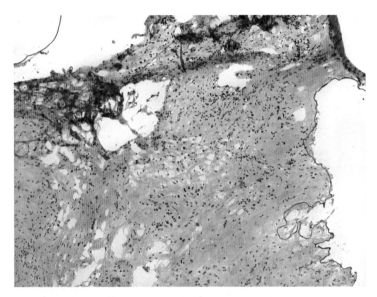

FIGURE 6.5 A frozen section of the retroperitoneal mass. Artifactual fold along the top border. Low-power view of a fibrofatty lesion with a seeming mononuclear infiltrate, possibly inflammatory.

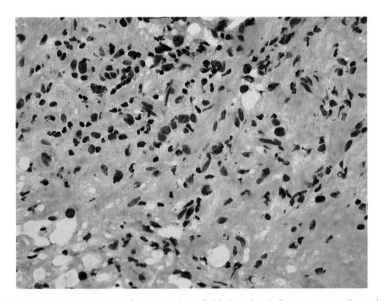

FIGURE 6.6 High-power view of the previous field showing inflammatory cells and larger polygonal cells focally growing in a single-file fashion, suggesting infiltrating lobular carcinoma.

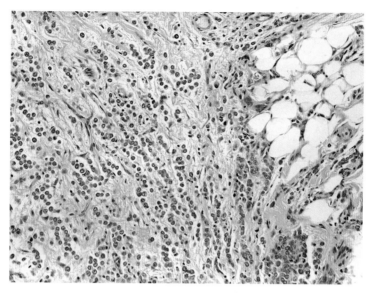

FIGURE 6.7 Permanently embedded section of the frozen section, showing infiltrating single files of malignant cells indicative of infiltrating lobular carcinoma. The history of a primary breast cancer with this diagnosis was later confirmed.

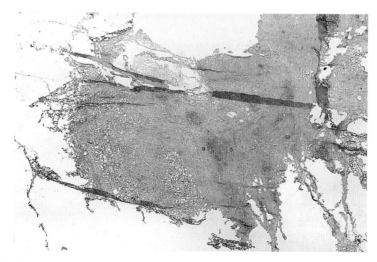

FIGURE 6.8 Low-power view of a frozen section of a breast mass in a 65-year-old woman with a history of left breast carcinoma with positive lymph nodes 3 years previously. She was postoperatively radiated. The frozen section of this ipsilateral mass was requested so that an immediate mastectomy could be done if it was malignant. The stellate shape is composed of dense fibrous tissue investing cords and nests of polygonal cells, simulating the growth of an infiltrating carcinoma.

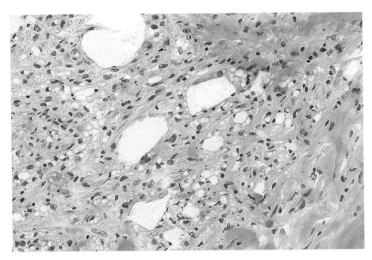

FIGURE 6.9 High magnification of the tumor, demonstrating sheets of polygonal cells with slightly atypical nuclei and abundant, pale to finely vacuolated cytoplasm. At the time of the frozen section analysis, these were interpreted to be histiocytes.

accepted that nodal involvement cannot be accurately predicted on clinical or imaging grounds alone, but histologic assessment is also required. In the past, every patient with an invasive breast cancer had at least a low axillary dissection in conjunction with a mastectomy or an excisional lumpectomy. However postoperatively, the clinical morbidity associated with this procedure included pain, limitation of motion, lymphedema, and infection. The concept of the sentinel node, first employed with respect to melanoma, has been effectively adapted to breast cancer and has evolved as part of breast conservation surgery.

A sentinel node is the first lymph node in a drainage basin to receive lymphatic fluid. As such, metastatic deposits are first anticipated in this location. In breast cancer, the sentinel node biopsy procedure allows for the preservation of function and cosmesis without compromising the necessary staging information (9–11). The sentinel node is identified by the injection of radioactive colloid and/or blue dye into the primary breast biopsy site. The affected node or nodes are then excised. The procedure is best applied to small primary tumors (<2 cm) and is well suited for mammographically discovered lesions. Patients with a positive sentinel node would require either a complete axillary dissection or radiation of the axilla.

The Sentinel Node and the Major Clinical Question

The major clinical question is deceptively simple, i.e., whether or not the sentinel node harbors a metastasis. Perhaps the question is best addressed as to whether the status of the sentinel node should be reported intraoperatively, i.e., immediately by frozen section analysis, or whether the diagnosis should be made under the routine circumstances of fixation and paraffin embedding. If the surgeon is immediately prepared to complete a low axillary dissection in light of a report of a metastatic deposit, then a frozen section can be justified. From the standpoint of the pathologist, the issues related to sentinel node examination concern the extent of gross sampling, the use of imprints or scrapes, the number of frozen or paraffin (permanent) sections to be examined, the spacing of those intervals, and the use of cytokeratin immunostaining on permanent preparations, to name a few. The assessment of tumor in a node has become more complex than just positive or negative and concerns the best way to recognize a metastasis, report it, and decide what to do about it (12).

The size of the metastasis further illustrates this complexity as it has itself become a source of controversy related to the question of the simple presence or absence of tumor. Most would agree that a metastasis of 2 mm or larger is clinically significant and should have a complete axillary dissection (Fig. 6.8). But the question is what constitutes a clinically significant metastasis, i.e., what is the significance of deposits between 0.2 and 2 mm as well as isolated microscopic tumor clusters smaller than 0.2 mm? Treating these very small and possibly insignificant lesions raises the issue of overtreatment and not treating them raises the issue of undertreatment. The frozen section focuses attention on the clinical relevance of the size of a metastasis. An agreement between the surgeon and the pathologist with respect to this issue needs to be worked out in advance of the procedure.

Since it is easier for the surgeon to complete the dissection at the time of the sentinel node excision, and if it is agreed that the presence of tumors of any dimension will influence the surgical procedure, a frozen section is reasonable. The actual detection of tumor is, in part, related to the expertise and technique of the examining pathologist. The reported 10% to 30% false-negative rate related to sentinel node frozen section may be due to sampling, i.e., failure to freeze the entire node or to cut more than one level for histologic evaluation (13,14). At the University of Chicago, sentinel node examination has increased since it began in 2000. Adding frozen section to this practice has been common since 2002 and has continued to the present (Table 6.2). Metastatic lesions are reported along with an estimation of size. Of more than 300 sentinel nodes examined on an annual basis since 2002, 30% to 40% have been initially examined by frozen section. There have been no false positives. There were six false negatives from 2002 to 2003 and six false negatives from December 2004 to August 2006. The false negatives in the latter period included only one missed micrometastasis. Other false negatives included artifacts of frozen section or sampling. The present practice among the surgeons is that if a frozen section demonstrates a metastasis of any size, the patient should have a low axillary dissection.

TABLE 6.2	Breast Cancer Sentinel Lymph Nodes[a]
Frozen section	
Negative	228
Positive	39
False-negative node	6
Obscured by tissue fold	
Obscured by fat	
Not on frozen section	
Tissue not completely frozen	
Atypical	
Missed micrometastasis	
Nonfrozen	
Negative	343
Positive	26

[a]University of Chicago (December 2004–August 2006).

The Sentinel Node Frozen Section and Its Interpretation

The gross examination is again key. Any macroscopically visible metastasis is clinically significant and care should be taken to make sure that area is mounted so that it will appear on the frozen section. Acknowledging that missing a small metastasis is much easier than finding it, freezing the entire node especially in the absence of a gross lesion is essential in dealing with the sampling issue. The standard reference point to justify reporting a metastasis should be detection of a tumor on an H&E-stained frozen section. While imprints and scrape preparations are important in other settings, tumor clusters demonstrated on such preparations in sentinel nodes without a histologic counterpart present a problem. While imprints of an obvious gross lesion (Fig. 6.10) can be quite useful (15), routine imprints of grossly negative nodes are not utilized. More than one level should be examined histologically, although there is no agreement on the number. Our practice is to examine at least two levels. The need to examine the entire node can be complicated by nodes of any size which are invested by fat which in turn can be difficult to trim. However, everyone involved should recognize that at some level sampling error is inherent in the accuracy of this procedure. The false negative is something to accept and to try to minimize, but it cannot be eliminated.

This is not an examination requiring anything other than a well cut and stained H&E section. The permutations in finding small lesions are many (Figs. 6.11, 6.12) and would also include tumor present on the frozen but not on the permanent section (still regarded as a positive).

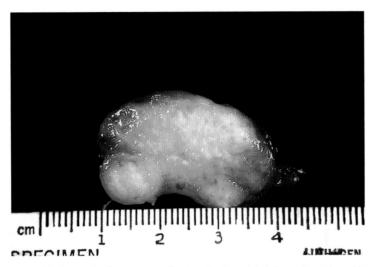

FIGURE 6.10 Photograph of a gross sentinel node almost totally replaced by white, poorly delineated tumor.

Another problem in this context concerns low-grade infiltrating lobular carcinoma, which occasionally simulates sinus histiocytosis. These cases are lessons in careful examination (Figs. 6.13, 6.14, e-Figs. 6.8–6.10). The identification of intracytoplasmic lumina in individual tumor cells has long been associated with lobular carcinoma, although not necessarily

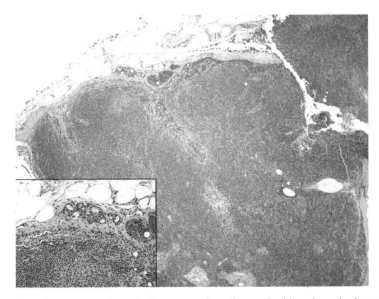

FIGURE 6.11 Low-power view of a frozen section of a sentinel lymph node demonstrating a few tumor clusters in the center capsular nodal tissue. *Inset*: High-power view of the capsular metastasis.

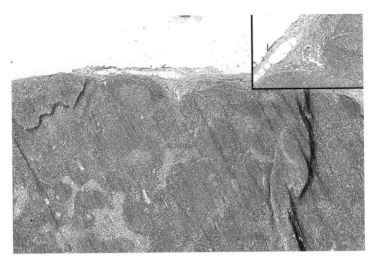

FIGURE 6.12 Low-power view of a frozen section of a sentinel node demonstrating a single intracapsular lymphatic cluster of tumor cells. *Inset*: High-power view of the intracapsular lymphatic group of tumor cells.

specific for this tumor type (Fig. 6.14). When present, they are helpful diagnostic adjuncts (16). Last is being aware of the sequelae of previous needle biopsy of axillary lymph nodes, occasionally done for clinically enlarged nodes to bypass formal sentinel node evaluation and proceed directly to an axillary dissection. The capsular reparative reaction includes

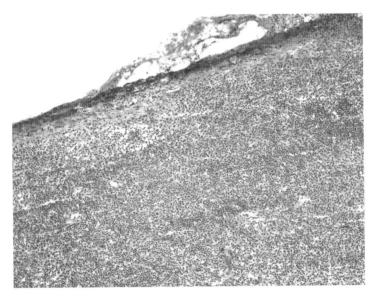

FIGURE 6.13 Low-power view of a frozen section of a sentinel lymph node from a patient with infiltrating lobular carcinoma. Subtle architectural distortion and a suggestion of cytologic atypia.

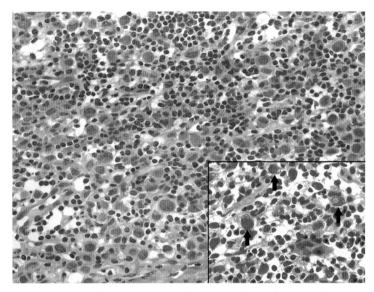

FIGURE 6.14   Frozen section. High-power view of a subcapsular area demonstrating diffuse infiltration by malignant cells. *Inset*: Frozen section. High-power view of the tumor cells demonstrating nuclear pleomorphism, pyknosis, and intracytoplasmic lumina. The latter is suggestive of infiltrating lobular carcinoma.

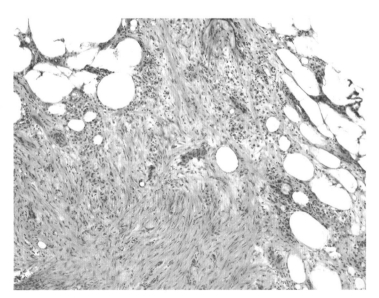

FIGURE 6.15   Frozen section of perinodal capsule and fat 1 week following a negative needle biopsy of this node. This field demonstrates an actively fibrotic background extending into the fat with associated chronic inflammation and prominent small vessels with atypical endothelial cells. The picture simulates a metastasis.

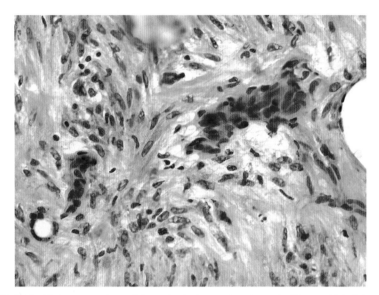

FIGURE 6.16 High-power view of two atypical vascular channels. The endothelial cells are enlarged and the lumina are virtually inapparent.

granulation tissue with endothelial enlargement and atypia as well as fibrosis that can be mistaken for desmoplasia (Figs. 6.15, 6.16, e-Figs. 6.11–6.13).

REFERENCES

1. Stewart FW. Tumors of the breast. In: *Atlas of Tumor Pathology* (Fascicle 34). Washington, DC: Armed Forces Institute of Pathology; 1950.
2. Cabioglu N, Hunt KK, Sahin AA, et al. Role for intraoperative margin assessment in patients undergoing breast conserving surgery. *Ann Surg Oncol.* 2007;14(4):1458–1471.
3. Laucirica R. Intraoperative assessment of the breast: guidelines and potential pitfalls. *Arch Pathol Lab Med.* 2005;129:1565–1574.
4. Ferreiro JA, Gisvold JJ, Bostwick DG. Accuracy of frozen section diagnosis of mammographically directed breast biopsies: results of 1,490 consecutive cases. *Am J Surg Pathol.* 1995;19:1267–1271.
5. Cheng L, Al-Kaisi NK, Liu AY, et al. The results of intraoperative consultations in 181 ductal carcinomas in situ of the breast. *Cancer.* 1997;80:75–79.
6. Troxel DB. Error in surgical pathology. *Am J Surg Pathol.* 2004;28:1092–1095.
7. Hall FM. Breast imaging and computer-aided detection. *N Engl J Med.* 2007;356: 1464–1466.
8. Oberman HA. A modest proposal. *Am J Surg Pathol.* 1992;16:69–70.
9. Schwartz GF, Giuliano AE, Veronesi U. Proceedings of the consensus conference on the role of sentinel lymph node biopsy in carcinoma of the breast. *Hum Pathol.* 2002;33: 579–589.
10. Reitsamer R, Peintinger F, Prokop E, et al. Sentinel lymph node biopsy alone without axillary lymph node dissection—follow up of sentinel lymph node negative breast cancer patients. *Eur J Surg Oncol.* 2003;349:546–553.
11. Vernesi U, Paganelli G, Viale G, et al. A randomized comparison of sentinel-node biopsy with routine axillary dissection in breast cancer. *N Engl J Med.* 2003;349:546–553.

12. Treseler P. Pathologic examination of the sentinel lymph node: what is the best method. *Breast J*. 2006;12(suppl 2):S143–S151.
13. Holck S, Galatius H, Engel U, et al. False-negative frozen section of sentinel lymph node biopsy for breast cancer. *Breast*. 2004;13:42–48.
14. Chao C, Abell T, Martin RCG II, et al. Intraoperative frozen section of sentinel nodes: a formal decision analysis. *Am Surg*. 2004;70:214–221.
15. Creager AJ, Geisinger KR, Shiver SA, et al. Intraoperative evaluation of sentinel lymph nodes for metastatic breast carcinoma by imprint cytology. *Mod Pathol*. 2002;15: 1140–1147.
16. Battifora H. Intracytoplasmic lumina in breast carcinoma: a helpful histopathologic feature. *Arch Pathol*. 1975;99:614–617.

7

URINARY TRACT (KIDNEY, UROTHELIUM, AND PROSTATE)

JEROME B. TAXY

INTRODUCTION: GENITOURINARY FROZEN SECTION

Requests for frozen section related to the genitourinary tract are infrequent; certain anatomic sites are seldom queried at all. Frozen section for a testicular tumor, for example, is used only rarely since the diagnosis of a mass lesion is made by clinical and imaging criteria. Violating the tumor capsule is considered suboptimal surgical technique. Under these circumstances, a radical orchiectomy is the standard procedure, and the cell type of a testicular tumor is most unlikely to influence the extent of surgery. Hence, testicular frozen sections are not discussed here. Adrenal tumors are also seldom submitted for frozen section, because the outcome of the frozen section is again unlikely to change the operative procedure. Adrenal cortical tumors are either small enough to be encompassed by an adrenalectomy, are thus unlikely to be considered malignant preoperatively and not a candidate for a wider, more radical resection, or are large and clinically obvious, possibly inoperable. Diagnostic samples from the latter are more amenable to fine needle aspiration and/or needle core biopsy and examined after conventional fixation and embedding. Cortical tumors of intermediate size with potentially indeterminate histologic features are likely to be deferred. Among adrenal medullary tumors, neuroblastoma is discussed in Chapter 5; pheochromocytoma is clinically established prior to surgery, typically a confined tumor, and subject to frozen section only under exceptional circumstances. This chapter will discuss frozen section as related to common lesions of the kidney, prostate, and urothelium, focusing on the urinary bladder. A review of intraoperative consultations for kidney and urinary bladder has recently appeared in the clinical literature (1).

Kidney: Introduction

Primary epithelial tumors of the kidney comprise approximately 3% of all solid neoplasms. The American Cancer Society estimates approximately 58,000 cases for 2009 with almost 13,000 deaths (2). These numbers, however, group renal cell carcinomas and carcinomas of the renal pelvis together. SEER data estimate that approximately 80% of the total numbers are renal cell carcinomas and 20% are urothelial carcinomas. Further, SEER data suggest an increase in renal cell carcinoma during the years 1975 to 1995 (3). The increase may reflect incidental imaging discoveries while pursuing a workup for other, possibly unrelated, intraabdominal complaints. As an inadvertent but clinically important consequence, treatment decisions have revisited the traditionally perceived biologic differences between renal cortical neoplasms, adenoma or renal cell carcinoma, especially the clear cell type, a distinction primarily based on tumor size. Since a solitary renal mass of whatever size discovered incidentally or not is presumed to be malignant and subject to surgical intervention, this distinction ceases to be theoretical and becomes a practical issue for the pathologist in the reporting context of a frozen section.

Surgical extirpation remains the primary accepted modality for treating renal cell carcinoma as it has been for more than 50 years. The standard procedure against which all others are measured is the open radical nephrectomy, that is, a wide excision of the kidney to include the perirenal fat, external investing (Gerota) fascia, and adrenal gland (4). In the past, partial nephrectomy for renal cell carcinoma was exceptional (5); however, in recent years, possibly related to the popularity of laparoscopic surgery, this procedure has become much more common. That partial nephrectomy has become an established procedure is perhaps indicated by a recent study summarizing more than 1,800 cases from 21 separate studies with results comparable to the standard radical nephrectomy, that is, low perioperative morbidity, preservation of renal function, and a low local recurrence rate (4,6).

KIDNEY: THE INTRAOPERATIVE QUESTIONS. Frozen section requests for lesions of the kidney generally focus on three major issues: (i) The identification, or confirmation, of tumor, (ii) the cell type of the tumor, (iii) the margin of resection pertaining to partial nephrectomy. With the sophisticated imaging techniques currently available, the preoperative diagnosis of a mass lesion, solid or cystic, is not usually problematic. The frozen section confirmation of an actual tumor may influence the nature of the surgical procedure, especially whether to remove the kidney, may suggest a benign or nonneoplastic condition, or may help to exclude a urothelial carcinoma, which would entail a nephroureterectomy. The interpretation of these frozen sections may assume greater clinical importance for those tumors close to the hilum or involving the renal pelvis. The cell typing data summarized in Table 7.1 summarizes the University of Chicago experience in both the confirmation of the presence of tumor as well as the cell type.

Nephron-sparing procedures, either open or laparoscopic, may require immediate pathologic evaluation of the parenchymal margin, and frozen section has been increasingly employed for this. The indications for partial nephrectomy have included the following:

TABLE 7.1 Kidney Frozen Section[a]	
FS Tumor Type	Number
RCC, nos	45
Clear cell	18[b]
Papillary	5
Chromophobe	1
Cystic	13
Urothelial	4
Oncocytoma	8[c]
Total	94

[a]University of Chicago 2000–2006
[b]One case deferred
[c]Three cases deferred
Total nephrectomies during this time: 571 (430 radical, 141 partial)
Total frozen section for margins: 105

1. A localized tumor in a patient who would be rendered anephric by the procedure (solitary kidney, atrophic or dysplastic contralateral kidney, irreversible benign contralateral disease, e.g., obstruction)
2. Bilateral kidney tumors
3. A comorbid condition compromising renal function (diabetes, hypertension, glomerulonephritis, reflux, recurrent infection)

The advisability of partial nephrectomy for those with a solitary, presumptively malignant, unilateral tumor and normal renal function is currently under discussion (6). In addition to potential complications of the immediate postoperative period, the clinical issues are recurrence related to multifocality and the extent to which recurrence predicts for metastatic disease and overall long-term survival. While multifocality is an issue in approximately 15% of sporadic renal cell carcinomas, occult multifocal tumors below the level of resolution of the imaging studies can obviously not be predicted. Nonetheless, in the metaanalysis by Uzzo, 5-year survivals between partial and total nephrectomy patients were virtually identical (4). Based on recurrence rates in the summarized large series of partial nephrectomy, the contribution of multifocal or multicentric tumors to subsequent recurrence or metastasis is probably small. Given this current understanding of the biologic behavior of renal cell carcinoma and the need to ensure complete excision of at least the dominant lesion, frozen sections in the context of partial nephrectomies are reasonable requests. It should be noted, however, that following some experience with this procedure, some investigators feel that frozen section for margins is not indicated (7,8).

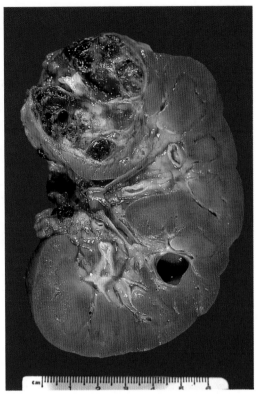

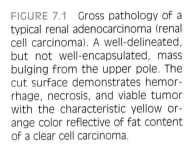

FIGURE 7.1 Gross pathology of a typical renal adenocarcinoma (renal cell carcinoma). A well-delineated, but not well-encapsulated, mass bulging from the upper pole. The cut surface demonstrates hemorrhage, necrosis, and viable tumor with the characteristic yellow orange color reflective of fat content of a clear cell carcinoma.

KIDNEY: FROZEN SECTION EXAMINATION. The typical gross pathology of renal cell carcinoma is a solitary circumscribed yellow to orange mass lesion. However it is widely recognized that the gross features of renal cell carcinoma vary widely (color, solid, cystic, hemorrhagic, necrotic, extrarenal extension). Instead of separate small biopsies being sent, it is optimal if the entire gross specimen with the lesion in place and not previously violated by the surgeon in the operating room is available for inspection. The degree of circumscription, extension of tumor beyond the kidney, and extent of infiltration of surrounding fat all impact on sampling, best accomplished by viewing the entire specimen (Figs. 7.1–7.3, e-Figs. 7.1–7.4).

While the histologic identification of specific cell type by frozen section has limited application, the presence of tumor is dependent on the ability to recognize specific cell types. In this regard, clear cell carcinoma is perhaps the most obvious with its characteristic highly vascularized, organoid growth of polygonal cells with clear cytoplasm (Fig. 7.4A). The cytoplasmic clarity of this predominant histologic subtype of renal cell carcinoma is due to accumulations of fat and/or glycogen. If the examiner feels the immediate need to further define the cytoplasmic content of a clear cell renal tumor, the presence of fat can be easily assessed at the time

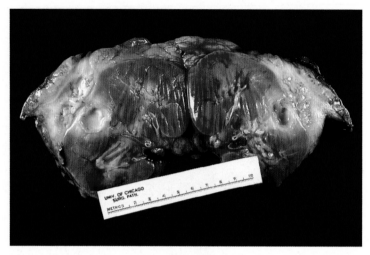

FIGURE 7.2   A clear cell renal cell carcinoma in the midportion of the kidney. The external fat overlying the tumor (Gerota fascia) has been inked before cutting. In this bivalved nephrectomy, the tumor involves the peripheral cortex and extends into the perinephric fat. The entire tumor is invested by broad bands of gray-white stroma and extends in wedge-type fashion close to a renal calyx.

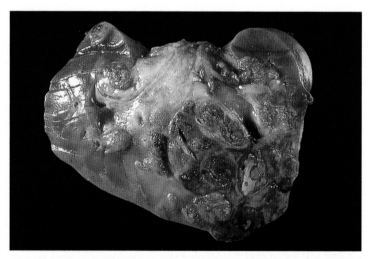

FIGURE 7.3   A poorly delineated renal tumor with multifocal distribution. Not a typical color for clear cell carcinoma, also involving the renal pelvis. This was a non-clear cell renal cell carcinoma.

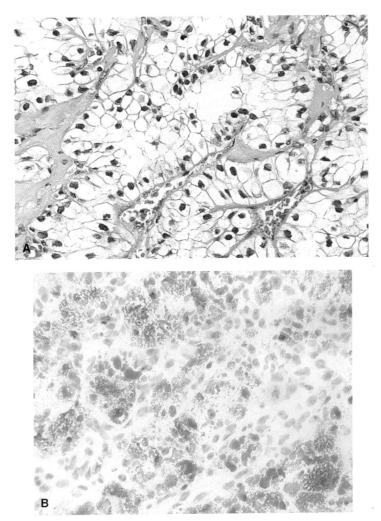

FIGURE 7.4 **A.** Histologic field of a clear cell renal cell carcinoma. Nests of polygonal cells with cytoplasmic clearing invested by a fine vascular stroma. **B.** Frozen section of the clear cell carcinoma in Figure 7.4 stained with oil-red-O. Globules of fat stain orange and are confined to the cytoplasm of the tumor cells.

of frozen section by doing an oil red O stain (Fig. 7.4B). Assessing glycogen requires PAS/PAS-D staining on paraffin material and would not be available in a frozen section setting. Chromophobe tumors are recognized by the pale, amphophilic cytoplasm and characteristic perinuclear halos (e-Figs. 7.5, 7.6).

Imprints are underutilized. Figure 7.5 (A and B) illustrates a gross specimen and the corresponding clinical radiograph with an obvious renal pelvic tumor. Imprints from this lesion stained with hematoxylin and eosin demonstrate syncytia of well-defined polygonal cells with nuclear

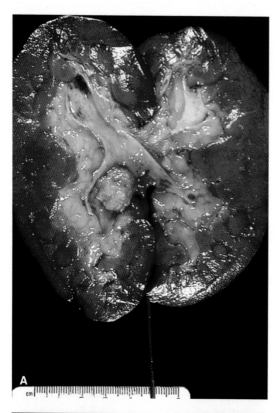

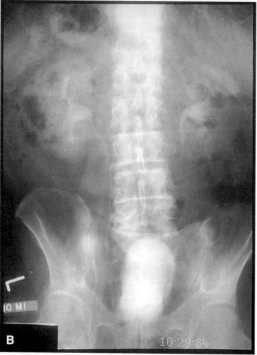

FIGURE 7.5 **A.** Bivalved kidney and attached ureter. In the mid-portion of the renal pelvis is an exophytic, rounded grayish tan mass highly suggestive of a urothelial carcinoma of the renal pelvis. **B.** Preoperative intravenous pyelogram demonstrating a renal pelvic filling defect in the left kidney.

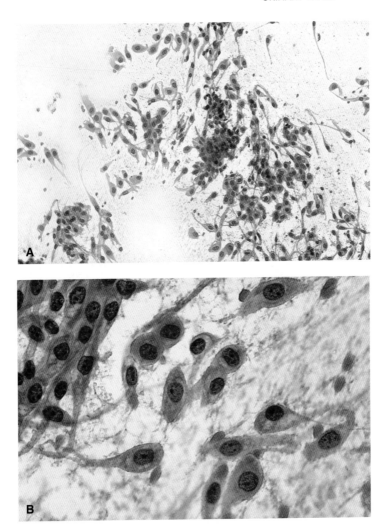

FIGURE 7.6 **A.** Low-power imprint of a renal pelvic tumor demonstrating syncytia of polygonal cells with polar processes, dense cytoplasm, and high-grade nuclei. **B.** High-power imprint highlighting the cytoplasmic process, well-defined cell borders, and cytoplasmic density. **C.** Histologic field of this tumor demonstrating typical papillary growth of high-grade urothelial carcinoma, cytologically similar to the imprint. (*continued*)

pleomorphism, abundant amphophilic to eosinophilic cytoplasm, and cytoplasmic processes, features commonly seen in urothelial tumors. These cytologic features (Fig. 7.6A and B) correspond histologically to urothelial carcinoma (Fig. 7.6C) and correlate with the gross examination.

Among the 94 cases summarized in Table 7.1 covering a $6^1/_2$-year period, the only diagnosis of a benign tumor was oncocytoma; a diagnosis of angiomyolipoma was not encountered. There were, however, four discrepant diagnoses (Table 7.2). In one instance, a renal pelvic tumor

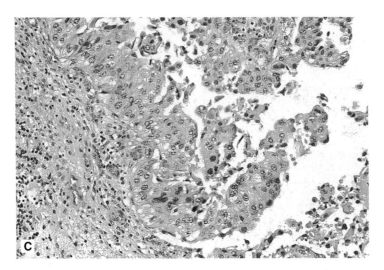

FIGURE 7.6 (*Continued*)

interpreted by frozen section as a urothelial carcinoma was changed on permanent section to papillary renal cell carcinoma. The non-clear cell nature of both tumors and the common feature of papillary growth accounted for the erroneous interpretation. Frozen section, like other modalities of morphologic assessment, is not perfect; there are hazards associated with immediate analysis, as this case emphasizes.

Diagnostic skills are not only challenged in discerning different cell types but in nonneoplastic tumor-like growths as well. Figure 7.7 is a gross photograph of a kidney from a 74-year-old male patient who was evaluated at another hospital with a presumptive diagnosis of a primary renal tumor at least partially affecting the renal pelvis. Upon referral, a laparoscopic nephrectomy was done with some difficulty because of local adhesions and scarring. The gross examination of the bivalved specimen demonstrated multiple grayish and orange-tinged masses of varying size partially involving the renal pelvis with associated calyceal dilatation and hemorrhage. No stones were present. The frozen section was requested to

---

TABLE 7.2 Frozen Section Discrepant Diagnoses[a]

1. FS diagnosis of urothelial carcinoma changed to papillary renal cell carcinoma
2. FS diagnosis of renal cell carcinoma, nos, changed to oncocytoma
3. FS diagnosis of chromophobe renal cell carcinoma changed to clear cell
4. FS diagnosis of benign cyst changed to papillary renal cell carcinoma[b]

[a]University of Chicago 2000–2006
[b]Separate lesions; papillary renal cell carcinoma not frozen

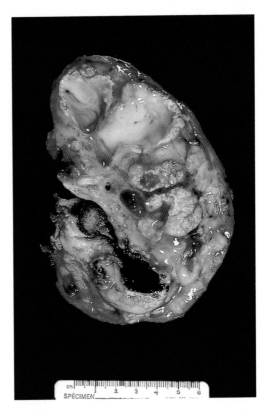

FIGURE 7.7 Xanthogranulomatous pyelonephritis. Gross photograph showing marked hydronephrosis and numerous poorly circumscribed deposits of yellow-gray tissue replacing renal parenchyma. Note hemorrhage in the lower pole calyx extending into the renal hilum, no stones.

rule out a urothelial carcinoma, which would have necessitated a completion ureterectomy. Microscopically, there were areas of inflammation and scarring with some brown pigment. Bits of irregular, blue-stained material suggesting a microlith were also present (Fig. 7.8). In the region of the renal pelvis, frozen section demonstrated a mixed inflammatory infiltrate with some foamy to clear histiocytes, creating some diagnostic uncertainty related to clear cell renal adenocarcinoma (Fig. 7.9). However, the gross and histologic features were not considered sufficient for a malignant diagnosis and frozen interpretation of probable xanthogranulomatous pyelonephritis was reported. This diagnosis was confirmed on examination of permanent material (e-Figs. 7.7–7.9). Xanthogranulomatous pyelonephritis is an unusual, but well-recognized, tumor-like lesion often associated with calculi and with the potential for diffuse organ replacement, extrarenal extension, and macroscopic resemblance to a malignancy (e-Figs. 7.10, 7.11).

Partial nephrectomy employs a sharp dissection of adjacent renal parenchyma to yield a rim of normal tissue around the tumor. The optimal amount of normal tissue is not an established figure. Having the entire gross specimen in this circumstance allows the inking of the parenchymal margin before the specimen is freshly cut. The question of whether to take

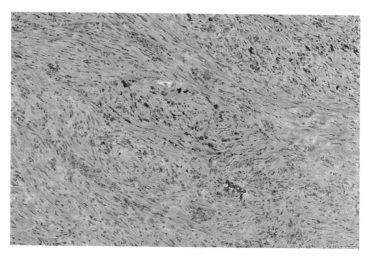

FIGURE 7.8   Frozen section. Low-power photomicrograph from a gross lesion demonstrating a fibroinflammatory infiltrate and a dense scar with a collection of pigmented cells, probably histiocytes. The associated blue-staining irregular body may represent a calcific focus, possibly from a microcalculus.

a "strip" margin or a representative section perpendicular to the inked edge at the point closest to the tumor has never been formally addressed. A perpendicular section may be better because the tissue section can then be taken from the point at which the tumor macroscopically most closely approaches the specimen edge. Given that the possible sources of confusion in this setting include sampling, detached atypical cells, crush artifact

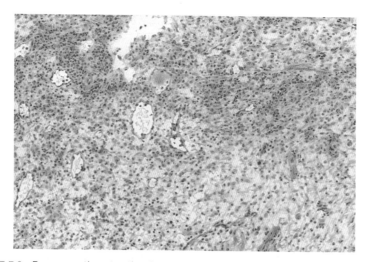

FIGURE 7.9   Frozen section. Another low-power area from the renal pelvis demonstrating a mixed inflammatory infiltrate with numerous polygonal cells with clear to coarsely vacuolated cytoplasm, probably histiocytes.

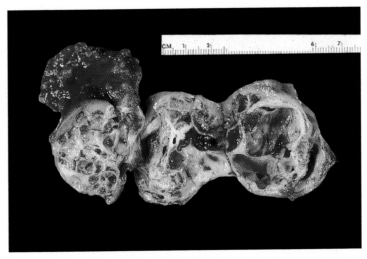

FIGURE 7.10 Partial nephrectomy, renal cell carcinoma. Circumscribed multiloculated cystic tumor with perinephric fat at upper left and thin parenchymal margin at upper right. Frozen section from upper right area.

and the misidentification of normal renal tubules for tumor (9,10), having secure gross landmarks is helpful.

Figure 7.10 illustrates a partial nephrectomy specimen from a patient with compromised renal function. This approximately 3-cm multiloculated cystic mass was removed in the usual fashion with what was grossly apparent as a very thin parenchymal margin. The frozen section sample should be taken from the closest margin after the tissue edge is marked with ink. Figures 7.11–7.13 are from a grossly similar case. The low-power

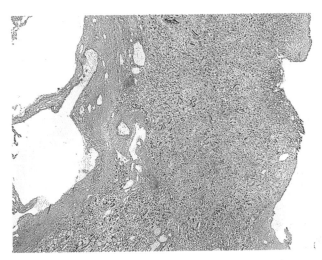

FIGURE 7.11 Frozen section, low-power of margin. Inked edge is separated from a tumor locule by a thin strip of uninvolved renal parenchyma.

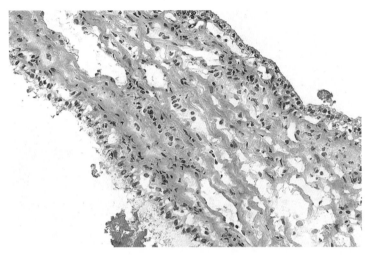

FIGURE 7.12 Frozen section showing the tumor cyst locules to be at least partially lined by clear epithelial cells. Even though in this field the cells are a single layer, this is sufficient for a renal cell carcinoma diagnosis.

examination demonstrates the cyst locules and a definite rim of normal renal parenchyma (Fig. 7.11). Further examination of the cyst walls demonstrates fibrous septations surfaced on both sides by a bland, but definite clear cell population of polygonal cells (Fig. 7.12). In other areas, invasion of the septae by the tumor cells was apparent (Fig. 7.13). A diagnosis of clear cell renal cell carcinoma with clear margins can be made, and the operation terminated.

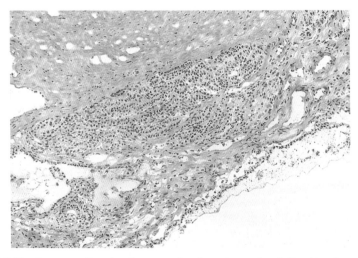

FIGURE 7.13 Frozen section. Another area showing a tumor locule lined by clear cells with a microscopic area of infiltration beneath.

Urothelial Carcinoma: Introduction

The urothelium is the most primitive of epithelia, both in its organization and in its individual cytologic characteristics. The simplicity of the cytoplasmic organization aptly suits the cells for fluid transport (11). In the past, this epithelium has been termed "transitional" epithelium, perhaps related to its transport function or possibly because of its ability under inflammatory and neoplastic conditions to demonstrate squamous and/or glandular differentiation. It is now accepted that these cells are not transitional in the sense they represent some intermediate phase of differentiation but do in fact represent a discrete form of epithelium. Hence, the current designation as urothelium.

The individual cell simplicity is also reflected in the histologic organization, since basal to surface maturation is subtle. The integrity and recognition of this polarity is essential to the interpretation of a frozen section. A key feature in the histologic assessment of urothelial organization is the preservation of the basal cell layer. Ideally, these are cells with a high nuclear to cytoplasmic ratio and a palisaded arrangement. The suprabasilar cells are more loosely arranged with minor increases in cytoplasm. These layers may only be a few cells in thickness. The presence of "umbrella cells", expansile cell processes and marked accumulations of cytoplasm, in the most superficial urothelial layer is not a reliable indicator of a normal maturation sequence since umbrella cells may persist over dysplastic urothelium.

UROTHELIAL CARCINOMA: INTRAOPERATIVE QUESTIONS. The pathobiology of urothelial carcinoma is linked to the multifocality or "field effect" inherent in its clinical manifestations. Although urothelial neoplasms occur from the renal pelvis to the bladder, perhaps the best examples of the frozen section issues in the intraoperative management of urothelial carcinoma are represented in the urinary bladder. A mass lesion may be accompanied by other similar lesions with grossly uninvolved intervening mucosa, the urothelium may be diffusely involved, or clinically inapparent intramucosal malignancy may be part of a process for which there is a dominant mass lesion (Figs. 7.14–7.16). In the past, radical cystectomy has been done when the tumor is both high grade and muscle invasive (e-Figs. 7.12–7.14). Those clinical criteria may be changing, so that radical cystectomy with curative intent may be undertaken for less than deeply invasive disease.

The major question related to surgical resection of urothelial carcinoma of the urinary bladder is the presence of dysplasia at the margins. It would be safe to say that the use of frozen section for ureteral margin assessment is currently at least controversial and possibly not indicated (12–18). While there is an understandable proscription related to cutting through invasive tumor, the examination of ureteral margins focuses on the detection of carcinoma not grossly apparent and confined to the mucosa. In this assessment, mucosa-confined carcinoma is regarded as synonymous with severe urothelial dysplasia. Frozen section examination

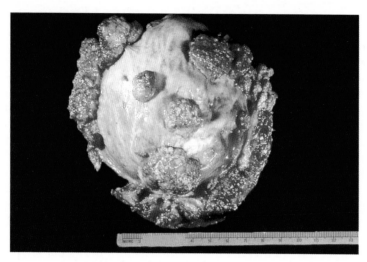

FIGURE 7.14 The inverted mucosa of a radical cystectomy demonstrating multiple, elevated friable tumors with intervening areas of uninvolved mucosa. This is a gross example of the multifocality ("field effect") anticipated in urothelial carcinoma.

of ureteral margins is clinically justified on the supposition that high-grade dysplasia is predictive for local recurrence and the development of upper tract tumors. Studies spanning the previous almost 20 years have indicated that frozen sections of ureteral margins during a radical cystectomy exhibit dysplasia of any degree in up to approximately 8% of cases; the presence of dysplasia is not predictive of local recurrence or subsequent upper tract recurrences which range from 2.4% to 17% (15,20).

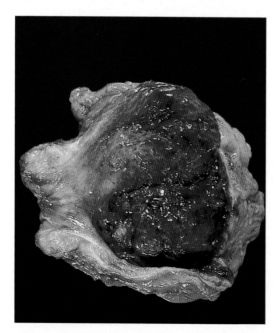

FIGURE 7.15 A radical cystectomy specimen (opened urethra to the left) with a diffuse hemorrhagic process involving most of the mucosal surface. A discrete mass is not apparent.

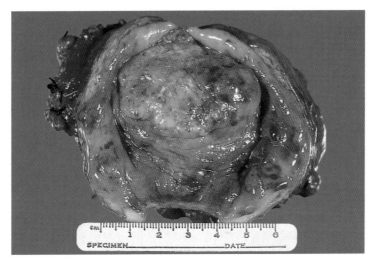

FIGURE 7.16 A radical cystectomy with a large dominant tumor in the posterior wall and dome.

Further, if frozen sections on ureteral margins are routinely re-quested, a urethral margin is not. Local urethral recurrences may occur in up to 10% of patients undergoing cystectomy but may be related more to local prostatic invasion than to urothelial dysplasia/carcinoma in situ at the distal margin (15,19,20). Assuming that the results of the frozen section will influence the intraoperative management, two additional questions should be raised: (i) Does the frozen section result actually in-fluence subsequent clinical behavior of the tumor? (ii) If not, then why do we do them? The issues of appropriate utilization and the dynamics of clinical decision-making in the context of frozen section in urothelial dis-ease are, therefore, not clear.

The circumstances for which frozen section may actually be indicated are (i) tumor involving the bladder neck, (ii) grossly apparent tumor multi-focality, (iii) extensive carcinoma in situ, (iv) involvement by tumor of the intramural ureter (15,20). As a matter of practice, however, the frozen sec-tion requests related to a radical cystectomy routinely only involve the (proximal) ureteral margins. These margins may be submitted separately or the pathologist may be asked to examine the proximal stumps on the cys-tectomy specimen. Most surgical pathologists would agree that it is difficult enough to assess urothelial dysplasia based on well-fixed and cut paraffin–embedded samples; doing this by frozen section can be extremely challeng-ing, especially if the distinction to be made is between something reactive/hyperplastic and a low-grade dysplasia. The recognition of dysplasia that is less than high grade is difficult because of the difficulty in recognizing the basal layer and the subtleties of urothelial maturation. In addition, degrees of dysplasia short of severe/carcinoma in situ may not be predictive of any-thing. Further, since there is no meaningful morphologic distinction between high-grade dysplasia and in situ carcinoma, the frozen section assessment should appropriately concern the presence of dysplasia and if present, whether it is low or high grade. High-grade dysplasia may be more easily appreciated because of more obvious nuclear pleomorphism, dyscohesion, and mitotic activity. Although immunohistochemistry for p53 is helpful in identifying some examples of carcinoma in situ, obviously this is not available for frozen section use. The intraoperative action taken as a result of these diagnoses is, ultimately, up to the surgeon. Whether the decision to submit additional margins is related to the degree of dysplasia and the long-term implication(s) of a negative or positive margin is uncertain.

UROTHELIAL CARCINOMA: FROZEN SECTION EXAMINATION. The mechanics of orienting the ureteral segment from a radical cystectomy require that the most proximal aspect of the ureter be mounted. The identity of the proximal aspect can be easily ascertained from a gross examination of the cystectomy specimen. If the distal end from a separately submitted ureteral segment is marked by the surgeon with a suture, the proximal end will be free from manipulation or crush artifact and it can then be amputated and embedded properly. Since this is a rounded structure with a central lumen of varying caliber, the freezing and cutting of the section will be optimized by ensuring that the tissue is evenly mounted and that embedding medium is evenly distributed including into the lumen. Excess fat should be trimmed off. A complete face of the ureter to include the mucosa, the muscular wall, and the surrounding connective tissue with a minimum of initial wasted sections is the objective. Nevertheless, it is almost impossible to prepare these frozen sections without some folding or cracking artifact, folds in the tissue, or an incomplete wall (Figs. 7.17, 7.18).

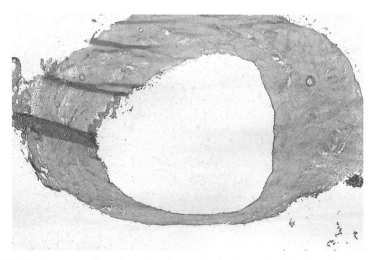

FIGURE 7.17 Frozen section of a ureteral margin. The lumen is dilated and the wall focally thinned, but the section demonstrates the entire circumference. The epithelium is very attenuated.

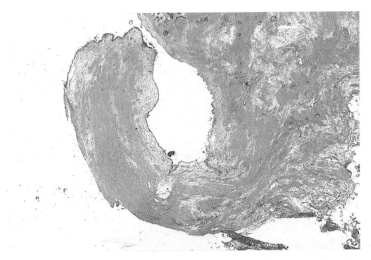

FIGURE 7.18 Frozen section of a ureteral margin. The mounting was not optimal in this sample, so the variable wall thickness is further complicated by incompleteness, as demonstrated in the upper left.

The spectrum of histologic and cytologic change is broad. At low magnification, reactive hyperplasia or low-grade dysplasia is characterized by a recognizable basal layer, suprabasilar layers of variable thickness with variable acquisition of cytoplasm. The very superficial layer may or may not exhibit umbrella cells (Fig. 7.19, e-Figs. 7.15, 7.16). Increasing degrees

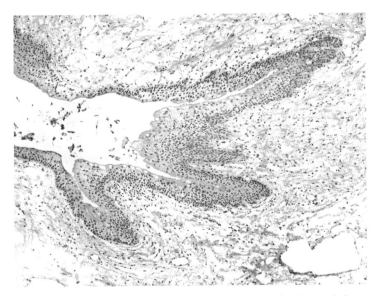

FIGURE 7.19 Frozen section of a ureteral margin demonstrating hyperplasia or perhaps low-grade dysplasia. There is preservation of the basal layer and some focal thickness of the urothelium with a tangential plane on the right side of the field. There is acquisition of cytoplasm in the more superficial layers, minimal nuclear atypia, no mitoses or necrosis.

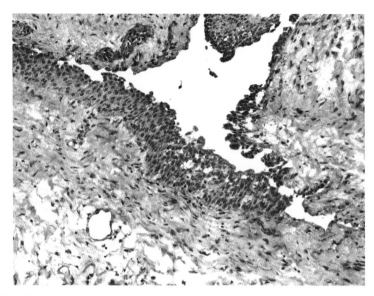

FIGURE 7.20   Frozen section of a ureteral margin showing high-grade (moderate) dysplasia. There is considerable variability in the thickness of the urothelium from one cell layer to several. The integrity of the basal layer is not readily apparent; there is little or no cytoplasmic accumulation. No nuclear pleomorphism or mitoses is present.

of atypia still show variable numbers of cell layers, but lose the basilar orientation as well as cytoplasmic accumulation (Fig. 7.20). Possible helpful clues to the high-grade nature of the dysplasia, in addition to the absence of cytoplasmic accumulations and the appearance of nuclear pleomorphism, are cytologic dyscohesion and mitotic activity (Figs. 7.21, 7.22).

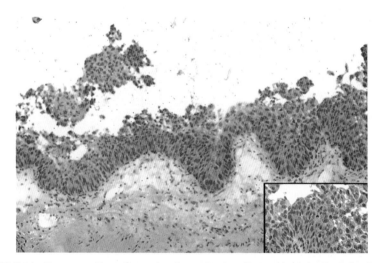

FIGURE 7.21   Frozen section of a ureteral margin showing marked dysplasia/in situ carcinoma. The cell layers are thick, the nuclei are large, and there is dyscohesion. Inset: Higher power of this frozen section demonstrating marked nuclear pleomorphism and a mitotic figure in the upper third of the epithelium.

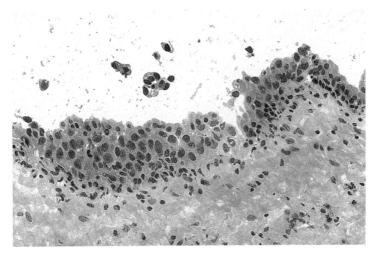

FIGURE 7.22 Low-power frozen section of marked dysplasia/in situ carcinoma. Basal layer architecture not apparent, marked nuclear pleomorphism and dyscohesive cell groups.

While not as common, invasive urothelial carcinoma at a margin is certainly encountered. The obvious disruption in the muscular architecture by tumor cells and attendant inflammation is apparent even at low magnification (Figs. 7.23, 7.24, e-Figs. 7.17, 7.18).

Prostate Cancer: Introduction

The development of PSA screening and radical prostatectomy has transformed the respective detection and treatment of prostatic adenocarcinoma.

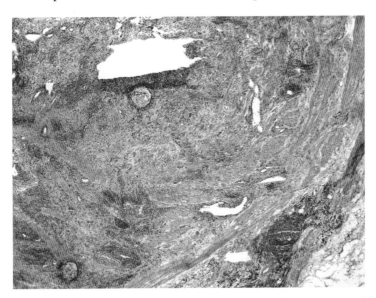

FIGURE 7.23 Low-power frozen section of ureter showing infiltrating urothelial carcinoma. Note the fold at the top complicating evaluation of the lumen. The infiltrating tumor nests are associated with inflammation.

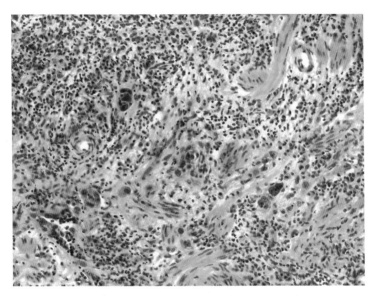

FIGURE 7.24 High-power frozen section of the ureter in Figure 7.23 demonstrating small nests of malignant cells and a marked inflammatory infiltrate.

Cancers are being detected in younger men and at earlier stages, although the Gleason grade has remained steady (21). The American Cancer Society estimates approximately 192,000 new cases of prostate cancer in 2009 with more than 27,000 deaths (2). It is the most common malignancy in men, and is the second leading cause of death from cancer. If a radical prostatectomy is done, however, a major goal is at least long-term local control, a factor directly related to the adequacy of resection, which depends on the status of the margins: peripheral capsular margins, apex, and base. The status of the margins is a major predictive factor in assessing the potential progression of the tumor (22). In one large series of approximately 7,300 cases equally divided between nerve-sparing and wide excision procedures, the incidence of positive margins (mostly apical and posterior) was about the same in both groups as was the progression-free survival (Table 7.3) (23). Therefore, at the time of surgery, if there is a palpable abnormality or unexpected bulge seen laparoscopically in the poles of the gland (apex or base) or in the peripheral capsule, a frozen section may be requested.

The most important complications of radical prostatectomy are urinary incontinence and impotence. The latter is related to the usual peripheral location for prostatic adenocarcinoma, the possibility for the tumor to penetrate the poorly defined capsular tissue as well as the known tumor tendency to track along the peripheral nerves. A resection of the neurovascular bundles ensures that the patient will be impotent. The nerve-sparing radical prostatectomy is designed to preserve potency without compromising extirpation of the tumor and ultimate local control. The

TABLE 7.3 Positive Margins in Radical Prostatectomy		
Procedure	Nerve-sparing	Wide Excision
N	3741	3527
+ Margin (overall)	27%	31%
Location (%)		
Apex	18	25
Posterior	16	19
Base	5	11
Urethra	2	5
Anterior	2	2

Modified from Ward JF, Zincke H, Bergstralh EJ, et al. The impact of surgical approach (nerve bundle preservation versus wide local excision) on surgical margins and biochemical recurrence following radical prostatectomy. *J Urol* 2004;172:1328–1332.

procedure is optimal for patients with clinically limited disease, intermediate Gleason scores on biopsy, and those who are preoperatively potent (23,24). Patients with a preoperative high histologic Gleason score are not necessarily excluded from having radical surgery (25).

The appreciation of the anatomic landmarks by the urologist is facilitated by laparoscopic surgery which, in increasing numbers, is being done robotically. However, the laparoscopic procedure has raised additional concerns over the potential for adequate resection of the gland because of the absence of tactile feedback for the surgeon and inadvertent capsulotomy related to the field of view. Frozen sections may be requested to assist in complete removal of the prostate gland as well as to assess whether tumor is present (26). A potential margin which is positive for tumor will result in additional tissue being submitted, and is likely to include a wide resection encompassing the neurovascular bundle, even though there is unlikely to be additional tumor. In one series of 101 patients undergoing nerve-sparing surgery with frozen section, 15 samples were positive, 12 of which demonstrated no tumor on additionally submitted tissue (26).

Inasmuch as preoperative staging cannot be consistently 100% accurate and as radical prostatectomy has a debatable role in the treatment of patients with metastatic disease, there is an advantage in detecting those patients who would not benefit from this form of treatment. In earlier years, it was common to do routine bilateral pelvic lymphadenectomies with frozen section analysis to identify such patients and not proceed to the prostatectomy if a metastasis were discovered. Unfortunately, no standardized method of examination was ever employed in the analysis of these nodes, such that the reported false-negative rate was as high as 70% in some series with very low sensitivities (27). In recent years, urologists have begun to use a panel of clinical and pathologic parameters to identify those patients who could undergo a radical prostatectomy without concurrent lymph node dissection. These parameters are clinical stage T2 or less, Gleason grade of 6 or less on biopsy, and serum PSA less than 10 ng/mL. Less than 4% of such patients are estimated to have a positive regional lymph node. Routine lymph node dissections therefore have disappeared. The role of frozen section in the evaluation of node dissections in selected patients is currently unsettled. With increasing numbers of radical prostatectomies being performed, the utilization of frozen section in the intraoperative management for both margins and lymph node status has occasioned debate in the clinical literature.

PROSTATE AND PELVIC LYMPH NODES: INTRAOPERATIVE QUESTIONS. In adenocarcinoma of the prostate, the use of frozen section is divided into two major areas: (i) margins of resection; (ii) status of the regional lymph nodes. While it is generally acknowledged that frozen section is accurate in determining neurovascular bundle preservation and eventual margin status (26,28,29), biochemical recurrence and a positive margin status may be similar in prostatectomies not examined by frozen section (26,29). It is certainly reasonable to question the use of frozen section in this context, since "if surgery is not going to be modified by the frozen section results, frozen section analysis should not be done" (27). Not surprisingly, therefore, one recent editorial argued against using frozen section for the determination of margin adequacy (30). The requests may be related to the surgeon's general experience with the open radical prostatectomy procedure, the equipment (if the procedure is done laparoscopically with or without robotic assistance), and the intramural retrospective study of institutional outcomes. With the steady increase of specimen submissions, the University of Chicago experience over approximately 6 years has resulted in more confidence on the part of the pathologist in the interpretation of these frozen sections and is summarized in Table 7.4. A comparison is made between those cases accessioned from 2000 to 2003 and those examined from 2004 to August 2006. This grouping parallels the increasing use of robot-assisted laparoscopic radical prostatectomy beginning around 2004. No false positives were discovered; there have been four false negatives over the entire time period.

The second major issue related to radical prostate surgery is the status of the regional lymph nodes. In the past, a lymph node with metastatic tumor was a reason to terminate the procedure (31). As indicated, the detection of nodal metastatic disease by frozen section is not a standardized procedure and as such, for grossly uninvolved nodes, the false-negative rate could be significant. In some studies, even metastases detected by frozen section did not preclude completion of the operation (27), thereby begging the question. In recent years, studies have shown that routine pelvic lymph node dissections are not only unnecessary but that frozen section of these nodes is also unnecessary, not predictive of

TABLE 7.4 Radical Prostatectomy: Prostate Frozen Sections[a]	
2000–2003	
Total radical prostatectomy	294
Total prostate frozen section	129
Apex	35
Base	27
Peripheral	67
Total positive	5 (4%)
2004–2006 (August)	
Total radical prostatectomy	677
Total prostate frozen section	429
Apex	163
Base	89
Peripheral	161
Other	16
Total positive	39 (9%)

[a]University of Chicago 2000–2006 (August)

biochemical relapse, and probably no more predictive of biologic behavior than the standard clinical nomogram (27,31–33).

The wide variation of the published experience related to lymph node frozen section is probably related to sampling. In the absence of grossly obvious metastatic disease, the pathologic analysis has varied from freezing everything, freezing a portion of the largest node, to imprinting all the nodes. The skills required to do a frozen section in this setting for metastatic disease are no different than those required, for example, for the sentinel lymph node for breast cancer, discussed earlier. No special expertise is required. However, the sentinel node concept has not been developed for prostate cancer; the node-bearing tissue is dissected en bloc by the surgeon and delivered as such to surgical pathology. The pelvic lymph nodes are multiple and while often sclerotic and microscopically calcific, are also often large, heavily invested by fat which cannot be trimmed. Making a complete examination by frozen section frequently yields qualitatively marginal preparations and is impractical. Besides the questionable utility of frozen section in this setting, two other factors related to routine pelvic lymphadenectomy are added costs and postoperative morbidity. The former could be of the nature of several thousand dollars; the latter could involve nerve and vessel injury sustained during the dissection, bleeding, infection, fistulas, and genital and lower extremity edema.

Presently, while routine intraoperative analysis of the lymph nodes for every case is not recommended, in the individualization of therapy

TABLE 7.5 Radical Prostatectomy and Pelvic Lymph Node Frozen Section[a]	
2000–2003	
Total radical prostatectomy	294
Total lymph node frozen sections	61
Total positive	3 (5%)
False negative	4 (7%)
2004–2006 (August)	
Total radical prostatectomy	677
Total lymph node frozen sections	299
Total positive	0
False negative	4 (1%)

[a]University of Chicago 2000–2006 (August)

such an examination may be deemed appropriate. A summary of the University of Chicago experience with pelvic lymph node frozen sections is in Table 7.5. From 2000 to 2003, 294 radical prostatectomies were done for which there were 61 requests for lymph node frozen sections. Since such requests are often multiple, the lymph node figure corresponds to a fewer number of patients. With the popularity of robot-assisted prostatectomy, between 2004 and August 2006, there were 677 prostatectomies with requests for lymph node examinations in 299 lymph nodes. The preoperative selection of patients is quite good and explains the very low frozen section positive rate. False negatives were also very low.

Urology residents with advanced training in laparoscopic as well as robot-assisted procedures are entering varies practice venues. Until the merits of and candidates for frozen section study are resolved, it is likely that frozen section requests will continue, though the utilization will be uneven. The interests of surgical pathologists will be well served by being prepared.

PROSTATE AND PELVIC LYMPH NODES: FROZEN SECTION EXAMINATION. The assessment of margins from an open prostatectomy specimen should be indicated by the surgeon based on a specific worrisome palpable abnormality. However, even in the context of a suspicious palpable abnormality, the gross appreciation of prostate cancer can be difficult, since firm, focally confluent nodules are part of the pathology of benign prostatic enlargement and often coexist with areas of malignancy (Fig. 7.25). The firm texture of diffuse and poorly circumscribed tumor growth is often accompanied by a yellow color (Fig 7.26, e-Fig. 7.19). For frozen section, the peripheral abnormalities in question are best examined by amputating a wedge of parenchymal and capsular tissues after the periphery has been

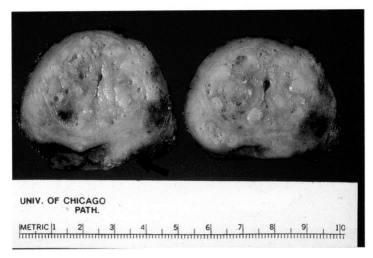

FIGURE 7.25 Two transverse sections from a radical prostatectomy demonstrating numerous central nodules replacing the gland. A small yellowish focus of carcinoma is apparent outside the prostatic capsule (arrow).

inked and before serial transverse sectioning of the gland. This wedge is then cut parallel to its long axis and mounted so that the nodule or area of firmness and the inked capsular tissue are included together (Fig. 7.27).

In laparoscopic resections, the margins cannot be felt. The tissue samples, therefore, will be unoriented biopsy fragments and all such fragments should be frozen. Adenocarcinoma is easy to spot if there is obvious

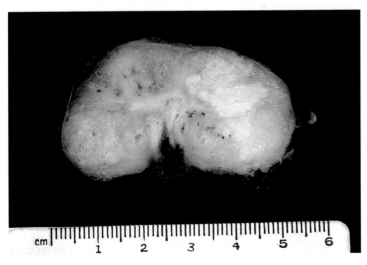

FIGURE 7.26 Transverse section from a radical prostatectomy demonstrating generally smooth surfaces with bilateral poorly circumscribed yellow areas indicative of adenocarcinoma.

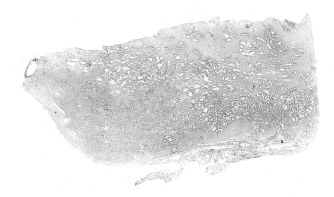

FIGURE 7.27 Low magnification view of a peripheral area of the prostate showing a poorly circumscribed cellular nodule of adenocarcinoma abutting the capsule, but not penetrating it, accounting for a firm texture palpated during open prostatectomy.

perineural invasion (Fig. 7.28); however, perineural infiltrates of artifactually distorted cells may be extremely difficult to recognize as adenocarcinoma (Fig. 7.29). Such artifactual distortion may not be appreciated as tumor until the permanent sections of the prostatectomy are available (e-Figs. 7.20 and 7.21).

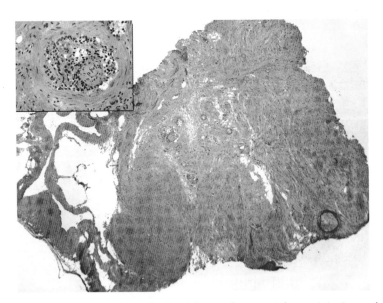

FIGURE 7.28 A tissue fragment submitted from a laparoscopic prostatectomy showing predominant fibromuscular tissue with a few glandular elements focally exhibiting perineural invasion, indicative of adenocarcinoma. Inset: High magnification of the glandular focus demonstrating clear-cut perineural invasion.

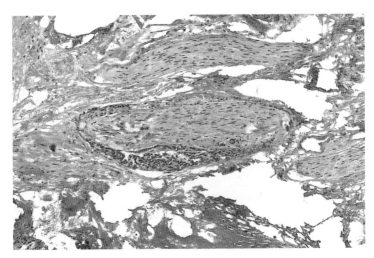

FIGURE 7.29   A tissue fragment from a laparoscopic prostatectomy in which a peripheral nerve is surrounded by artifactually distorted cells, suspicious for adenocarcinoma.

Fragments exhibiting cellular glandular proliferation may not be recognizable at all as adenocarcinoma on a frozen section (Fig. 7.30). An "atypical" diagnosis may create a dilemma for the surgeon. A difficult dissection and apparent adhesions of the prostatic capsule to the pelvic sidewall may create a suspicion of infiltrating carcinoma. In this context, the presence of granulomatous prostatitis should be remembered (Fig. 7.31).

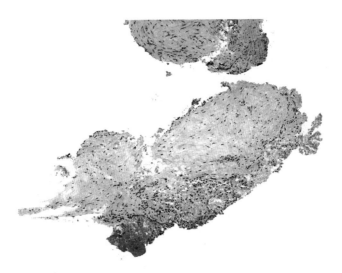

FIGURE 7.30   Tissue fragments from a laparoscopic prostatectomy with a cellular glandular proliferation, suspicious but not definitive for adenocarcinoma.

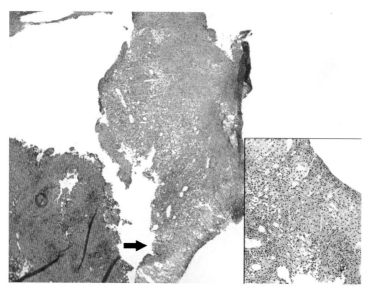

FIGURE 7.31 Tissue fragments from a laparoscopic prostatectomy in which there were adhesions of the gland to the peripheral pelvic soft tissue. This diffusely cellular fragment consists of inflammatory cells with multinucleated giant cells, indicative of granulomatous prostatitis. Inset: High magnification of a focus of granulomatous prostatitis.

In the examination of pelvic lymph nodes, unless there is a node already marked as suspicious or positive or one which can be grossly identified by the pathologist as such, a positive frozen section may represent a random event. The tumor may be present in small nodes and not in the expected large ones (Fig. 7.32).

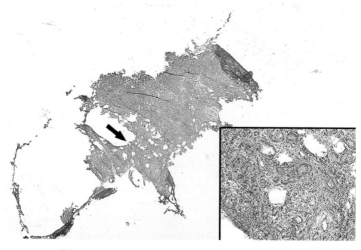

FIGURE 7.32 A small lymph node totally replaced by adenocarcinoma. Inset: High magnification of adenocarcinoma as seen in the frozen section.

REFERENCES

1. Truong LD, Krishnan B, Shen SS. Intraoperative pathology consultation for kidney and urinary bladder specimens. *Arch Pathol Lab Med.* 2005;129:1585–1601.
2. American Cancer Society, Cancer Facts and Figures 2009, Atlanta: American Cancer Society; 2009, p. 4.
3. Chow WH, Devesa SS, Warren JL, et al. Rising incidence of renal cell cancer in the United States. *JAMA.* 1999;281:1628–1631.
4. Uzzo RG, Novick AC. Nephron sparing surgery for renal tumors: indications, techniques and outcomes. *J Urol.* 2001;166:6–18.
5. Marshall FF, Taxy JB, Fishman EK, et al. The feasibility of surgical enucleation for renal cell carcinoma. *J Urol.* 1986;135:231–234.
6. Pahernik S, Roos F, Hampel C, et al. Nephron sparing surgery for renal cell carcinoma with normal contralateral kidney: 25 years of experience. *J Urol.* 2006;175:2027–2031.
7. Kubinski DJ, Clark PE, Assimos DG, et al. Utility of frozen section analysis of resection margins during partial nephrectomy. *Urology.* 2004;64:31–34.
8. Duvdevani M, Laufer M, Kastin A, et al. Is frozen section analysis in nephron sparing surgery necessary? A clinicopathological study of 301 cases. *J Urol.* 2005;173:385–387.
9. McHale T, Malkowicz SB, Tomaszewski JE. Potential pitfalls in the frozen section evaluation of parenchymal margins in nephron-sparing surgery. *Am J Clin Pathol.* 2002; 118:903–910.
10. Krishnan B, Lechago J, Ayala G, et al. Intraoperative consultation for renal lesions: implications and diagnostic pitfalls in 324 cases. *Am J Clin Pathol.* 2003;120:528–535.
11. Battifora H, Eisenstein R, McDonald JH. The human urinary bladder mucosa: an electron microscopic study. *Inv Urol.* 1964;1:354–361.
12. Johnson DE, Wishnow KI, Tenney D. Are frozen-section examinations of ureteral margins required for all patients undergoing radical cystectomy for bladder cancer? *Urology.* 1989;33:451–454.
13. Lebret T, Herve JM, Barre P, et al. Urethral recurrence of transitional cell carcinoma of the bladder: predictive value of preoperative latero-montanal biopsies and urethral frozen sections during prostatocystectomy. *Eur Urol.* 1998;33:170–174.
14. Schoenberg MP, Carter HB, Epstein JI. Ureteral frozen section analysis during cystectomy: a reassessment. *J Urol.* 1996;155:1218–1220.
15. Stenzl A, Bartsch G, Rogatsch H. The remnant urothelium after reconstructive bladder surgery. *Eur Urol.* 2002;41:124–131.
16. Schumacher MC, Scholz M, Weise ES, et al. Is there an indication for frozen section examination of the ureteral margins during cystectomy for transitional cell carcinoma of the bladder? *J Urol.* 2006;176:2409–2413.
17. Osman Y, El-Tabey N, Abdel-Latif M, et al. The value of frozen-section analysis of ureteric margins on surgical decision-making in patients undergoing radical cystectomy for bladder cancer. *BJU Int.* 2007;99: 81–84.
18. Lee SE, Byun SS, Hong SK, et al. Significance of cancer involvement at the ureteral margin detected on routine frozen section analysis during radical cystectomy. *Urol Int.* 2006;77:13–17.
19. Lebret T, Herve JM, Barre P. Urethral recurrence of transitional cell carcinoma of the bladder: predictive value of preoperative latero-montanal biopsies and urethral frozen sections during prostatocystectomy. *Eur Urol.* 1998;33:170–174.
20. Stein JP, Clark P, Miranda G. Urethral tumor recurrence following cystectomy and urinary diversion: clinical and pathological characteristics in 768 male patients. *J Urol.* 2005;173:1163–1168.
21. Crawford ED. Epidemiology of prostate cancer. *Urology.* 2003;62 (suppl 6A):3–12.
22. Epstein JI, Partin AW, Sauvageot J, et al. Prediction of progression following radical prostatectomy: a multivariate analysis of 721 men with long-term follow-up. *Am J Surg Pathol.* 1996;20:286–292.
23. Ward JF, Zincke H, Bergstralh EJ, et al. The impact of surgical approach (nerve bundle preservation versus wide local excision) on surgical margins and biochemical recurrence following radical prostatectomy. *J Urol.* 2004;172:1328–1332.

24. Sokoloff MH, Brendler CB. Indications and contraindications for nerve-sparing radical prostatectomy. *Urol Clin N Am.* 2001;28:535–543.

25. Donohue JF, Bianoc FJ Jr, Kuroiwa K, et al. Poorly differentiated prostate cancer treated with radical prostatectomy: long-term outcome and incidence of pathological downgrading. *J Urol.* 2006;176:991–995.

26. Goharderakhshan RZ, Sudilovsky D, Carroll LA, et al. Utility of intraoperative frozen section analysis of surgical margins in region of neurovascular bundles at radical prostatectomy. *Urology.* 2002;59:709–714.

27. Beissner RS, Stricker JB, Speights VO, et al. Frozen section diagnosis of metastatic prostate adenocarcinoma in pelvic lymphadenectomy compared with nomogram prediction of metastasis. *Urology.* 2002;59:721–725.

28. Fromont G, Baumert H, Cathelineau X, et al. Intraoperative frozen section analysis during nerve sparing laparoscopic radical prostatectomy: feasibility study. *J Urol.* 2003;170:1843–1846.

29. Eichelberg C, Erbersdobler A, Haese A, et al. Frozen section for the management of intraoperatively detected palpable tumor lesions during nerve-sparing scheduled radical prostatectomy. *Eur Urol.* 2006;49:1011–1018.

30. Solway MS. Frozen sections for positive margins? *Eur Urol.* 2006;49:950–951.

31. Link RE, Morton RA. Indications for pelvic lymphadenectomy in prostate cancer. *Urol Clin N Am.* 2001;28:491–498.

32. Kakehi Y, Kamoto T, Okuno H, et al. Per-operative frozen section examination of pelvic nodes is unnecessary for the majority of clinically localized prostate cancers in the prostate-specific antigen era. *Int J Urol.* 2000;7:281–286.

33. Weckermann D, Goppelt M, Dorn R, et al. Incidence of positive lymph nodes in patients with prostate cancer, a prostate-specific antigen (PSA) level of <10 ng/ml and biopsy Gleason score of <6 and their influence on PSA progression-free survival after radical prostatectomy. *BJU Int.* 2006;97:1173–1178.

8

HEAD AND NECK

ADRIANA ACURIO AND JEROME B. TAXY

INTRODUCTION

Intraoperative consultation in head and neck cancer management concerns tumor diagnosis, margin evaluation, and nodal status, one or all of which help to determine the extent of surgery. These issues will be addressed here related to conventional mucosal squamous carcinoma and salivary gland tumors. Tissue artifacts commonly encountered on frozen sections and the effects of (neo)adjuvant therapy as possible pitfalls in interpretation will also be discussed. In addition, we will discuss the relatively recent application of frozen section to the management of acute invasive fungal rhinosinusitis as a guide for surgical debridement, which is an essential part of the therapy for this disease. Studies on the accuracy of frozen section in head and neck cancers suggest it is reliable, with an accuracy rate of 98% and a sensitivity and specificity of 89% and 99%, respectively (1).

Mucosal Lesions of the Head and Neck: Indications and Intraoperative Questions

AN IMMEDIATE DIAGNOSIS ON A PRIMARY LESION. While most primary diagnoses of squamous cell carcinoma rely on routinely processed endoscopic biopsies, a request for an immediate specimen evaluation reflects a set of clinical circumstances specific to each patient. An intraoperative diagnosis of squamous cell carcinoma on an untreated primary mucosal lesion, or a posttreatment persistent/recurrent lesion, may be requested to ensure adequacy or to justify proceeding with an immediate wide resection (Fig. 8.1). A frozen section may be helpful not only to establish a diagnosis but, if in situ carcinoma is identified, to confirm that the lesion is primary (Fig. 8.2). The presence of carcinoma may also initiate an immediate neck dissection.

Most difficulties in frozen section analysis of mucosal biopsies center on differentiating neoplastic from reactive lesions, such as pseudoepitheliomatous hyperplasia or flat lesions simulating dysplasia but associated with infections, prior treatment, chronic ulcers, or even some benign neoplastic lesions. Crush artifact, especially in intensely inflamed areas or involving minor tonsillar tissue, is a potential source of confusion, and

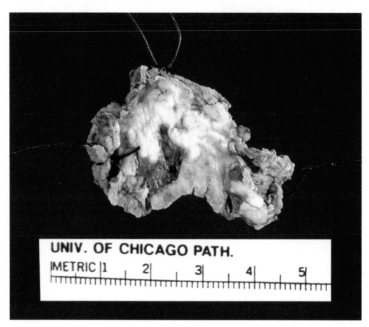

FIGURE 8.1 Gross photograph of a poorly circumscribed ulcerated white lesion of the retromolar trigone, excised and appropriately marked with sutures.

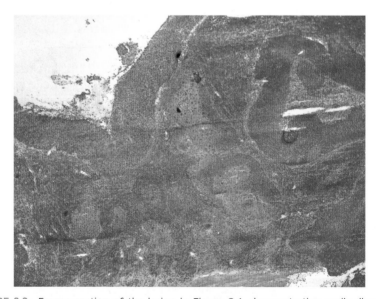

FIGURE 8.2 Frozen section of the lesion in Figure 8.1, demonstrating easily discernible surface in situ squamous carcinoma and an infiltrating, keratinizing component. In situ disease helps to verify the lesion as a primary tumor.

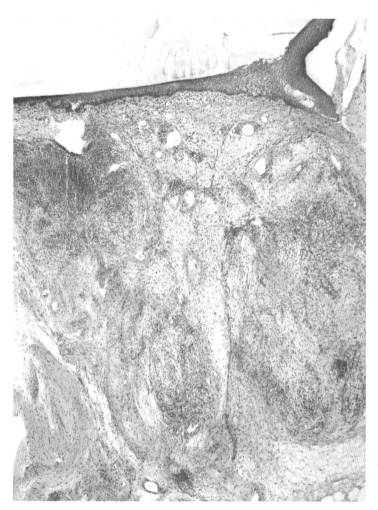

FIGURE 8.3 Frozen section of palatal mucosa after treatment. The surface epithelium is attenuated, the cells are somewhat crowded but not pleomorphic nor mitotically active. The submucosal tissue is edematous and inflamed. There is no tumor identified.

interpretation of such areas should be avoided (e-Fig. 8.1). Potentially confusing surface mucosal changes include edema and chronic inflammation (Fig. 8.3) or ulceration with the association of prominent atypical (probably inflammatory) stromal cells and granulation tissue (Fig. 8.4), reflective of prior treatment. In conjunction with these features, there may be isolated nests of squamous epithelium highly suggestive of infiltrating cancer (e-Fig. 8.2). It may be diagnostically uncertain at the time of the frozen section that such areas are reactive related to prior treatment or a solitary focus of residual/persistent cancer. The pathologist may be reluctant to establish a malignant diagnosis based on such an isolated observation, especially if a radical procedure will be the result. These

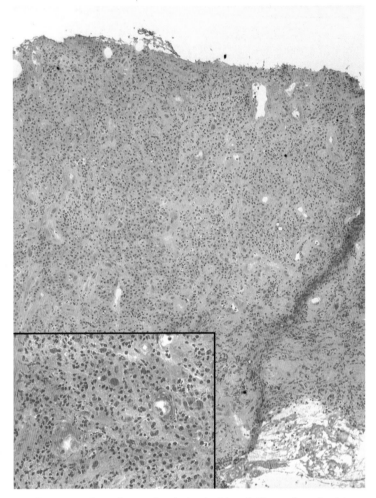

FIGURE 8.4 Frozen section of a previously treated tonsil. The surface (top) is completely ulcerated. The tissue is replaced by abundant chronic inflammatory cells and active granulation tissue with the small vessels lined by fibrinous debris. This is early treatment effect. Inset: Treatment effect. Higher-power view of the granulation tissue seen in Figure 8.4, vessels lined by fibrinous material, and intervening inflammatory infiltrate. Note the scattered large cells.

circumstances are common enough such that the frozen section might best be reported descriptively as "atypical," serving to alert the surgeon to obtain additional samples not to be frozen. The pathologist will also then have time to study the permanent material and arrive at a secure diagnosis.

Additionally related to the assessment of surface changes and the appreciation of changes in the underlying stroma is the presence of infiltrating scar tissue and prominent blood vessels suggesting desmoplasia (e-Fig. 8.3). Especially difficult in this regard are the changes in minor salivary gland tissue reflective of previous treatment. These changes histologically

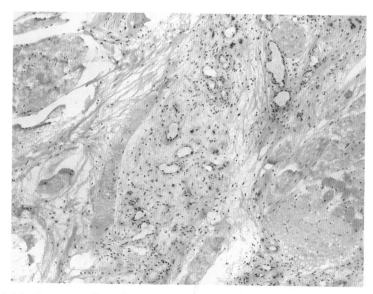

FIGURE 8.5 Frozen section of submucosal palatal tissue demonstrating minor salivary gland tissue with partial lobular atrophy. There is stromal edema and early fibrosis. The epithelial structures show occasional nuclear enlargement. This is early treatment-related sialometaplasia.

simulate the changes of necrotizing sialometaplasia (Fig. 8.5, 8.6, e-Figs. 8.4, 8.5) and are principally characterized by the preservation of the lobular growth pattern, despite the nuclear atypia and squamoid features. Given the potential consequences, a frozen section diagnosis of infiltrating cancer should be unequivocal, demonstrating irregular growth patterns and a desmoplastic reaction (Fig. 8.7, e-Fig. 8.6).

THE STATUS OF A MUCOSAL RESECTION MARGIN. While the histologic changes in the margins are similar to what has been described earlier for primary mucosal lesions, at stake is whether additional tissue needs to be excised if the margin is involved. The more basic questions should be the following: what constitutes involvement, and what quantitatively is an adequate margin? That the answers to these questions are not readily apparent nor are they likely to be adequately resolved by frozen section study does not prevent them from being frequently asked with a plethora of specimens (2).

The known multifocality ("field effect") of squamous carcinoma and its dysplastic precursors in the upper aerodigestive tract, the uncertain predictive value of dysplasia related to the subsequent development of invasive cancer, and the lack of agreement as to what constitutes an adequate or involved ("positive") margin makes it arguable whether preinvasive dysplasia should be reported in an intraoperative setting. Being aware of the treatment algorithm is critical in this regard. It is easy to understand that surgeons have an aversion to cutting across invasive tumor and to

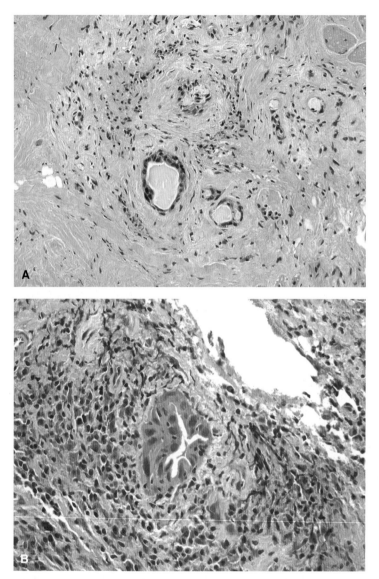

FIGURE 8.6 **A.** Frozen section after treatment. The lobular atrophy remains, the stroma is more fibrotic and the epithelial atypia in the remaining ducts/acini is more pronounced with some squamous metaplasia. This should not be interpreted as pseudoglandular squamous carcinoma. **B.** Frozen section. A remaining salivary gland duct with marked surrounding inflammation and marked nuclear atypia with the suggestion of squamous differentiation.

agreeing that this observation should be reported. Indeed, in an extensive review of the literature, Batsakis (3) suggests that only involvement by invasive carcinoma should be reported as positive. The clinical significance of preinvasive dysplasia related to local recurrence and survival is debatable (2–5) even as it has been suggested that approximately 75% of

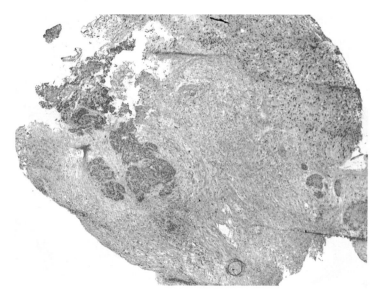

FIGURE 8.7 Frozen section of a margin from a tongue resection, demonstrating an infiltrating, desmoplastic focus of squamous carcinoma (left). These characteristic morphologic features should be the reference points for the frozen section diagnosis. To the right and top is treatment change manifested in the skeletal muscle of the tongue showing atrophy and nuclear crowding.

patients with positive surgical margins will either develop local recurrence or demonstrate residual disease upon reoperation (6). The most widely accepted, albeit arbitrary, designation of a close margin is tumor within 5 mm of the inked surgical margin (7), risking more local recurrences and poorer overall prognosis. The 5-mm designation is modified for extralaryngeal sites, such as the oral cavity and oropharynx where a 10-mm margin of normal tissue is considered more appropriate (5). It is possible that the increased numbers of lymphovascular spaces in these sites predispose for local spread and recurrence and therefore determine the need for wider margins.

Although there are suggestions that frozen sections for margins in head and neck cancers be abandoned (8), presently this might be a tough case to make to the surgeons given the many samples frequently submitted from patients undergoing a definitive resection. The morphologic challenge is that even with properly fixed and embedded samples, there is difficulty in differentiating ordinary squamous or pseudoepitheliomatous hyperplasias from intramucosal squamous dysplasia, not to mention grading it. Tangential sections and treatment effect can easily complicate the recognition of invasive tumor as discussed earlier. Frozen section, especially in the context of prior treatment, adds to the potential for interpretative uncertainty but its execution cannot be allowed to compromise the eventual complete permanent evaluation.

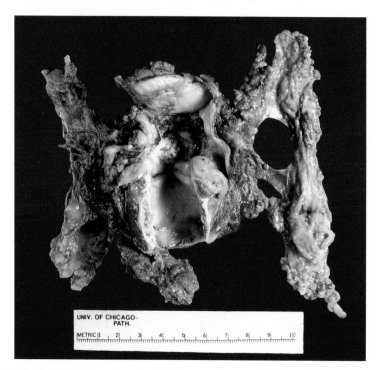

FIGURE 8.8 Gross photograph of a total laryngectomy with bilateral neck dissections. A complicated specimen such as this needs to be oriented with the surgeon prior to any frozen section sampling. This specimen has been opened posteriorly, clearly demonstrating a supraglottic, ulcerated tumor extending on to the lower aspect of the epiglottis. The inferior tracheal margin is grossly free of tumor. Both contiguous neck dissections are spread out for easy recognition. This patient had been previously radiated, so the soft tissues of the neck are scant and lymph node recovery would be expected to be diminished.

In addition to awareness of the treatment algorithm, margin assessment should ensure that the pathologist has some knowledge of or actually is able to examine the gross specimen. Given the inherent complexity of head and neck anatomy, orientation of the resection specimen by the surgeon in person, by diagram, or in the form of suture designations is essential. In addition, measurements, photographs, and/or specimen diagrams should be prepared before samples are taken for frozen section (Fig. 8.1, 8.8, 8.9, e-Figs. 8.7, 8.8). From large specimens, the manner in which the tissue is mounted and sectioned may vary. Right angle or perpendicular gross sectioning best allows for thorough macroscopic analysis including measurement of the distance from the lesion to the nearest surgical margin (e-Fig. 8.8). The selected area for frozen section analysis should be visually closest to the margin. Parallel or en face sectioning does provide a larger area for microscopic examination, potentially the entire margin. However, this method does not allow for gross appreciation of the tumor or an accurate assessment of the distance between the lesion and the nearest margin.

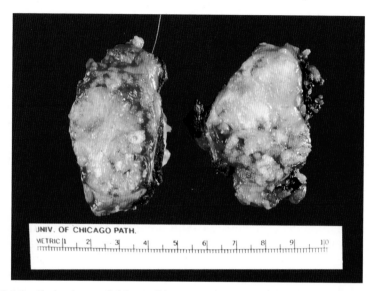

FIGURE 8.9 Bivalved superficial parotidectomy with a pleomorphic adenoma. Note the edges that have been inked prior to sectioning. Also, a single suture emanates from one end, designated by the surgeon as the superior and lateral edge. The tumor is generally well circumscribed except for the inferior aspect and does grossly extend to the edges of the sample. A gross examination in this case could justify taking additional inferior tissue.

Alternatively, the surgeon may submit samples from the resection bed resulting in the simultaneous arrival of large numbers of specimens to the surgical pathology laboratory for immediate examination. In this event, the mucosal surface needs to be identified and the specimen mounted so that the microtome knife will cut perpendicular to this plane. Spiro et al. (6) reported an 89% diagnostic accuracy rate for frozen section of oral cancer irrespective of, whether the margins were obtained from the patient or from the surgical specimen. A major limitation in margin analysis and correction is the ability to relocate the harvest site following frozen section diagnosis. A recent study assessing the adequacy of current techniques used for relocating frozen section specimens to the defect cavity showed a difference of more than 1 cm in 32% of cases (9). These findings highlight the need to accurately trace the position of frozen sections if samples that subsequently prove positive are to be used to greatest effect.

Assuming that the tissue sample has been properly embedded and the tissue block appropriately faced, there is no standard number of levels to examine. Our practice is to examine two frozen sections at two different but relatively close levels from each block. Additional deeper sections can be cut as necessary. Two levels decrease the sampling error and ensure against loss of time incurred by a section inadvertently falling off the slide or being wiped off if the cover slip is erroneously placed on the wrong side. Sectioning the frozen sample to the depletion of the tissue block is occasionally justified but is not standard practice, as advocated by some

(10). Depletion of the sample could create a reconciliation problem with the subsequent paraffin embedding ("frozen control"), even though the diagnostic area seen on the frozen does not have to be present on the permanently embedded "control" for the diagnosis to be maintained.

THE COMPLICATING EFFECTS OF PREVIOUS TREATMENT. The histologic changes induced by radiation and/or chemotherapy may be misinterpreted as squamous carcinoma and therefore are potential pitfalls. Surface ulceration and regeneration, sialometaplasia, and stromal cell atypia have been partially illustrated earlier (Figs. 8.3–8.6). The major morphologic manifestations of treatment often encountered at frozen section are as follows:

(a) *Ulceration and epithelial hyperplasia.* Although the ulcers are morphologically nonspecific, the adjacent epithelium may exhibit basal layer expansion with less definition of its palisading and some nuclear enlargement with nucleoli. Compensatory squamous hyperplasia, occasionally in the form of pseudoepitheliomatous hyperplasia, demonstrates expansion but maintenance of orderly maturation (Fig. 8.10). Mitoses restricted to the basal layer may signify regeneration. The major diagnostic dilemma, even when examining such specimens, which have not been frozen, is true dysplasia in which there is loss of maturation toward the surface and suprabasilar mitoses. Uncertainty in this assessment should generate a deferred diagnosis and/or a request for more tissue.

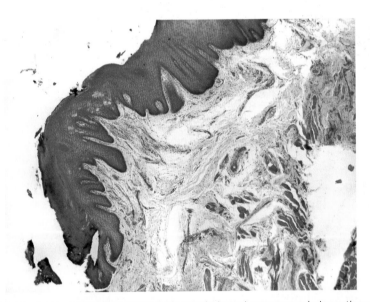

FIGURE 8.10 A margin showing epithelial hyperplasia and pronounced elongation of the rete ridges simulating pseudoepitheliomatous hyperplasia. Underlying stromal edema and accentuation of the separation of the skeletal muscle fibers. No tumor.

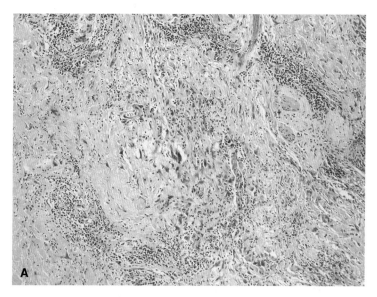

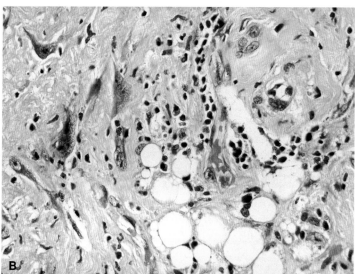

FIGURE 8.11 **A.** Frozen section of posttreatment stromal changes in soft tissue. In an in-flamed and fibrotic background, there is edema, granulation tissue and clusters of stellate-shaped markedly atypical cells with enlarged, hyperchromatic nuclei. The cells are nonco-hesive. **B.** A group of these atypical cells with stellate shape, hyperchromatic nuclei with internal vacuolization and the fibroinflammatory background. These cells could be misin-terpreted as malignant.

(b) *Stromal changes* manifested by varying degrees of cytologic atypia involving a single cell or groups of cells (Fig. 8.11). Chiefly, these cells are fibroblasts ("radiation" fibroblasts), characterized by their large size and abundant basophilic cytoplasm with irregular stellate

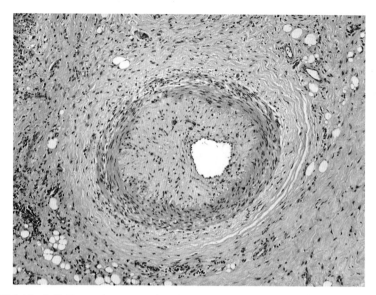

FIGURE 8.12   Soft tissue demonstrating later treatment changes affecting the vascular supply. Note the marked arterial thickening with subintimal fibrous proliferation and lumen compromise. These changes contribute to the ischemic tissue changes seen clinically (ulceration and edema) and possibly to the development of sialometaplasia encountered histologically.

ends. The nuclei are hyperchromatic and irregular but may also be vacuolated. These changes are accompanied by hyalinized fibrosis and fibrin deposits.

(c) *Vascular changes* seen earlier in radiation injury are characterized by proliferation of telangiectatic, asymmetric capillaries with intraluminal fibrin (Fig. 8.4). Intimal proliferation with luminal narrowing and the presence of foamy macrophages within the intimal layer are some of the most common delayed responses to radiation injury (Fig. 8.12). The latter changes are readily seen in frozen sections several weeks following treatment.

(d) *Treatment-related sialometaplasia* (Figs. 8.5, 8.6, e-Figs. 8.4, 8.5). The characteristic histologic features are atrophic acini, ductal dilatation, and squamous metaplasia of the residual acinar and ductal elements. The lobular architecture is maintained but partially distorted by therapy-related inflammation and fibrosis. The metaplastic lobules vary in size and are often surrounded by granulation tissue and focally intense acute and chronic inflammation. With regeneration, mitotic activity, individual cell necrosis, enlarged nuclei, and prominent nucleoli may be present. The morphology of this injury to minor salivary glands is not necessarily specific to radiation or a particular cytotoxic drug. The mechanism, however, may be influenced by ischemia related to the vascular changes described above as well as to direct cytotoxic effect.

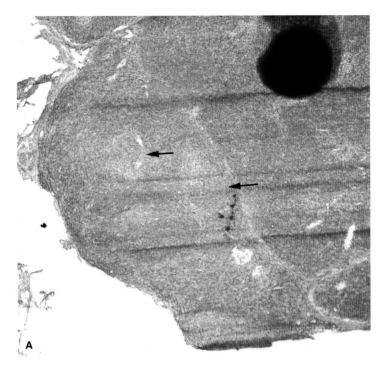

FIGURE 8.13   **A.** Lymph node with the abnormal area marked by a blue dot by the pathologist who did the frozen section. Microscopic deposits of tumor (arrows) are admixed with reactive germinal centers. **B.** The areas of tumor are highlighted in this view. Note the pigment artifact as a marker from **A.** The permanent preparation of this block was negative for tumor, a procedural hazard in doing any lymph node frozen section. **C.** To resolve this problem, one H&E frozen section was destained and restained by immunohistochemistry for cytokeratin, establishing without doubt the original diagnosis. The "disappearance" of a diagnostic focus on the permanent section does not invalidate the original observation. (*continued*)

IDENTIFICATION OF NODAL METASTASIS. The immediate identification of nodal metastases may initiate the performance or extent of a neck dissection. The intraoperative diagnosis of carcinoma in lymph nodes is for the most part nonproblematic (11,12). However, finding small metastases, false positives, and false negatives are as present here as in the evaluation of lymph nodes from other organ systems. If a small lesion is identified, calling attention to it by dotting the area is especially helpful to a subsequent examiner, especially in the event the focus disappears on the permanent sections (Fig. 8.13). To this must be added the possibility of treatment effects in the form of xanthogranulomatous and fibrotic reactions. In some studies, frozen section analysis of sentinel lymph nodes demonstrates a sensitivity of 93% and a negative predictive value of 94% (13). Frozen section of lymph nodes is contraindicated in cases where lymphoproliferative lesions are suspected, since no therapy is imminent and

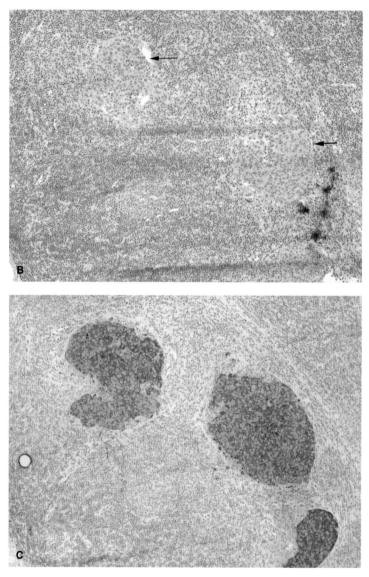

FIGURE 8.13 *(Continued)*

valuable tissue is wasted. However, the submission of fresh tissue is needed for triage purposes (flow cytometry, cytogenetics and imprints).

Salivary Gland Tumors: Indications and Intraoperative Questions

The major indications are similar to those involving mucosal lesions: tumor identification and margin status. As in other settings, frozen section should not be initiated unless the reported diagnosis will directly influence surgical action. The detailed histopathologic features of the many benign and malignant salivary gland tumors are beyond the scope of this discussion and are best covered in standard texts of surgical pathology or in specialty texts on head and neck pathology. While the argument can be made that detailed knowledge of the histopathologic features of the major tumor types (both benign and malignant) is essential in intraoperative evaluation, it may be more productive to pay attention to patterns of growth and infiltration as well as cytologic features, which are generically indicative of benign or malignant tumors. Therefore, the intraoperative setting allows a certain relaxation in the exactness of classification of individual salivary gland tumors and relies foremost on the recognition of a benign or malignant lesion. Imprints in this setting are very helpful.

Primary tumors of the parotid gland comprise the largest number of salivary gland tumors and most of these are benign. Eighty percent of parotid tumors, fifty percent of submandibular and sublingual tumors, and twenty percent of minor salivary gland tumors are benign. The most common tumor is pleomorphic adenoma followed by Warthin tumor. In the United States, salivary gland malignancies are uncommon, accounting for 6.0% of all head and neck cancers and 0.3% of all malignancies. Common malignant tumors include mucoepidermoid carcinoma, adenoid cystic carcinoma, carcinoma expleomorphic adenoma, and polymorphous low-grade adenocarcinoma. The frozen section recognition of salivary gland tumors varies and may be related to the relative infrequency of these entities overall and their acknowledged innate histological heterogeneity.

SPECIMEN HANDLING. The gross examination of salivary gland tumors is critical, even if determinations of benign or malignant cannot be made. To this end, orientation of the specimen by the surgeon is an advantage, and if this is provided, the specimen should be inked appropriately. This examination not only directs the sites of possible frozen section samplings, but also directs attention to those areas that must be studied on the routine permanent sections. Anatomically, the parotid gland lobes are delineated by being lateral (superficial) or medial (deep) to the facial nerve. Since most parotid gland tumors are located laterally, superficial lobectomies are the most common specimens. Tumors involving the sublingual or submandibular glands are usually treated by complete excision; intraoral minor salivary gland lesions are resected similarly to defined mucosal lesions.

Benign and malignant tumors of the major salivary glands do not consistently follow rules of gross representation that indicate their biologic behavior especially regarding circumscription and local invasion. Figure 8.9 shows an oriented superficial lobectomy of a pleomorphic adenoma (mixed tumor) with multilobulation but without uniform circumscription, a somewhat worrisome feature for a benign tumor. Gross features such as this could be related to a recurrence of an incompletely or improperly resected tumor in the past. In e-Figure 8.9, the circumscribed lesion is an acinic cell carcinoma (a diagnosis not established at frozen section), which extends to the inked edge of the specimen. Although this is a superficial lobectomy, there is gross involvement of the margin, easily communicated in an intraoperative setting. A frozen section is not required to advise the removal of additional subcutaneous tissue. The high-grade mucoepidermoid carcinoma grossly depicted in e-Figure 8.10 not only extends to the inked edge but is not well circumscribed, extending into the adjacent salivary gland and soft tissue. Since the diagnosis of malignancy had been established previously by fine needle aspiration (FNA), the surgeon was satisfied by a gross examination of the margins.

FROZEN SECTION EXAMINATION. Masses in the head and neck, including salivary gland lesions, are easily accessible to FNA, which is widely accepted as a first-line diagnostic procedure because it is minimally invasive, virtually lacks complications, and is done in an outpatient setting. So even prior to the receipt of the specimen in surgical pathology, the surgeon may have a specific diagnosis or at least a general idea of the diagnosis. The accuracy of FNA may be quite comparable to that of intraoperative frozen section (14); the use of both techniques may provide a useful redundancy in successful surgical management. It is, therefore, advantageous for the pathologist to at least know the FNA results, better to have the slides available for review concurrent with the frozen section.

Benign tumors The most common major or minor salivary gland neoplasm is pleomorphic adenoma comprising 60% of all benign salivary gland tumors. A slowly growing, firm painless mass, it most frequently occurs in the superficial lobe where a major hazard is compromise of the facial nerve by extrinsic compression. Grossly, tumors in the parotid often have a capsule while those originating in the minor salivary glands do not. The cut surface is tan white and uniform. Local recurrences are typically associated with previous attempts at enucleation. The recurrences, although histologically benign, are often multifocal, randomly scattered through remaining salivary gland and adjacent soft tissue (Fig. 8.9).

The cytomorphologic diversity of pleomorphic adenoma is well known and is related to the dual cellular components of epithelial and myoepithelial cells. The latter contributes to a fibrocollagenous, myxoid, and chondroid matrix. In the frozen section setting, the amount of each component is highly variable, not predictable, and the source of potential diagnostic problems. Sampling to demonstrate both cell components is not consistently successful.

The major reason to establish the diagnosis of pleomorphic adenoma is to limit the operation to a superficial lobectomy in the case of a parotid location or a simple excision in the case of a minor salivary gland location. This is especially true in the absence of a preoperative FNA. A malignant diagnosis could result in a wider excision and sacrifice of the facial nerve. The diagnostic challenges are confronted in tumors more cellular than usual, raising the differential diagnosis of mucoepidermoid carcinoma or

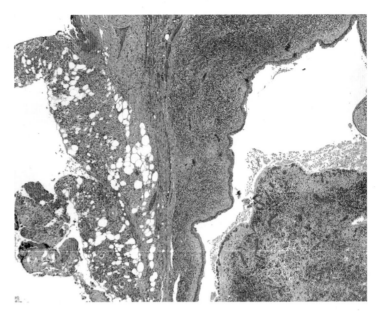

FIGURE 8.14 Frozen section of a typical Warthin tumor. Uninvolved salivary gland tissue (left) is adjacent to a partially cystic tumor, the spaces of which are lined by oncocytes and abutted by dense lymphoid tissue. Blue ink denotes the specimen margin.

carcinoma ex-pleomorphic adenoma. Occasional cribriform architecture raises the possibility of adenoid cystic carcinoma.

The second most common tumor in the major salivary glands, primarily in the parotid, is the Warthin tumor. The gross appearance consists of a poorly circumscribed, soft, and fluid-filled brown to tan tumor. Histologically, the typical features are oncocytes directly apposed to dense collections of lymphocytes with germinal center formation. The histologic diagnosis by frozen section is generally not difficult (Fig. 8.14). Difficulty may arise if the frozen section demonstrates the squamous metaplasia occasionally seen in these tumors (15). The metaplasia may be spontaneous, secondary to in vivo fluid extravasation or possibly to previous FNA attempts, but should not be misinterpreted as squamous carcinoma (Fig. 8.15).

Malignant tumors The critical role of frozen section in salivary gland tumor management may be in the assessment of both margin status and the distinction of a benign from a malignant tumor. Frozen sections for margin assessment should be taken from the closest margin as determined by gross examination through serial cuts. There is no magic quantitative distance agreed upon to constitute an adequate or close margin, so an actual measurement may be optimal. A positive margin should consist of tumor actually abutting the inked edge. Figure 8.16 illustrates an adenoid cystic carcinoma histologically extending to the inked margin. In this case,

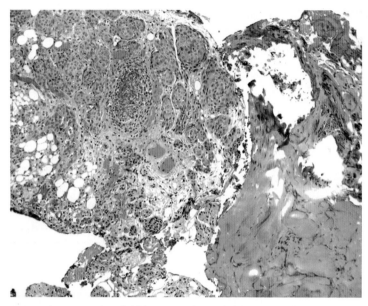

FIGURE 8.15   A frozen section field from another Warthin tumor. The inked edge is mixed with cautery artifact denoting the edge of the specimen. The central portion is marked by nests of metaplastic squamous epithelium adjacent to small salivary gland acini. Squamous metaplasia is common in Warthin tumors and oncocytomas. This should not be misinterpreted as squamous carcinoma.

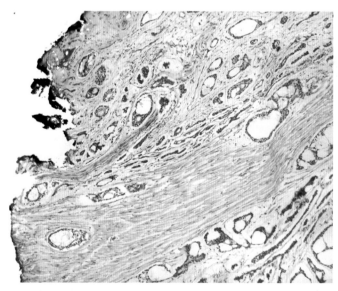

FIGURE 8.16   A frozen section of an inked margin. Tumor typing can be accomplished since the architectural features and perineural invasion are typical of adenoid cystic carcinoma. Tumor clearly extends to the inked margin.

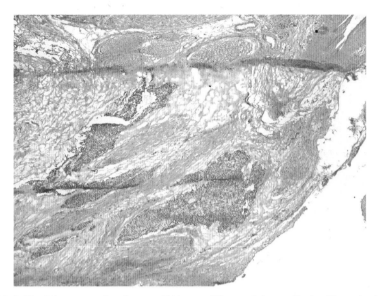

FIGURE 8.17 A frozen section from soft tissue of the neck in a patient with a prior history of high-grade mucoepidermoid carcinoma. The tumor was not available for review at the time of the frozen. Obvious irregular nests of malignant tumor invading soft tissue and nerve. A specific tumor type could not be established at the frozen but is not required under these circumstances.

a good gross examination led to proper tissue selection. The tumor type was also easily recognized morphologically.

Successfully subclassifying the tumor is a bonus. Recognizing the process as malignant may be a more important pathologic assessment. In a patient whose mucoepidermoid carcinoma had been excised 13 years previously, a maxillary recurrence was being "mapped" by frozen section. A soft-tissue biopsy from the neck was submitted. There was no opportunity to review the previous material but, in this instance, simple identification of a high-grade malignant process was indicated (Fig. 8.17). Patients with high-grade salivary gland lesions commonly demonstrate locally invasive growth, vascular or neural invasion. Simply being alert to these aspects of tumor growth as well as cytologic features of malignancy may be the key to intraoperative management (e-Fig. 8.11). Final tumor classification and margin assessment can await permanent preparations.

Invasive Fungal Sinusitis

Acute invasive fungal sinusitis is a life-threatening disease. The surgical treatment for these patients is emergent operative debridement with the goal being marginal tissue free of organisms. The literature related to the use of frozen section is scant (16,17). The patients are uniformly immunologically compromised secondary to diabetes or undergoing treatment for an underlying malignancy. The organisms that are typically

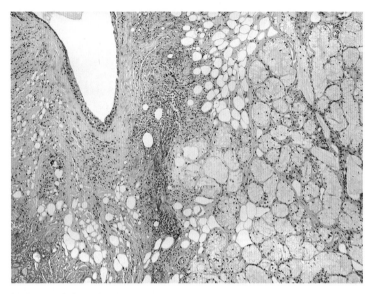

FIGURE 8.18 Nasal sinus tissue from a patient with acute invasive fungal sinusitis. A portion of metaplastic squamous mucosa and underlying minor salivary gland tissue are separated by a focus of inflammation and a small colony of broad-based nonseptate hyphae, proven *Mucor* by culture.

associated with these infections, for example, *Aspergillus* and *Mucor* species, exhibit soft tissue, vascular and neural invasion–producing extensive necrosis, and purulence in the paranasal sinuses (Figs. 8.18, 8.19). However, the organisms are easily recognized by standard hematoxylin and eosin stains on both frozen and permanent sections. Tissue sections demonstrate organisms invading paranasal sinus soft tissue, blood vessels, and nerves (e-Fig. 8.12). Occasionally, tissue smears or sections stained by Diff-Quik will be effective in demonstrating organisms (e-Fig. 8.13). The mortality rate in the short term from acute fungal sinusitis is approximately 80%.

Contraindications for Head and Neck Frozen Section

1. Evaluation of small tissue samples when additional sampling for routine processing is not planned.
2. Evaluation of samples that do not directly impact the immediate surgical management of the patient.
3. Evaluation of cutaneous lesions clinically suspicious for primary melanoma.
4. Diagnostic lymph node biopsies, especially for hematopoietic disease. Lymph nodes should, however, be submitted in the fresh state for appropriate triage for necessary special studies, that is, flow cytometry, imprints, microbiology.
5. Evaluation of fat or heavily calcified or ossified tissue.

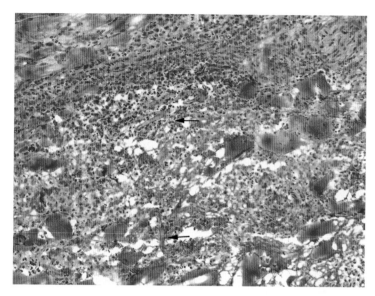

FIGURE 8.19   An abscess in the paranasal sinus soft tissue, exhibiting necrotic skeletal muscle and broad-based predominantly nonseptate fungi (arrows), proven *Mucor* by culture.

In the head and neck, as elsewhere, the potential for misuse of limited material, the misconstruing of the frozen section as a shortcut to well-fixed and processed tissue, or the improper triage of diagnostic samples are the contraindications for frozen section. It is axiomatic that what we do as pathologists must have clinical relevance and the information we deliver must serve the patients' best interests. Head and neck cancers are a challenge in this regard and require collaboration but not contention with our surgical colleagues.

REFERENCES

1. Jones AS, Hanafi ZB. Do positive resection margins after ablative surgery for head and neck cancer adversely affect prognosis? A study of 352 patients with recurrent carcinoma following radiotherapy treated by salvage surgery. *Br J Cancer.* 1996;74:128–132.
2. Brandwein-Gensler M, Teixeira M. Oral squamous cell carcinoma: histologic risk assessment, but not margin status, is strongly predictive of local disease-free and overall survival. *Am J Surg Pathol.* 2005;29:167–178.
3. Batsakis J. Surgical excision margins: a pathologist's perspective. *Adv Anat Pathol.* 1999;6:140–148.
4. Ribeiro NFF, Godden DRP, Wilson GE, et al. Do frozen sections help achieve adequate surgical margins in the resection of oral carcinoma. *Int J Oral Maxillofacial Surg.* 2003;32:152–158.
5. Sutton DN, Brown JS, Rogers SN. The prognostic implications of the surgical margin. *Int J Oral Maxillofacial Surg.* 2003;32:30–34.
6. Spiro RH, Buillamondegui O, Pulino AF, et al. Pattern of invasion and margin assessment in patients with oral tongue cancer. *Head Neck.* 1999;5:103.
7. Vilram B, Strong EW, Shah JP. Failure at primary site following multimodality treatment in advanced head and neck cancer. *Head Neck.* 1999;21:408–413.

8. Frable WJ. Accuracy of frozen sections in assessing margins in oral cancer resection. *J Oral Maxillofacial Surg.* 1997;55:669–671.

9. Kerawala CJ, Ong TK. Relocating the site of frozen sections—is there room for improvement? *Head Neck.* 2001;23:230–232.

10. Cooley ML, Hoffman HT, Robinson RA. Discrepancies in frozen section mucosal margin tissue in laryngeal squamous cell carcinoma. *Head Neck.* 2002;24:262–267.

11. Luna MA. Uses, abuse and pitfalls of frozen section diagnoses of diseases of the head and neck. In: Barnes L, ed. *Surgical Pathology of the Head and Neck.* New York: Macel Dekker; 2000, pp. 2–12.

12. Asthana S, Deo SV, Shukla NK, et al. Intraoperative neck staging using sentinel node biopsy and imprint cytology in oral cancer. *Head Neck.* 2003;25:368–372.

13. Tschopp L, Nuyens M, Stowffer E, et al. The value of frozen section analysis of the sentinel lymph node in clinically. No squamous cell carcinoma of the oral cavity and oropharynx. *Otolaryngol Head Neck Surg.* 2005;132(1):99--102.

14. Wong, DSY. Frozen section during parotid surgery revisited: efficacy of its applications and changing trend of indications. *Head and Neck.* 2002;24:191--197.

15. Taxy JB. Necrotizing squamous/mucinous metaplasia in oncocytic salivary gland tumors: a potential diagnostic problem. *Am J Clin Pathol.* 1992;97:40–45.

16. Hofman B, Castillo L, Betis F, et al. Usefulness of frozen section in rhinocerebral mucormycosis: diagnosis and management. *Pathology.* 2003;35:212–216.

17. El-Zayaty S, Langerman A, Taxy JB. Utility of frozen section diagnosis in the management of invasive fungal sinusitis. *Mod Pathol.* 2008;21(suppl 1):234A, USCAP Abstract #1073, Denver.

9

THYROID AND PARATHYROID

ADRIANA ACURIO AND JEROME B. TAXY

INTRODUCTION: THYROID FROZEN SECTION

Historically, intraoperative consultation by frozen section has been used to establish a definitive diagnosis in the surgical treatment of thyroid nodules. The justification of this practice has been that a frozen section diagnosis of malignancy allows for an immediate completion thyroidectomy, thus avoiding an additional procedure. The advent of fine needle aspiration (FNA) has changed the management of thyroid nodules by providing a preoperative method for identifying some malignancies, for example, papillary and medullary carcinomas, and for recognizing most benign follicular processes, for example, colloid nodules and thyroiditis, therefore possibly avoiding surgery altogether (1). Since a diagnosis of follicular carcinoma is not possible by FNA, cellular follicular lesions unaccompanied by concomitant quantities of colloid, that is, "follicular neoplasm," are surgically approached. The questions, however, remain: (i) How necessary is an immediate diagnosis? (ii) What constitutes the thoroughness of sampling for that tissue diagnosis to represent good patient care?

Experience has shown that there are diagnostic challenges in thyroid histopathology even when paraffin-embedded sections of an entire lesion are available. For pathologists, a frozen section of a mass lesion in the thyroid represents a technically less than ideal histologic preparation of inherent limited sampling but with potentially major clinical consequences. Attempting a diagnosis under these circumstances may appear ill advised, and it may occasionally seem to the pathologist that the clinical physicians caring for patients with thyroid disease do not adequately grasp this. It is not surprising, therefore, that there is occasional contention between surgeons and pathologists and even among pathologists about the appropriate use of intraoperative diagnosis in thyroid surgery.

It is acknowledged that the diagnostic utility of frozen section is limited for cellular follicular lesions (1,2), an aspect frequently cited as an example of inaccuracy and a reason to avoid frozen section in this context (3). However, it could also be argued that the combination of FNA and frozen section generally provides the greatest level of intraoperative diagnostic accuracy. The preoperative FNA diagnosis and the limitations of frozen section notwithstanding, definitive surgical treatment is still based on a tissue examination. And, irrespective of one's opinion on this issue, frozen section requests are a reality of daily practice. This chapter will not resolve this controversy but will discuss the indications, limitations, and diagnostic challenges encountered in the intraoperative examination of thyroid and parathyroid lesions.

Thyroid Frozen Section: Intraoperative Questions

The frozen section in thyroid disease concerns these major areas.

- Confirmation and tissue diagnosis of a clinical thyroid mass, possibly identified preoperatively by FNA
- Examination of a regional lymph node for the presence of metastatic disease
- Identification of unanticipated neck masses, for example, thymic remnants, aberrant parathyroids, or enlarged lymph nodes

Each point relates to the potential for altering the surgical procedure. Confirmation of a malignant thyroid tumor commits the patient to a total thyroidectomy, much easier to do in an unoperated neck than in a previously explored and possibly fibrotic neck. Regional node metastases are arguably less pressing since formal neck dissections are not indicated in thyroid cancer, but the presence or absence of a nodal metastasis may suggest stopping or expanding the procedure. The identification of unanticipated masses may further individualize the surgical treatment.

Thyroid Frozen Section: Gross Specimen Handling

The best initial examination is that of the gross specimen. A lobectomy is the most common surgical approach to a thyroid mass and regards the lesion as potentially malignant. Enucleations and needle core biopsies are of controversial appropriateness and are fortunately uncommon. The specimen is routinely inked, weighed, and serially sectioned perpendicular to the long axis of the lobe ("breadloaf" fashion), carefully maintaining the capsular integrity over the lesion and maximizing views of the capsular–parenchymal interface. Important gross features that guide the histologic sampling include the sizes and colors of the lesion(s); circumscription; the presence of cysts, hemorrhage, stellate shape, fibrous components, or necrosis. For example, a solitary circumscribed mass is consistent with a follicular adenoma; a solid brown lesion with a central scar is highly compatible with a Hurthle cell tumor (oncocytoma) (Fig. 9.1, e-Fig. 9.1). A stellate gritty gray mass, with or without encapsulation and occasionally quite small, is suggestive of papillary carcinoma (Fig. 9.2, e-Figs. 9.2, 9.3). The best sample to take for frozen section study is one that includes the tumor–parenchymal interface and the peripheral external surface.

The Thyroid: Frozen Section and Its Interpretation

Total or subtotal thyroidectomy specimens for cancer are generally accompanied by a preoperative diagnosis of carcinoma per FNA. In such

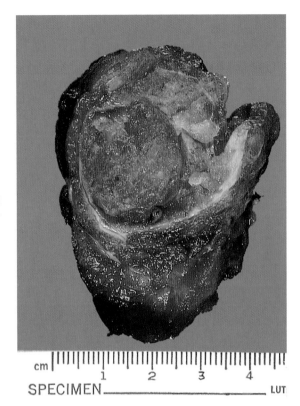

FIGURE 9.1 Hurthle cell tumor. Brown, well-circumscribed, and partially encapsulated lesion demonstrating a central scar.

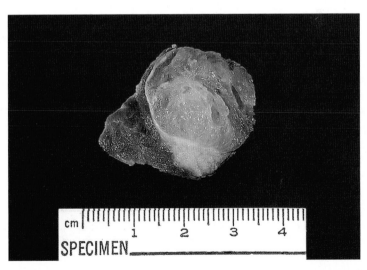

FIGURE 9.2 Papillary carcinoma. Partially encapsulated colloid nodule with a firm gray white, noncircumscribed mass extending away from the thin fibrous capsular band.

cases, the need for intraoperative consultation is less imperative and probably not indicated since the definitive surgical procedure has already been done. For lobectomy specimens that lack a definitive preoperative diagnosis, frozen section examination may be useful.

If a frozen section is to be done, a simultaneous cytologic imprint preparation is recommended (4,5). The imprint provides cytomorphologic features that are less well represented on the frozen preparation, such as the nuclear grooves and pseudoinclusions characterizing papillary carcinoma. To prepare an imprint slide, a fresh cut through the tissue is made. Excess blood or fluid is blotted off and the tissue is firmly touched against a glass slide. If the slide is to be stained by H&E, it must be fixed immediately in alcoholic formalin to avoid drying artifacts. This type of staining best maintains nuclear detail. When using Diff-Quick or Giemsa staining, the slide is air-dried first. This staining may not as effectively enhance the nuclear detail; however, it preserves acellular background material such as colloid and amyloid. Employing both stains does require some visual adjustments but is redundantly beneficial. Imprint preparations are reviewed concurrently with the frozen section and further increase the diagnostic accuracy, especially in cases of papillary carcinoma. In benign colloid nodules or thyroiditis, the imprint findings reflect similar features as seen in the FNA. In the case of follicular neoplasms, cytologic preparations will not distinguish between follicular adenoma and follicular carcinoma, since the diagnosis depends on the histologic recognition of vascular invasion. Small lesions (<5 mm) should have imprints made but should not be frozen.

Colloid Nodules and Follicular Neoplasms

Colloid nodules are grossly multiple and may result in an enlarged or goitrous gland. On cross section, there is often partial encapsulation of the nodules (Fig. 9.3). Degenerative changes in the form of hemorrhage, calcification, cyst formation, and fibrosis are common (e-Fig. 9.4A–C). These areas should be avoided for frozen section sampling (6,7). Imprint preparations show relatively scant bland follicular cells and abundant background colloid (Fig. 9.4). Occasional admixtures of oncocytes (Hurthle cells) are also common (Fig. 9.5). The histologic picture is varied and technically complicated by tissue folds or the tendency of colloid to exhibit "chatter" artifact. Dilated follicles are lined by flat atrophic cells and alternate with smaller follicles lined by plumper cells (Fig. 9.6A–C). Occasionally, there are also benign papillary-like formations that protrude toward the center of a cystically dilated follicle. The foci of cellular stratification may lead to consideration of papillary carcinoma; however, the typical nuclear features required to make this diagnosis are not present. These morphologic features reflect the reaction of the thyroid gland to fluctuations of TSH, which is part of the genesis of colloid nodules.

While the histologic distinction between an individual colloid nodule and a true follicular neoplasm may be difficult, follicular neoplasms

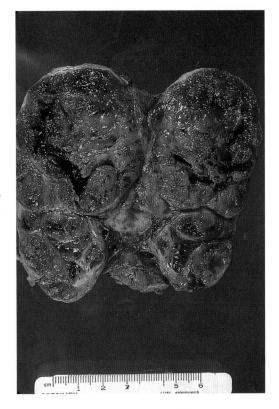

FIGURE 9.3 Colloid nodules. Bi-valved lobectomy with multiple nodules of varying sizes and circumscription in an enlarged gland.

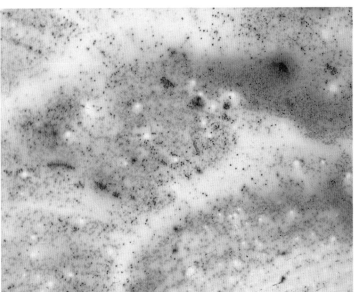

FIGURE 9.4 Colloid nodule (Diff-Quik imprint preparation). Abundant background colloid and limited cellular elements similar to FNA features.

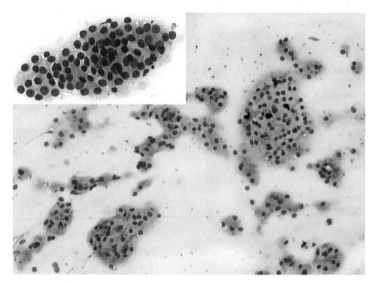

FIGURE 9.5   Colloid nodule (Diff-Quik imprint). Clusters of cells with oncocytic (Hurthle cell) features.

are grossly typically solitary (Fig. 9.1, 9.7, e-Fig. 9.1). Imprints show bland to cytologically atypical follicular cells, increased in number compared to colloid nodules, with a background of colloid, which is less abundant than in colloid nodules (e-Fig. 9.5A, B). Histologically, peripheral

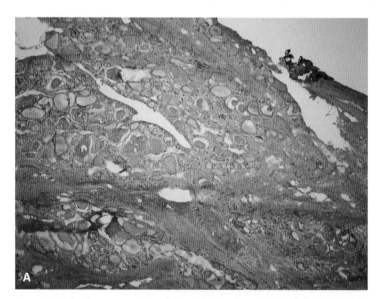

FIGURE 9.6   Colloid nodule. **A.** Frozen section with dilated follicles of varying sizes containing colloid, subdivided by bands of fibrous tissue. **B.** Frozen section showing colloid-containing follicles lined by flattened epithelium. **C.** Frozen section showing variably sized follicles, one dilated but with cellular stratification. (*continued*)

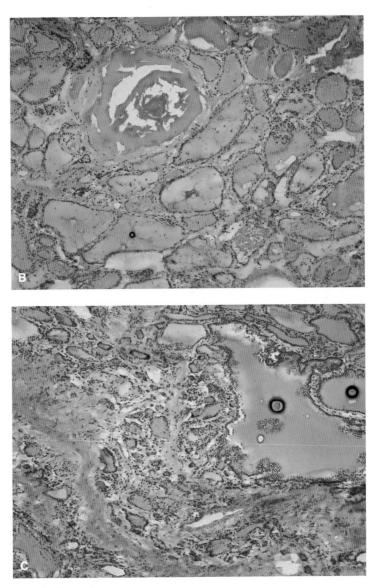

FIGURE 9.6 (*Continued*)

neoplastic follicles tend to be smaller, more densely packed with scant or absent intraluminal colloid. Since nuclear pleomorphism and atypia are not reliable features of malignancy in the thyroid, the demonstration of capsular and/or vascular invasion are required for a diagnosis of carcinoma (Fig. 9.8). Although this phenomenon is seldom encountered by frozen section, finding it requires a sample from the interface between the capsule and the uninvolved thyroid. In most instances, a frozen section diagnosis of a solitary follicular lesion will be either benign or deferred,

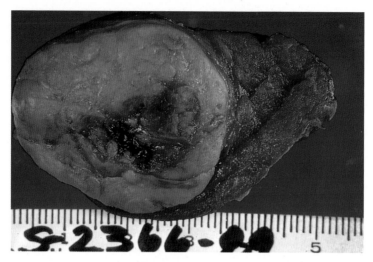

FIGURE 9.7   Follicular neoplasm (adenoma): Gross photo of a solitary, circumscribed, and encapsulated mass with central hemorrhage, possibly secondary to prior FNA.

with the final diagnosis dependent on a thorough examination of the lesion after appropriate fixation.

From the foregoing statement, it is apparent that follicular carcinoma is rarely established by frozen section (8), supporting those who argue against frozen sections in this regard. Surgeons who request frozen sections on follicular lesions should understand that follicular neoplasms appearing grossly encapsulated may show only a partially penetrated capsule microscopically and thereby constitute a diagnostic dilemma in the intraoperative setting (Fig. 9.8). Experience suggests that missing an area of vascular invasion is far more likely than recovering it. It is neither

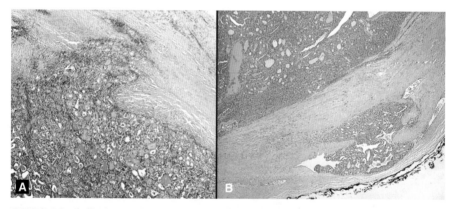

FIGURE 9.8   Follicular carcinoma frozen section. Partial capsular penetration (**A**) and vascular invasion (**B**) rarely encountered in the intraoperative setting.

practical nor cost effective to submit multiple tissue sections for frozen section study to determine the presence of such invasion. In addition, consideration must be given to the potentially complicating influence of the post-frozen artifacts in the permanent sections. Assuming that the gross differences between follicular adenoma and minimally invasive follicular carcinoma are subtle even under the best of circumstances, the frozen section evaluation of follicular thyroid lesions are likely to fall short of a definitive malignant diagnosis.

Additional confounding factors by frozen section include encapsulated thyroid tumors that exhibit involutional changes or exhibit vascular proliferative changes within the capsular and pericapsular vessels, mimicking vascular invasion. In particular, the various changes associated with FNA-induced or spontaneous bleeding common in colloid nodules can exhibit distention of the vessel lumina by a proliferative cellular infiltrate (6,7). Given the inherent processing difficulties, potential technical artifacts (tissue folds, knife marks, etc), as well as possible capsular disruption, a diagnosis even on the permanent sections could be significantly compromised.

In the case of widely invasive follicular carcinoma, intraoperative diagnosis is less problematic since it is also clinically quite apparent. Histologically, capsular invasion is extensive and vascular infiltration can be often seen in large caliber vessels. The intraoperative question in this circumstance is the documentation of diagnostic tissue prior to closing, as the patient may be unsuitable for a potential curative procedure.

Lymphocytic Thyroiditis

The formation of mass lesions in thyroiditis is common because of the ongoing inflammation and fibrosis. However, the diagnosis of thyroiditis may not be established until there has actually been tissue examination. Although a preoperative FNA is commonly done, given the scattered distribution of the lymphoid aggregates and follicles, the diagnostic spectrum of cytologic polymorphism may not be adequately represented. The aspirated nodule may be a mixture of follicular cells, Hurthle cells, and variable numbers of lymphocytes. Since true neoplasms do occur in the setting of thyroiditis, surgical exploration may be indicated to better characterize a mass lesion or to provide relief from the inflammatory sequelae of tracheal or esophageal compression. The workup for possible lymphoma can be initiated at this setting (e-fig. 9.6).

Grossly, there is diffuse possibly asymmetrical enlargement of the gland with multiple focally confluent nodules separated by fibrous bands (Fig. 9.9). On imprint preparations, in addition to a scattered background of mature and focally stimulated lymphocytes, the follicular epithelium may exhibit oxyphilic changes with nuclear enlargement and hyperchromasia. Histologically, the main components are follicular epithelium with varying degrees of nuclear atypia, oncocytes either singly distributed (Ashkenazy cells) or in clusters (Hurthle cells), and a mature lymphocytic

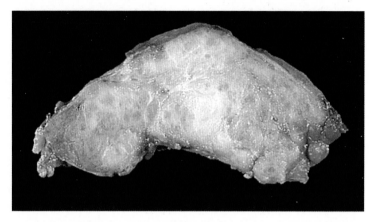

FIGURE 9.9 Lymphocytic thyroiditis. Gross photograph demonstrating multiple small nodules and broad areas of dense white fibrous tissue.

infiltrate with occasional germinal center formation (Figs. 9.10, 9.11, e-fig. 9.6). The disruption in architecture often complicates the assessment of the presence of tumor especially in distinguishing between hyperplastic nodules and oncocytic (Hurthle cell) tumors.

Papillary Thyroid Carcinoma

As the most common thyroid malignancy, the typical gross representation of papillary carcinoma ranges from stellate, unencapsulated, and small to

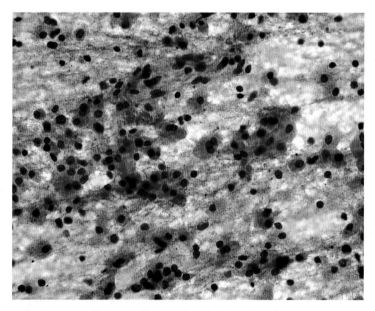

FIGURE 9.10 Lymphocytic thyroiditis: H&E imprint showing clusters of bland oncocytes (Hurthle cells) and a background of mature small lymphocytes.

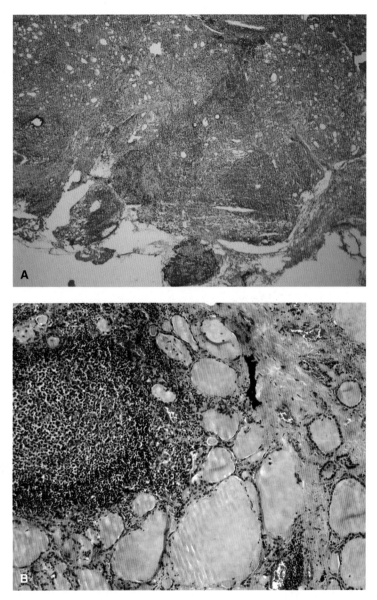

FIGURE 9.11 Lymphocytic thyroiditis. **A.** Frozen section showing thyroid parenchyma with a dense lymphocytic infiltrate. **B.** Frozen section with a prominent germinal center.

poorly demarcated, gray, and gritty mass (Fig. 9.2, e-Figs. 9.2, 9.3). Larger lesions are accompanied by fibrosis accounting for the palpable firmness and gritty sensation upon cutting. Larger papillary carcinomas may have incomplete circumscription, and because they have been clinically palpated have commonly been identified preoperatively by FNA. Incidentally

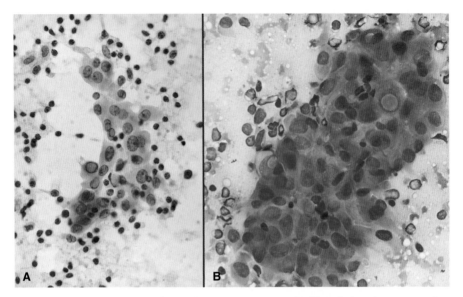

FIGURE 9.12 Papillary thyroid carcinoma. FNA (**A**) and Diff-Quik imprint preparation (**B**) demonstrate nuclear crowding, overlap, and numerous intranuclear cytoplasmic pseudoinclusions.

discovered lesions (found during surgery for a different clinically apparent mass) are relatively common, often small (<1 cm), and accompanied by dense fibrosis. Although an astute observer will grossly recognize small or occult papillary carcinomas, their biologic potential is unclear. Small lesions also raise the issue of multifocality, a well-recognized feature of the disease. The intraoperative setting cannot resolve either of these problems. Following a frozen section diagnosis of papillary carcinoma irrespective of tumor size, the surgeon must decide whether to complete the thyroidectomy.

The diagnosis of papillary carcinoma is based on a spectrum of features centering on the nuclear morphology of the thyroid follicular cell (9). Although no single feature is pathognomonic, the combined use of imprints (Fig. 9.12, e-Fig. 9.7) and frozen section (Fig. 9.13) facilitates the recognition of as many nuclear changes as possible (Table 9.1). Papillary growth and psammoma bodies are two parameters unfortunately not always present. The relationship of the fibrosis, either as a capsular structure or subdividing the tumor, is an important feature as well as a potential diagnostic hazard, since both fibrous patterns are present in colloid nodules. Also, the sclerosis is potentially problematic histologically, since it results in diminished numbers of and isolation of follicles or tumor groups. Although the enlargement of the nuclei is appreciated on tissue sections by the crowding and overlap within the papillae or follicles, the nuclear features of this tumor are best brought out by cytologic techniques, either

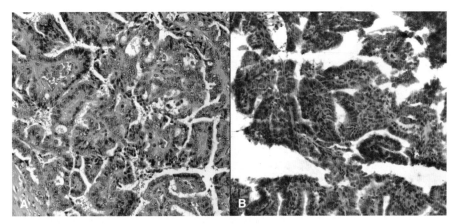

FIGURE 9.13 Papillary thyroid carcinoma. **A.** Characteristic architecture and nuclear features are readily observed on permanent H&E sections. **B.** Frozen section demonstrates papillary architecture and nuclear crowding, but often fails to demonstrate the characteristic nuclear membrane changes.

preoperative FNA or imprints prepared in concordance with the frozen section. Papillary clusters are tightly packed groups of cells with considerable nuclear overlap. The nuclear membrane irregularities are seen light microscopically as nuclear grooves and/or pseudoinclusions. These are poorly represented on actual frozen sections (Fig. 9.13). In either typical papillary or the follicular variant, architectural format, some nuclear features, such as chromatin clearing ("Orphan Annie eye" nuclei) are artifacts related to fixation and are best seen in permanent paraffin-embedded sections, not on frozen sections. In the follicular growth pattern ("follicular variant") of papillary carcinoma, the absence of the typical papillary growth pattern forces reliance on an appreciation of the nuclear features by a cytologic method. Mitotic activity is usually minimal and is generally diagnostically unimportant in the intraoperative or final diagnosis of this tumor.

TABLE 9.1 **Histologic and Cytologic (Nuclear) Features of Papillary Carcinoma As Seen by Frozen Section**

Architectural Features	Nuclear Features
Papillary architecture	Enlarged nuclei (usually larger than normal follicular nuclei)
Capsular invasion	Nuclear crowding/overlap
Dense fibrosis	Numerous nuclear grooves
Psammoma bodies	Intranuclear cytoplasmic pseudoinclusions

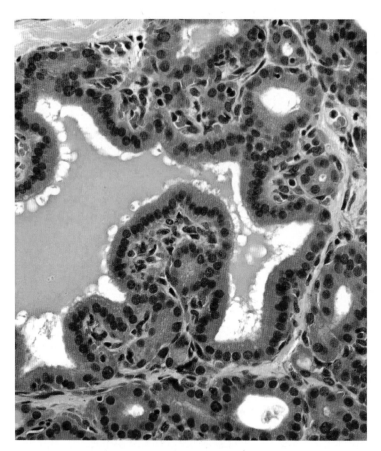

FIGURE 9.14 Graves disease (frozen section) with pseudopapillary infoldings and nuclear crowding, but not the typical nuclear features of papillary carcinoma.

Some of the architectural and cytomorphologic features of papillary thyroid carcinoma are simulated by artifacts of the frozen section, such as intranuclear bubbles as a fixation artifact, frozen crystallization artifact simulating pseudoinclusions, or presence of pseudopsammoma bodies in Hurthle cell tumors, among others. In addition, benign conditions such as nodular hyperplasia with papillary proliferations encountered either in colloid nodules or in patients previously treated for Graves disease or the nuclear enlargement in thyroiditis may cause confusion with papillary carcinoma (Fig. 9.14) (6). Attention to the typical nuclear changes will avoid erroneous interpretation, although in a patient with Graves disease, it is implied that medical therapy has failed and the patient is committed to total thyroidectomy, which is a cancer operation anyway.

Medullary Carcinoma

Medullary carcinoma is histologically diverse, potentially aggressive, and a diagnostic challenge. Grossly, the primary tumors range in size from

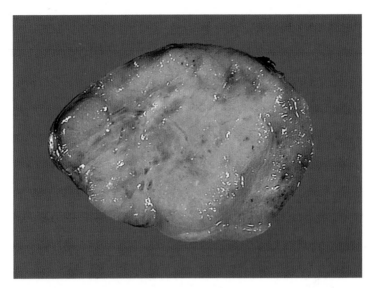

FIGURE 9.15   Medullary carcinoma. Firm unencapsulated lesion with tan-pink cut surface.

clinically occult to masses that occupy variable portions of the thyroid gland. They are firm and generally light tan or gray (Fig. 9.15, e-Fig. 9.8). Typically, encapsulation is not a prime feature. The first clinical manifestation of disease may be a neck metastasis, having been previously excised or recovered by FNA, originating in a small or occult primary tumor. The eosinophilic cytoplasm is granular and focally intense both on imprints and on frozen sections (Fig. 9.16). Histologically, medullary carcinoma

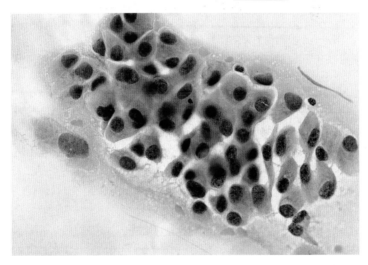

FIGURE 9.16   H&E imprint preparation of medullary carcinoma exhibiting finely granular cytoplasm and characteristic "salt-and-pepper" chromatin pattern with inconspicuous nucleoli.

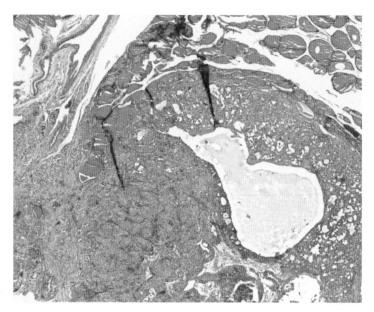

FIGURE 9.17 Medullary carcinoma (frozen section) demonstrating organoid (nested) growth and a focal desmoplastic reaction (left). Interface with thyroid is without a fibrous capsule.

typically demonstrates nested or trabecular architecture with at least a focally desmoplastic background. The tumor cells are polygonal, spindle shaped, or both, with a "salt-and-pepper" evenly distributed chromatin pattern and inconspicuous nucleoli (Fig. 9.17). There are, however, follicular, anaplastic, pigmented, and even mucin-containing variants. In its primary location in the thyroid, encapsulation may be incomplete with invasion into the adjacent thyroid parenchyma. Larger lesions may exhibit necrosis and hemorrhage as well as calcifications or even psammoma bodies. Although hyalinized bands of dense eosinophilic material indicative of amyloid are readily found in permanent histologic sections (10). However, this feature is less apparent on frozen section. Since medullary carcinoma may require the analysis of permanent sections with immunohistochemical determination for calcitonin for definitive diagnosis, an intraoperative identification of a malignant tumor may be sufficient for initial therapeutic purposes.

Nodal Metastasis, "Lateral Aberrant Thyroid," and Autoamputation

As a presenting clinical sign, lymph node metastases are common in thyroid cancer and may be seen in more than 50% of patients with papillary carcinoma at the time of diagnosis. In papillary carcinoma, recent studies have demonstrated that nodal involvement in patients 45 years or older is a significant prognostic indicator of future local and regional recurrence

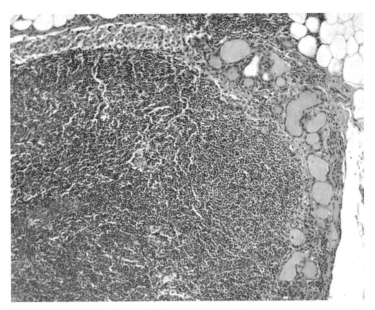

FIGURE 9.18 Frozen section. Metastatic papillary thyroid carcinoma in a cervical lymph node. Despite its bland histology, it represents metastatic disease.

(10,11). If there is a lymph node exploration, it is generally performed at the time of primary operation and nodes may be submitted for frozen section study. The same caveats related to lymph nodes as described elsewhere (Chapters 6 and 7) concerning false negatives apply here as well, especially related to occult metastases. Occult primary papillary or medullary carcinoma with clinically apparent metastatic disease is well known.

Some disagreement exists regarding the presence of histologically benign thyroid inclusions within lymph nodes or soft tissues of the neck (12). "Lateral aberrant thyroid" indicates the presence of apparently normal thyroid tissue within a lymph node of the lateral neck. In the past, this was thought to represent some wayward embryologic rest. However, these foci should be regarded as metastases from thyroid cancer (Fig. 9.18, 9.19).

In patients with colloid goiter or thyroiditis, nodules of thyroid tissue may occasionally detach from the main thyroid lobe possibly because of ongoing inflammation and fibrosis. The autoamputated thyroid nodule then appears as an anatomically distinct soft tissue nodule simulating a lymph node. Before making a diagnosis of metastatic cancer, it is important to recognize architectural features such as a subcapsular sinus that identify a specific structure as a lymph node. Additionally, if there is thyroiditis in the independent nodule, it should also be present in the main thyroid gland. The distinction between this phenomenon and metastatic thyroid carcinoma is particularly difficult and may not be easily resolved by frozen section.

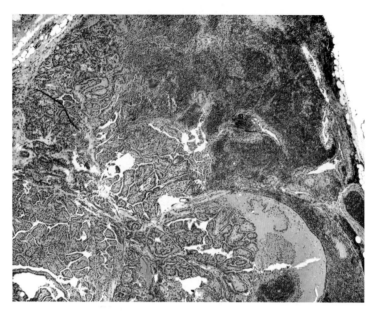

FIGURE 9.19   Frozen section. Extensive involvement of cervical lymph node by papillary thyroid carcinoma, architecturally typical.

Intraoperative Diagnosis of Thyroid Gland Lesions: How Appropriate Is It?

The intraoperative examination of thyroid lesions continues to be frequently requested in an attempt to complete surgical therapy during a single operation. Whether this is a reasonable request has yet to be settled. Frozen section is applicable to mass lesions that are either obviously benign (colloid nodules) and amenable to unilateral lobectomy or obviously malignant, which will result in a completion thyroidectomy, even if preoperatively unanticipated. Malignancies that are potentially identifiable during an intraoperative consultation include conventional types of papillary carcinoma (both papillary and follicular variants), floridly invasive follicular carcinoma, anaplastic carcinoma, and medullary carcinoma (13,14). The utilization issue centers on the use of frozen section in the diagnosis of encapsulated and less than grossly obviously malignant follicular neoplasms. For diffuse abnormalities that have failed medical therapy, such as Graves disease or thyroiditis, a complete thyroidectomy is done in one operation and does not require a frozen section.

Especially related to follicular lesions, frozen section may be questioned by the frequent preoperative utilization of FNA and the real accuracy of a frozen section diagnosis. Callcut et al. reported on the accuracy and utility of frozen section in the evaluation of benign versus malignant follicular thyroid lesions. Of 152 surgical resections, frozen section was reported as benign in 32%, malignant in 4%, indeterminate in 2%, and in 62% of the cases the diagnosis was deferred to permanent sections. It was

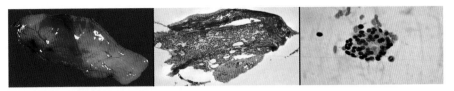

FIGURE 9.20 Parathyroid composite. On the left is the external aspect of a 300-mg soft light brown parathyroid. A thin focally hemorrhagic but otherwise transparent capsule is present. The middle panel is a low-power frozen section showing the typical small follicular arrangement. The right panel is an H&E imprint of a follicle of chief cells from an enlarged parathyroid gland.

found that when the diagnosis of follicular thyroid carcinoma is made in frozen section, it has a sensitivity of 67%, specificity and positive predictive value of 100% each, and an accuracy of 96%. However, in the majority of cases (64%), a definitive diagnosis on frozen section was not achieved, making routine use of frozen section for follicular lesions not cost effective (15). Certainly, it may be argued that if the outcome of the frozen section has no bearing on the ultimate operative procedure, it is not useful nor is it appropriately employed. Deferral rates notwithstanding, until there is an agreed uniform management for patients with thyroid nodules, it is likely that intraoperative evaluation of thyroid lesions will remain common and will continue to play a role in patient management.

PARATHYROID

Parathyroid: Gross Specimen Handling

The average normal gland weighs approximately 35 mg, with an upper limit of normal reaching as high as 80 mg in some studies (16). In routine practice, glands weighing more than 40 mg are considered pathologic (17). Adherent fat should be trimmed, and a careful gross assessment made of color, consistency, and external appearance (Fig. 9.20). The gland's weight is preferably determined on an analytical balance. The gland is typically bivalved, the gross surfaces are inspected, and an imprint made. Excised parathyroid glands are not routinely inked, unless there are surrounding adherent structures suggesting a malignancy. A representative section of the gland to include the external surface should be submitted.

Parathyroid Adenoma and Parathyroid Hyperplasia: Frozen Section Analysis

The surgical management of hyperparathyroidism entails neck exploration with the removal of enlarged glands. Grossly, parathyroid glands may be confused with thyroid nodules, small lymph nodes, aberrant thymic tissue, or even fat. Simple histologic identification settles this issue. Histologic confirmation of parathyroid tissue is usually straightforward and can be

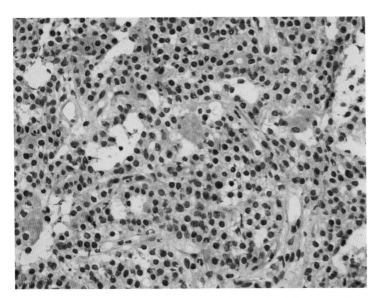

FIGURE 9.21 Parathyroid. Frozen section from an enlarged gland demonstrating small follicles and solid nests of chief cells with uniform dark nuclei, amphophilic to vacuolated cytoplasm.

easily made from frozen section and/or cytologic imprints (Figs. 9.20, 9.21) (18). What diagnosis, however, should the pathologist report?

Since parathyroid carcinoma is very rare, the usual intraoperative question is whether the enlarged gland represents hyperplasia or adenoma. There is an expectation that the pathologist is able on morphologic grounds to distinguish between an adenoma and hyperplasia. As a practical matter, an adenoma is a solitary lesion and hyperplasia involves more than one gland, reflective of a systemic condition such as chronic renal insufficiency. However, the traditional morphologic criteria for each condition, that is, normal rim tissue for an adenoma, increased intraglandular/intracellular fat (demonstrable by oil-red-O staining) in hyperplasia, are not consistently present and therefore not reliable. Therefore, if the surgeon indicates that there is one dominant gland with hard-to-find or very small remaining glands, the diagnosis of adenoma should be established. The improved imaging techniques that have facilitated the preoperative localization of presumed abnormal glands and the intraoperative monitoring of PTH levels are also diagnostically useful.

Theoretically, the distinction of hyperplasia from adenoma has clinical relevance since hyperplasia, by definition, will recur or persist if only one gland is removed. Several criteria have been proposed for the diagnosis of adenoma, including the presence of a rim of normal parathyroid tissue, small amounts of stromal fat, confirmation of at least one remaining normal parathyroid gland, normal or diminished size of the three remaining glands. There are occasional instances, however, of multiple adenomas. Hyperplastic glands, on the other hand, are typically multinodular and diffusely hypercellular, composed of more than one cell type, although chief cells predominate, with a greater component of stromal fat. Rim tissue may be present in both conditions but a rim of normal parathyroid tissue is seen in only 30% to 50% of frozen sections. Even with a coexisting histologically normocellular gland, hyperplasia cannot be excluded since some patients initially present with only one enlarged gland, that is, asymmetric and unequal hyperplasia.

Cellularity and stromal fat content have been proposed in the past as histologic criteria in distinguishing parathyroid adenoma from hyperplasia. Normal parathyroid glands have a reported stromal fat content representing approximately 25% to 50% of the gland. It is now thought that stromal fat is not a reliable feature for determining normal versus abnormal glands primarily because it fluctuates with illness or stress. Another observation used by some in the assessment of normal versus abnormal parathyroid is the amount of intracellular fat content. First proposed by Roth and Gallagher, normal glands and those suppressed by a functional adenoma have an increased intracellular fat content when compared with adenomas and hyperplastic glands (19). However, intracellular fat content is not a reliable feature since parathyroid adenomas may have significant intracellular fat. The use of Sudan IV, oil-red-O stain, or osmium carmine at the time of frozen section has been incorporated in some laboratories to highlight the differences in intracellular lipid content. As an alternative, some have suggested Wright-Giemsa–stained cytologic preparations to evaluate cytoplasmic lipid content. The use of these techniques during intraoperative consultation has proven laborious and operator dependent.

The consistent and accurate histologic distinction between adenoma and hyperplasia in a single gland is virtually impossible. Therefore, a diagnosis of parathyroid adenoma or hyperplasia on frozen section is unnecessary and should be supplanted instead by descriptively confirming the presence of parathyroid tissue, for example, "enlarged parathyroid gland," with a weight. This information should be correlated with intraoperative parathyroid hormone levels to arrive at a definitive diagnosis.

REFERENCES

1. Abboud B, Allam S, Chacra LA, et al. Use of fine-needle aspiration cytology and frozen section in the management of nodular goiters. *Head Neck.* 2003;25:32–36.

2. Alonso N, Lucas A, Salinas I, et al. Frozen section in a cytological diagnosis of thyroid follicular neoplasm. *Laryngoscope.* 2003;113:563–566.

3. Lumachi F, Borsato S, Tregnaghi A, et al. Accuracy of fine-needle aspiration cytology and frozen-section examination in patients with thyroid cancer. *Biomed Pharmacother.* 2004;58:56–60.

4. Basolo F, Ugolini C, Proietti A, et al. Role of frozen section associated with intraoperative cytology in comparison to FNA and FS alone in the management of thyroid nodules. *Eur J Surg Oncol.* 2007;33:769–775.

5. Taneri F, Poyraz A, Salman B, et al. Using imprint and frozen sections in determining the surgical strategies for thyroid pathologies. *Endocr Regul.* 2001;35:71–74.

6. Baloch ZW, LiVolsi VA. Cytologic and architectural mimics of papillary thyroid carcinoma. Diagnostic challenges in fine-needle aspiration and surgical pathology specimens. *Am J Clin Pathol.* 2006;125(suppl):S135–S144.

7. Tse LL, Chan I, Chan JK. Capsular intravascular endothelial hyperplasia: a peculiar form of vasoproliferative lesion associated with thyroid carcinoma. *Histopathology.* 2001; 39:463–468.

8. Leteurtre E, Leroy X, Pattou F, et al. Why do frozen sections have limited value in encapsulated or minimally invasive follicular carcinoma of the thyroid? *Am J Clin Pathol.* 2001;115:370–374.

9. Barnes L, ed. *Surgical Pathology of the Head and Neck.* Vol. 3. Pittsburgh, PA: Marcel Dekker Inc; 2001.

10. LiVolsi VA. *Surgical Pathology of the Thyroid.* Vol. 1. Philadelphia: Saunders; 1990, p. 422.

11. Shindo M, Wu JC, Park EE, et al. The importance of central compartment elective lymph node excision in the staging and treatment of papillary thyroid cancer. *Arch Otolaryngol Head Neck Surg.* 2006;132:650–654.

12. Rosai J, Kuhn E, Carcangiu ML. Pitfalls in thyroid tumour pathology. *Histopathology.* 2006;49:107–120.

13. Anderson CE, McLaren KM. Best practice in thyroid pathology. *J Clin Pathol.* 2003; 56:401–405.

14. LiVolsi VA, Baloch ZW. Use and abuse of frozen section in the diagnosis of follicular thyroid lesions. *Endocr Pathol.* 2005;16:285–293.

15. Callcut RA, Selvaggi SM, Mack E, et al. The utility of frozen section evaluation for follicular thyroid lesions. *Ann Surg Oncol.* 2004;11:94–98.

16. Saffos RO, Rhatigan RM, Urgulu S. The normal parathyroid and the borderline with early hyperplasia: a light microscopic study. *Histopathology.* 1984;8:407–422.

17. Elliott DD, Monroe DP, Perrier ND. Parathyroid histopathology: is it of any value today? *J Am Coll Surg.* 2006;203:758–765.

18. Westra WH, Pritchett DD, Udelsman R. Intraoperative confirmation of parathyroid tissue during parathyroid exploration: a retrospective evaluation of the frozen section. *Am J Surg Pathol.* 1998;22:538–544.

19. Roth SI, Gallagher MJ. The rapid identification of "normal" parathyroid glands by the presence of intracellular fat. *Am J Pathol.* 1976;84:521–528.

10

GASTROINTESTINAL TRACT

REBECCA WILCOX AND AMY NOFFSINGER

INTRODUCTION: GASTROINTESTINAL FROZEN SECTION

There are only a few indications for intraoperative frozen section in the evaluation of gastrointestinal disorders. These include determination of the extent of spread of a tumor, the adequacy of tumor resection usually through evaluation of resection margins, and determination of a diagnosis in cases where an unusual finding is encountered at the time of surgery. Often the question that the surgeon has regarding the specimen can be answered by careful gross examination. As a result, close communication between the surgeon and the pathologist is necessary for optimal specimen evaluation and patient care.

Frozen sections should never be performed on endoscopic biopsy specimens since the procedure may introduce artifacts into the specimen that may compromise the pathologist's ability to make an accurate diagnosis, and the small amount of tissue present in such biopsies may be completely exhausted as a result of the procedure. In addition, a frozen section diagnosis rendered on an endoscopic biopsy specimen would not result in an immediate action on the part of the endoscopist solely on the basis of the histologic diagnosis. In addition, since small biopsy specimens can often be rapidly processed, a definite diagnosis may be provided in emergent cases within a few hours of the endoscopic procedure. In cases where possible perforation of a viscus is suspected as a result of the endoscopy, the decision regarding whether or not to take the patient to the operating room for treatment should be based on symptoms, not the results of frozen section, since these are often not definitive and can in some situations be misleading (Fig. 10.1).

Esophagus: Major Intraoperative Questions

There are only a few indications for frozen section evaluation of esophageal resection specimens. Most often, the pathologist is called upon to determine the adequacy of resection of an esophageal or gastroesophageal junction tumor. Less frequently, a definitive diagnosis for a submucosal or intramural mass lesion is requested.

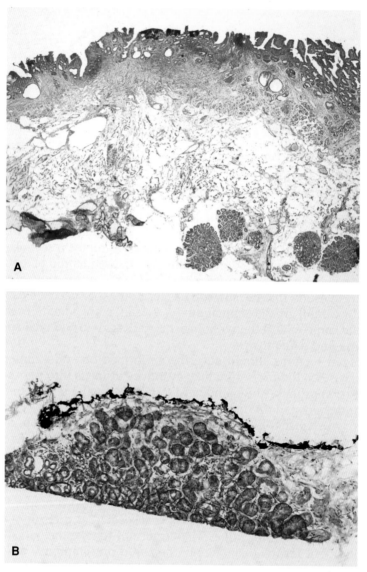

FIGURE 10.1 Endoscopic mucosal resection (EMR). **A.** Esophageal EMR specimen from a patient with Barrett's esophagus and high-grade dysplasia. The patient developed severe chest pain immediately following the procedure, and was clinically felt to have esophageal perforation. **B.** Higher-power view of the deep margin of the EMR specimen showing a submucosal gland, but no muscularis propria. **C.** Permanent section from the same specimen showing the submucosal glands abutting the inked margin. In this section, the muscularis mucosa is easily seen as a single layer (arrow). **D.** Section from another EMR in which thickening, duplication, and disarray of the muscularis mucosae is present. This is a common finding in Barrett's esophagus patients, and should not be misinterpreted as representing muscularis propria. (*continued*)

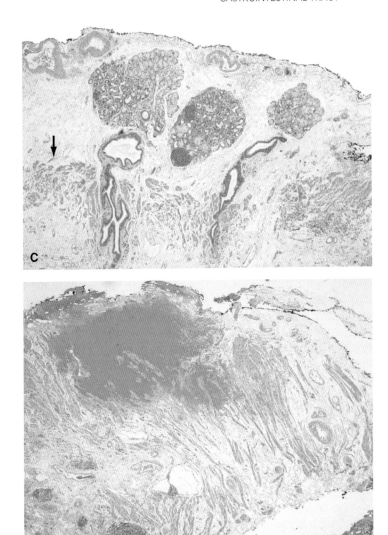

FIGURE 10.1 (Continued)

Esophagus: Interpretation of the Frozen Section

EVALUATION OF RESECTION MARGINS. *Esophagectomy or esophagogastrectomy specimens* are indicated in patients with invasive squamous cell or adenocarcinoma of the esophagus or carcinoma of the gastroesophageal junction. In the past, esophageal resection was also undertaken for treatment of patients with high-grade dysplasia arising in the setting of Barrett's esophagus. Currently, however, this radical approach to treatment of high-grade dysplasia is becoming less common since newer, less invasive endoscopic techniques have been shown to be of equal value in the treatment of preinvasive or early invasive Barrett's-associated neoplasia (1–3) (Fig. 10.1).

In the case of esophagectomy or esophagogastrectomy, the pathologist is most often called upon to evaluate the adequacy of the resection margin. In such specimens, the gastric portion of the resection is usually sufficiently generous, and the tumor far enough away, that the distal margin can be evaluated grossly. In one study of 189 resections for esophageal or gastroesophageal junction carcinoma, a microscopically positive distal resection margin was found in 24 cases (4). In the patients with positive distal margins, the median distance of the distal margin from the tumor was 1 cm, with a range from 0.5 to 4.5 cm. The authors of this study suggest that a grossly measured distance of 5 cm between the tumor and the distal margin is sufficient to ensure an adequate resection.

The proximal esophageal margin is often closer to the tumor, and therefore will more likely require frozen section for evaluation. For patients with squamous cell carcinomas of the esophagus, a proximal margin of at least 3 cm is recommended (5). It is important to note that esophageal squamous cell carcinomas may be multifocal, and therefore, simple gross examination of the resection margin may not be adequate to determine if the margin is free of tumor (6,7). In addition, squamous dysplasia may occasionally be encountered at the margin of resection, but may not be identified grossly.

Studies suggest that 5 to 8 cm of grossly negative proximal esophagus should be resected in patients with gastroesophageal junction adenocarcinomas (8,9). Adenocarcinomas may on occasion extend proximally in the submucosa, leaving the overlying squamous epithelium intact (Fig. 10.2). Such submucosal invasion may extend for a considerable distance, with one reported case reaching upward for as much as 8 cm (10). Such submucosal extension is not grossly recognizable, and could therefore be easily missed without frozen section evaluation. Some studies suggest that frozen section need only be performed in cases where the primary cancer is deeply invasive (T3 or T4), since the risk for a positive proximal resection margin is small in superficial lesions, but increases significantly with increasing depth of invasion by the primary tumor (11).

When margins for Barrett's-associated adenocarcinoma are being evaluated, it is important to determine not just whether the margin is free of invasive carcinoma, but also that there is no Barrett's-associated dysplasia present. It is also important to report whether nondysplastic Barrett's mucosa is present at the margin since the goal of most Barrett's-associated cancer resections is to remove not only the tumor, but also all of the Barrett's mucosa which may be at risk for later neoplastic transformation (Fig. 10.3).

Preoperative radiation therapy is now used in the majority of patients with esophageal carcinomas of both squamous and glandular origin. As a

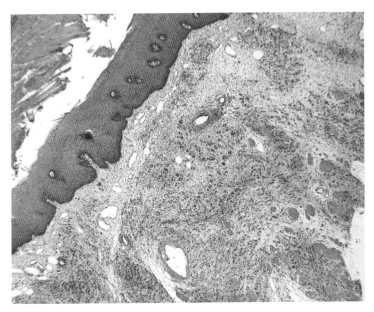

FIGURE 10.2 Distal esophageal or gastroesophageal junction adenocarcinomas often extend proximally under the squamous mucosa. In this photomicrograph, the squamous mucosa is intact, overlying an infiltrating adenocarcinoma, causing the surface to appear grossly normal. In such cases, a positive margin could be missed if the specimen was only inspected grossly without a frozen section.

result, frozen sections performed for evaluation of the resection margin commonly show evidence of radiation injury. The fact that the patient has undergone such treatment is often not conveyed to the pathologist, and may result in misinterpretation of radiation atypia as neoplasia on frozen section (Fig. 10.4).

Both radiation- and chemotherapy-associated esophagitis result in large, bizarre-appearing squamous epithelial cells with increased cytoplasmic volume and enlarged nuclei. Bizarre (radiation) fibroblasts and vascular changes in the lamina propria are also common and suggest that radiation has been given preoperatively (Fig. 10.4). Epithelial hyperplasia develops in an effort to reepithelialize areas of erosion or ulceration. Mitotic figures may appear higher in the mucosa than normal, and the regenerating epithelium may show features simulating dysplasia.

Histologic examination in the later stages of radiation injury shows acanthosis, parakeratosis, hyperkeratosis, hyalinized blood vessels, submucosal and muscular fibrosis, and muscular degeneration. Fibrosis and degeneration affect the deeper esophageal tissues rather than the mucosa. The myenteric plexus becomes inflamed and fibrotic. The muscularis propria appears degenerated. Atypical fibroblasts may be embedded in dense collagenous tissue. Submucosal glands become atrophic, with acinar loss and dilatation, and inspissation of the ductular contents. Squamous

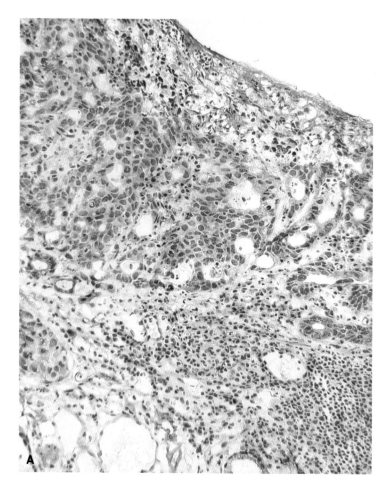

FIGURE 10.3   Resection for Barrett's-associated adenocarcinoma. **A.** The proximal margin is not involved by invasive adenocarcinoma, but Barrett's-associated high-grade dysplasia is present. The glands have a complex back-to-back architecture, and are lined by cells with large, irregular nuclei. **B.** Section from another patient showing low-grade dysplasia and adjacent nondysplastic Barrett's epithelium (arrow). (*continued*)

metaplasia of the ducts of these glands and the presence of radiation-induced atypia may simulate invasive squamous cell carcinoma (Fig. 10.4).

Endoscopic Mucosal Resection Specimens

The pathologist may rarely be asked to determine adequacy of the margins of endoscopic mucosal resection (EMR) specimens. EMR is increasingly being used to treat patients with Barrett's-associated dysplasias and intramucosal carcinomas because the risk for nodal metastasis in these lesions is extremely low (12,13). In addition, the technique is minimally invasive, and is associated with potentially lower morbidity and mortality than is esophagectomy. In addition, many patients who develop Barrett's-associated neoplasia

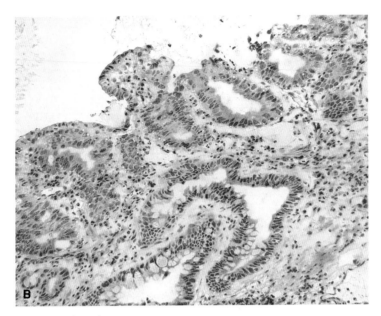

FIGURE 10.3 (*Continued*)

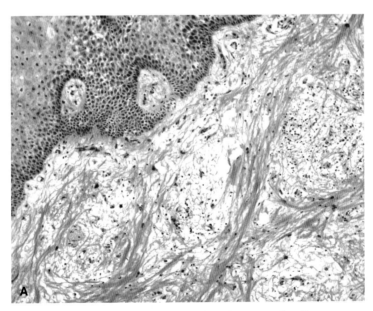

FIGURE 10.4 Radiation atypia. **A.** Low-power view demonstrating the presence of scattered large, atypical-appearing stromal cells in a patient who has undergone preoperative radiation therapy. **B.** Higher-power view of a so-called radiation fibroblast. (*continued*)

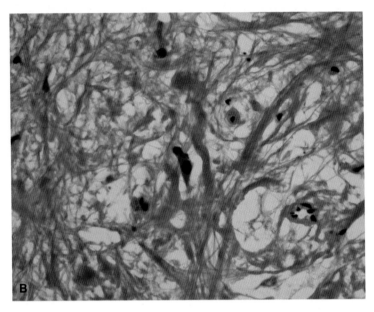

FIGURE 10.4 (*Continued*)

are elderly and may have other medical conditions that make them poor candidates for major operative procedures like esophagogastrectomy. Current endoscopic techniques, however, may be limited in their ability to recognize the extent of dysplasia present, although newer modalities such as narrow band imaging are making endoscopic identification of dysplasia more accurate (14,15). As a result, histology remains the gold standard for dysplasia diagnosis. Endoscopic ultrasound is able to accurately identify periesophageal lymph nodes, but is less useful for determining the depth of invasion of a tumor (16,17). As a result, some investigators have begun to advocate the use of frozen sections in evaluating EMR specimens. In a recent study, Prasad et al. examined 30 consecutive EMR cases using frozen section, and attempted to determine whether or not invasive carcinoma was present, the degree of dysplasia present, as well as the status of the deep and peripheral margins of the specimen (18). There was very little interobserver variation (as determined by κ scores) between the frozen section and permanent section diagnoses for both degree of dysplasia/carcinoma and margin adequacy in this study. Endoscopic ultrasound may not be accurate in determining the depth of invasion of an esophageal neoplasm, and the diagnosis of invasive adenocarcinoma on frozen section evaluation of the EMR specimen could allow the endoscopist to resect less tissue, and therefore prevent possible procedure-related complications, since the presence of invasion is an indication for esophagectomy. In addition, the identification of a positive resection margin could allow the endoscopist to resect additional tissue to ensure complete removal of all dysplastic mucosa. It is currently unclear, however, if the additional time and expense required to perform frozen section evaluation of such EMR specimens would actually contribute significantly to patient care, and frozen sections may introduce artifacts into the tissue that make their evaluation on final permanent section more difficult. In addition, endoscopy, unlike surgery, is noninvasive, and can be easily repeated in the case of a positive margin. In fact, all EMR patients with Barrett's dysplasia undergo routine follow-up endoscopy regardless of the adequacy of their resections because even nondysplastic Barrett's mucosa continues to be at risk for neoplastic transformation as a result of the field defect that affects the esophageal mucosa of these patients.

TUMOR IDENTIFICATION AND DIAGNOSIS. Frozen section is rarely used for the diagnosis of epithelial neoplasms of the esophagus since the majority of these are diagnosed preoperatively by endoscopic biopsy. Frozen sections, however, are sometimes requested for mesenchymal or submucosal tumors to determine their type, and to predict their behavior (benign vs malignant) and hence, the type of operation the surgeon will perform. Unexpected mucosal lesions may also occasionally be encountered by the surgeon and may sometimes be biopsied and sent for frozen section (Fig. 10.5).

The most common mesenchymal tumor of the esophagus is a leiomyoma. Esophageal leiomyomas typically occur in adults, and often represent incidental findings at surgery. On gross examination, leiomyomas typically

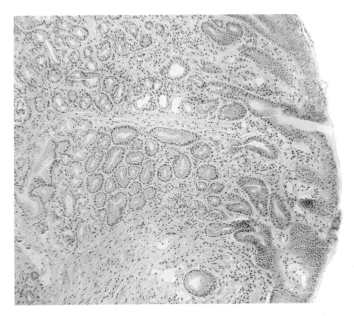

FIGURE 10.5 Esophageal inlet patch. A pink velvety lesion was seen by the surgeon in the proximal esophagus. An inlet patch is a benign tissue rest comprised of normal-appearing gastric mucosa.

appear pale pink, are firm or rubbery in consistency, and may appear lobulated. They are usually round or oval with a whorled appearance resembling their uterine counterparts. Microscopically, leiomyomas are low to moderately cellular tumors containing interlacing fascicles of bland spindle-shaped smooth muscle cells. The nuclei generally appear elongated or cigar shaped, usually without significant pleomorphism. Mitotic activity is minimal or absent.

In contrast, gastrointestinal stromal tumors (GIST) are rare in the esophagus, and most occurring in this location are malignant. Grossly, they may be intramural or polypoid, and often resemble smooth muscle tumors. They exhibit a cellular spindle cell pattern, or show areas of epithelioid differentiation. The histologic pattern varies, ranging from sheets of cells to areas with nuclear palisading and myxoid change. A definite diagnosis of GIST is often not possible on frozen section, since GISTs often resemble other spindle cell tumors. In such cases, the diagnosis should be deferred until permanent sections can be made because of the significant difference in behavior of most GISTs compared with benign leiomyomas.

Granular cell tumors also arise in the esophagus. Grossly, these tumors usually appear as smooth, sessile, and yellow to grayish white lesions. They arise in the submucosa or muscularis propria and are usually covered by a normal-appearing, intact mucosa. Esophageal granular cell tumors resemble similar tumors arising elsewhere in the body (Fig. 10.6). Pseudoepitheliomatous hyperplasia of the overlying squamous epithelium

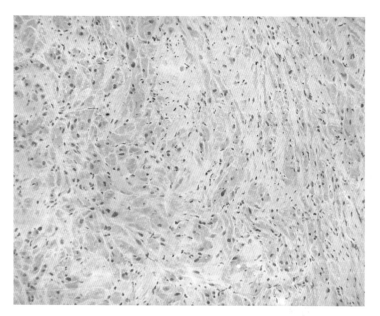

FIGURE 10.6 Granular cell tumor. The tumor is composed of polygonal cells with ill-defined cell borders and abundant eosinophilic granular cytoplasm. The nuclei are small and show mild pleomorphism. No mitotic figures are identified.

occurs in esophageal lesions as it does in granular cells tumors underlying the skin. In some cases, an extensively infiltrating pattern may be seen, a feature that does not rule out a benign lesion. Granular cell tumors, however, can be malignant, although the malignant variety is rare. Features that raise the suspicion of a malignant lesion include large size (>5 cm), increased cellularity, tumor necrosis, tumor cell spindling, increased nuclear size, nuclear pleomorphism, large nucleoli, and identification of greater than two mitoses per ten high-power fields (19). Granular cell tumors may histologically resemble melanoma, carcinoma, or GIST (20) (Fig. 10.7). However, the bland cytologic features should suggest that the lesion is benign. In cases where the tumor predominantly appears to be composed of spindled cells, however, a definite distinction from GIST or other spindle cell tumors may not be possible on frozen section, and the diagnosis may need to be deferred to permanent sections. Areas of pseudoepitheliomatous hyperplasia and the clinical impression of a mass may cause granular tumors to be misinterpreted as squamous carcinomas, particularly if only a small superficial sample is examined. The epithelial cells of pseudoepitheliomatous hyperplasia generally lack cytologic atypia and the connective tissue interface is far more complicated in invasive squamous cell carcinoma than in pseudoepitheliomatous hyperplasia.

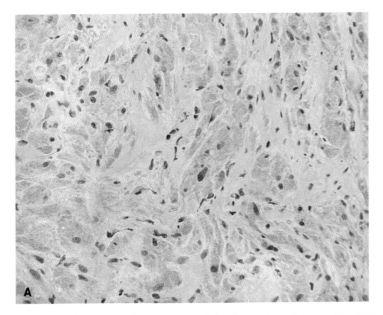

FIGURE 10.7   **A.** Higher-power view of an esophageal granular cell tumor. The tumor cells are variable in size and shape and contain granular cytoplasm. **B.** Frozen section of an epithelioid GIST for comparison. The cells appear more uniform and cohesive, and do not have the same granular quality to their cytoplasm as does the granular cell tumor. (*continued*)

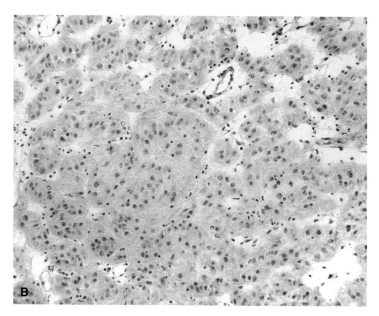

FIGURE 10.7 (*Continued*)

Stomach: Major Intraoperative Questions

As in the esophagus, the surgeon performing either a partial or total gastrectomy may sometimes request frozen section evaluation of the margins of resection. Such resections are most commonly carried out for gastric carcinomas or GISTs. Evaluation of resection margins to determine the adequacy of antrectomy in patients with atrophic autoimmune gastritis or hypergastrinemia-associated gastric endocrine tumors may also be an indication for frozen section.

Frozen sections may be requested to confirm suspected cases of gastric cancer prior to resection when biopsies taken endoscopically were negative. Intraoperative diagnosis may additionally be performed for definitive diagnosis of intramural lesions not accessible by endoscopic biopsy, or in patients with perforated gastric ulcers.

Some recent studies have suggested that surgery for gastric carcinoma, in particular for early gastric cancer, can be minimized or individualized based on the presence of absence of metastasis in a sentinel lymph node (21,22). As a result, pathologists may increasingly be called upon to evaluate sentinel lymph nodes in gastric cancer patients intraoperatively. This may be done either by frozen section or touch imprint cytologic examination (23). Sentinel node biopsy, though standard care in breast cancer and melanoma, has not yet been validated in gastric cancer however, and therefore at the present time is infrequently performed other than in clinical trials.

Stomach: Interpretation of the Frozen Section

EVALUATION OF RESECTION MARGINS. Frozen section interpretation of resection margins is generally straightforward. However, difficulties may be encountered when the resection is being undertaken for a diffuse or signet ring cell gastric adenocarcinoma. The tumor cells comprising these lesions are sometimes quite small, inconspicuous, and may resemble histiocytes, plasma cells, or lymphocytes (Fig. 10.8). In addition, the neoplastic cells are not cohesive, and therefore do not form glandular structures of nests that can be more easily recognized on frozen section. It is critical that the pathologist be aware of the histology of the carcinoma that is being resected before the adequacy of resection can be determined. Rapid immunostaining for cytokeratin or rapid mucin stains have been proposed by some as aids in interpretation of frozen sections taken from patients with diffuse gastric carcinomas (24–27). The utility of such stains in actual daily practice, however, is yet to be determined.

Difficulties may also be encountered in interpretation of resection margin adequacy in patients with autoimmune gastritis. Patients with autoimmune atrophic fundic gastritis commonly develop carcinoid tumors

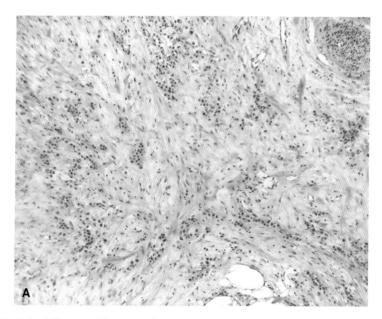

FIGURE 10.8 Diffuse gastric cancer. **A.** Frozen section of a perigastric mass in a patient undergoing gastrectomy for poorly differentiated adenocarcinoma. At low power, the neoplastic cells often resemble inflammatory cells or histiocytes. **B.** On frozen section, reactive vessels may sometimes resemble small infiltrating glands similar to those seen in some poorly differentiated gastric cancers. The endothelial cells lining such vessels may even appear cytologically atypical if significant inflammation is present. **C.** High-power view demonstrating plasmacytoid neoplastic gastric adenocarcinoma cells. **D.** Cytokeratin stain highlighting the infiltrating tumor cells. (*continued*)

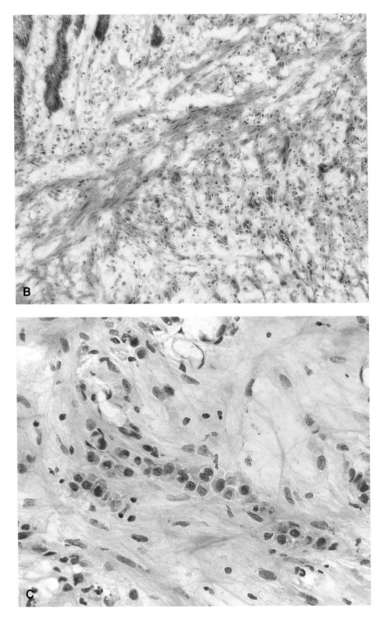

FIGURE 10.8 *(Continued)*

as a result of the hypergastrinemia that accompanies their disease. Achlorhydria results in stimulation of antral G cells to release gastrin, and over time, the development of antral G-cell hyperplasia. The gastrin has a trophic effect on enterochromaffin-like cells in the body of stomach, resulting in enterochromaffin-like cell hyperplasia, and ultimately in the

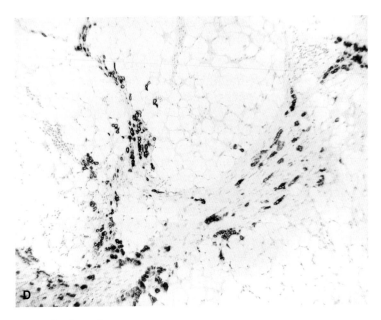

FIGURE 10.8 (*Continued*)

formation of macroscopic carcinoid tumors. This form of carcinoid tumor is designated type I carcinoid, and is relatively indolent, rarely invading deeply or metastasizing (28–31). The treatment of choice for patients with single type I carcinoids is endoscopic removal of the lesion. However, in patients with type I tumors that are too large for endoscopic resection, or those that are recurrent or multiple, antrectomy may be performed (32).

The goal of surgical treatment of type I carcinoid tumors is to remove all of the gastrin-secreting G cells in the antrum, and thereby reverse the patient's hypergastrinemia (32,33). Return of serum gastrin levels to normal results in regression of the carcinoid tumors in the body of the stomach (34–36). Therefore, the pathologist may be called upon to examine the margins of an antrectomy specimen to determine the adequacy of the resection. The distal margin of resection should be comprised solely of duodenal tissue. The proximal margin should demonstrate only oxyntic mucosa, however, since the patients have atrophic fundic gastritis, normal parietal cells are not present. The margin may show the features of atrophic fundic gastritis including plasma cell and lymphocytic infiltrates in the lamina propria and intestinal metaplasia. Such changes should not be seen in antral tissue from these patients, and therefore the presence of such atrophic gastritis confirms that the resection has been extended into the body of the stomach. In the absence of definite atrophic gastritis, the pathologist should look for evidence of G-cell hyperplasia in the necks of the gastric glands. This finding should be confirmed by immunohistochemical staining for gastrin on permanent sections. The presence of a carcinoid tumor at the proximal margin is not of consequence since the tumors should regress postoperatively.

TUMOR IDENTIFICATION AND DIAGNOSIS. Gastric carcinomas may be difficult to diagnose when they are of the poorly differentiated and diffuse or signet ring cell histologic types (as discussed earlier in the chapter). Mesenchymal tumors are also not easy to differentiate from one another on frozen section since many appear as bland spindle cell lesions. The stomach is the most common site for GISTs to arise. Two morphologic phenotypes exist. The first is a cellular spindle cell tumor characterized by fascicles of spindle cells, often with pronounced palisades, monotonous and uniform nuclei, and perinuclear vacuoles that indent the nucleus (Fig. 10.9). Occasional large nuclei may occur. Nuclear palisading resembling that seen in peripheral nerve sheath tumors may be a prominent histologic feature (Fig. 10.10). Hyalinization and myxoid degeneration are common. Epithelioid GISTs also commonly occur in the stomach. These tumors contain round epithelioid cells with prominent clear cytoplasm and cytoplasmic perinuclear vacuolization (Fig. 10.11). The tumor cells lie in sheets or packets rather than in fascicles; they tend to be oriented in a perivascular pattern.

Spindle cell GISTs must be differentiated from other gastric spindle cell tumors including leiomyomas, leiomyosarcomas, peripheral nerve sheath tumors, and inflammatory fibroid polyps. This distinction often requires the use of a panel of immunostains, and therefore, may be difficult or impossible on frozen section. As a result, it is best to diagnose such lesions as a "spindle cell proliferation," and defer the final diagnosis to permanent sections. In some cases, the pathologist may be able to diagnose the lesion as a "malignant spindle cell proliferation" when there is abundant mitotic activity and nuclear pleomorphism. One should never, however, classify a gastric spindle cell lesion as definitely "benign" on frozen section, since further sampling of the tumor on permanent sections may show features predictive of more aggressive behavior.

Small Intestine: Major Intraoperative Questions

Most frozen section requests related to small intestinal pathology are for evaluation of mass lesions. Primary neoplasms most commonly encountered in the small bowel include adenocarcinomas, endocrine tumors (carcinoids), lymphomas, and GISTs. Frozen sections may also commonly be requested in patients with tumors metastatic to the small bowel.

Resection margins for neoplastic processes involving the small intestine are infrequently evaluated by frozen section. Occasionally, the pathologist may be asked to examine a specimen intraoperatively from a patient with a nonneoplastic small intestinal disease, such as diverticulosis or inflammatory bowel disease. This is most often done to exclude the possibility of carcinoma or dysplasia involving a strictured segment of intestine,

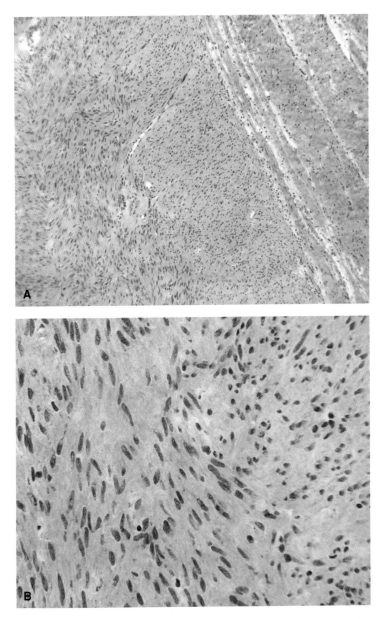

FIGURE 10.9 Spindle cell gastrointestinal stromal tumor (GIST). **A.** Low-power photomicrograph demonstrating a GIST arising in the muscularis propria. The tumor (left) is more cellular than the adjacent smooth muscle (right) and is less eosinophilic. **B.** Spindle cell GISTs are typically comprised of monotonous cells with minimal nuclear pleomorphism. **C.** Significant nuclear atypia is more commonly seen in leiomyosarcomas. **D.** Strong diffuse CD117 staining in a GIST. Immunohistochemical staining is often necessary to make a definitive diagnosis of GIST. On frozen section, "spindle cell neoplasm consistent with GIST" is generally the best diagnosis to render. (*continued*)

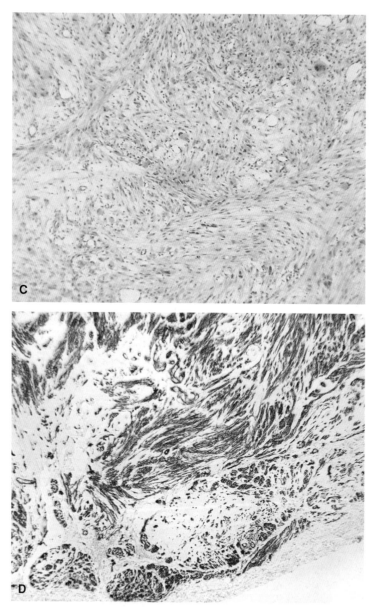

FIGURE 10.9 (*Continued*)

or in the area of a perforated diverticulum. In such cases, the differential diagnosis is between an inflammatory mass and an invasive neoplasm.

Frozen sections of resection margins from inflammatory bowel disease patients should not be performed as these have no clinical value. Numerous studies have demonstrated that microscopic evidence of active Crohn's disease at a resection margin has no influence of the risk for later

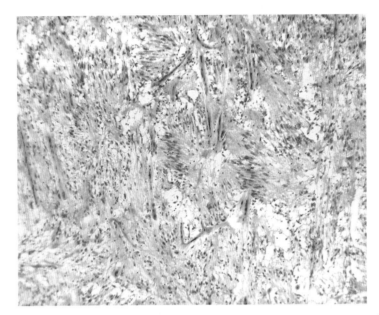

FIGURE 10.10   GIST. This GIST shows prominent palisading reminiscent of a peripheral nerve sheath tumor. This feature is commonly seen in GISTs, and should not be misinterpreted on frozen section as schwannoma or other neural neoplasm.

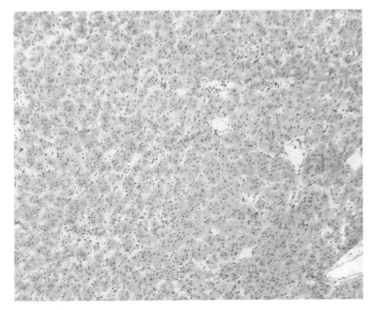

FIGURE 10.11   Epithelioid GISTs are often composed of monotonous polygonal cells with eosinophilic cytoplasm and monomorphic nuclei. They may resemble hepatoid carcinomas or granular cell tumors on frozen section and in routine H&E-stained permanent sections.

disease recurrence (37–42). It is reasonable, however, for the surgeon to request that the margins of a small bowel resection be evaluated grossly at the time of surgery for the presence of macroscopic disease, as gross margin involvement may have an influence on surgical outcome.

Small bowel: Interpretation of the Frozen Section

Most frozen sections performed on small bowel resections do not pose significant diagnostic difficulties. It may sometimes be difficult to distinguish the fibrosis associated with a perforated diverticulum, a fistula tract in a patient with Crohn's disease, or other inflammatory mass lesion with a spindle cell neoplasm (Figs. 10.12–10.14). The presence of significant inflammation in the lesion suggests that it is more likely inflammatory in nature. However, in some cases, it may be necessary to defer diagnosis until permanent sections are available.

The most common indication for frozen section evaluation of a small intestinal lesion is characterization of a mass lesion. Both nonneoplastic and neoplastic lesions occur, and are generally not difficult to diagnose. High-grade lymphomas may be diagnosed with a combination of frozen section and touch imprint examination (Fig. 10.15), but low-grade lesions may require deferral of the diagnosis until permanent sections can be prepared. Occasional nonneoplastic masses may contain glandular elements

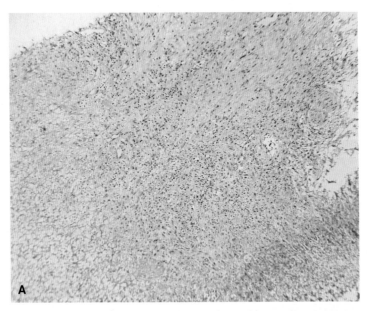

FIGURE 10.12 Crohn's stricture. **A.** Low-power view showing fibrosis, necrosis, and chronic inflammation. **B.** Higher power demonstrating a dense infiltrate of mononuclear cells. These cells must be differentiated from the infiltrating malignant cells of a signet ring cell adenocarcinoma. **C.** Identification of a granuloma is helpful in establishing the diagnosis of Crohn's disease. (*continued*)

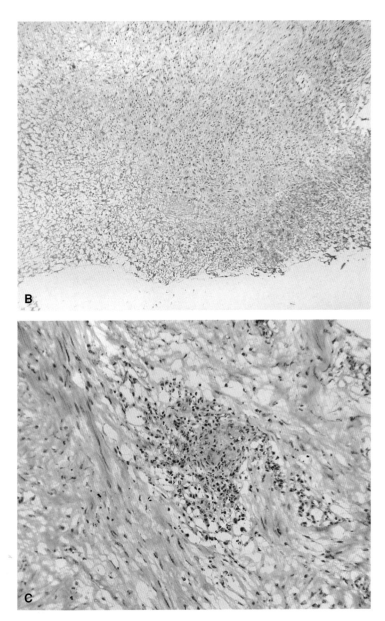

FIGURE 10.12 (Continued)

that could potentially be confused with adenocarcinoma. Such lesions include heterotopic pancreas and cases of enteritis cystica profunda.

Grossly, heterotopic pancreas usually appears well demarcated, and
has a solid tan or cystic lobular appearance on cut section, depending on
whether or not the pancreatic ducts are dilated. The lesion may lie in
the mucosa, the submucosa, or on the serosa, or may sometimes be

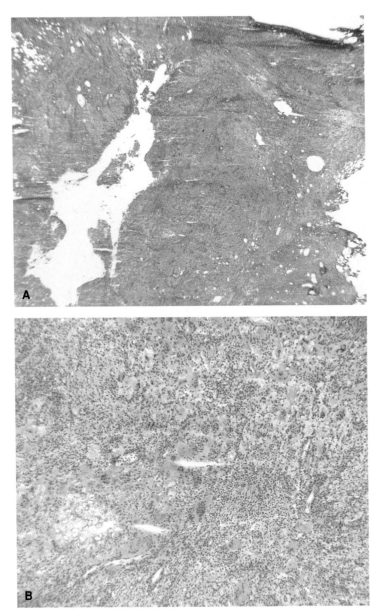

FIGURE 10.13 Perforated diverticulum. This specimen was sent for frozen because of the presence of a mass lesion concerning for a neoplastic process. **A.** Low-power view showing a densely cellular apparent inflammatory mass. **B.** Higher-power view demonstrating the intense inflammatory infiltrate present. **C.** Vegetable material is identifiable, suggesting a perforation. (*continued*)

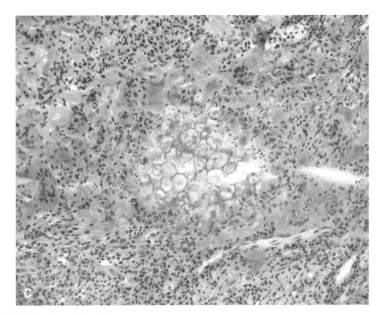

FIGURE 10.13 (*Continued*)

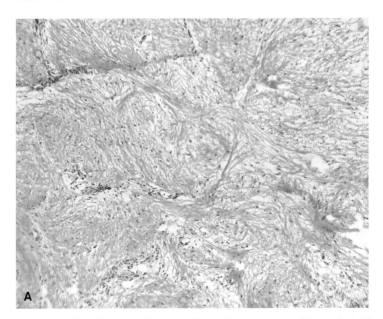

FIGURE 10.14 Spindle cell lesions of the small bowel. **A.** Mesenteric fibromatosis (desmoid). This lesion is hypocellular and comprised predominantly of collagen with interspersed fibroblast-like cells. The low cellularity of this lesion makes the diagnosis of GIST unlikely, although treated GISTs may also appear hypocellular. **B.** Small intestinal GIST. Low-power view of a spindle cell lesion arising in the muscularis propria of the small intestine (right). **C.** Higher-power view showing a moderately cellular spindle cell proliferation. There is minimal cytologic atypia, a feature that often characterizes both benign and malignant GISTs. **D.** Leiomyosarcoma. This spindle cell lesion demonstrates more prominent nuclear pleomorphism than does a typical GIST. Bizarre tumor giant cells are scattered throughout the tumor. (*continued*)

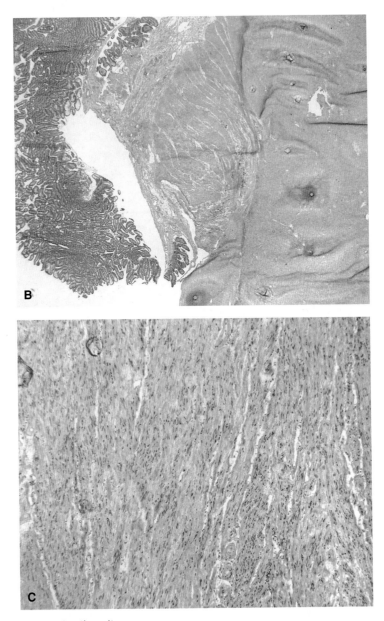

FIGURE 10.14 (*Continued*)

transmural. Histologically, pancreatic acini, ducts, or islets occur alone or in combination with one another (Fig. 10.16). When the lesion contains only ducts surrounded by the circular and longitudinal muscles, they are sometimes erroneously referred to as adenomyomas. However, the orderly arrangement of the two muscle layers around the ducts distinguishes the

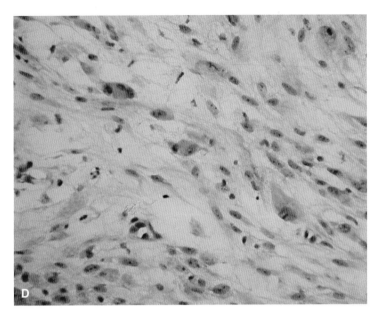

FIGURE 10.14   (*Continued*)

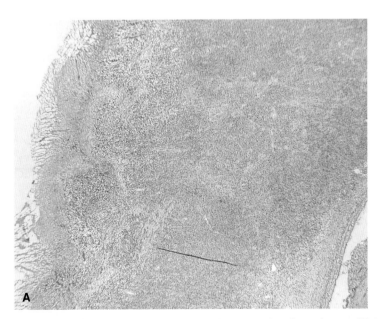

FIGURE 10.15   Small bowel lymphoma. **A.** Full-thickness section through a small intestinal mass lesion demonstrates a densely cellular infiltrate invading all layers of the bowel. **B.** High-power view demonstrating a diffuse infiltrate comprised of atypical lymphoid cells. (*continued*)

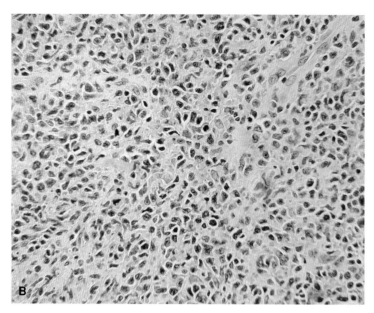

FIGURE 10.15 *(Continued)*

two lesions. In contrast to adenocarcinomas, the ducts of heterotopic pancreas are arranged in a lobular configuration that is readily appreciated on low-power examination. On higher power, these lesions lack the cytologic atypia that characterizes most adenocarcinomas. It is important to keep in mind, however, that heterotopic pancreas can, on rare occasions, become inflamed or undergo neoplastic transformation.

It is not uncommon to encounter displaced epithelium in resection specimens from patients with Crohn's disease. This entity is referred to as enteritis cystica profunda when it affects the small bowel. In enteritis cystica profunda, displaced epithelium is implanted into the submucosa, muscularis propria, or serosa following mucosal ulceration or the formation of mucosal microdiverticula. Mucosal repair leaves the detached epithelium buried in the deeper layers of the bowel wall. Displaced epithelium may also be the consequence of epithelialization of fissures or fistulous tracts.

Grossly, the bowel wall affected by enteritis cystic profunda appears thickened, and the cut surface often shows the presence of numerous cystic submucosal spaces. These are often quite prominent and glisten because of their mucinous content. The mucosa overlying such lesions usually shows evidence of active or healed Crohn's disease. Histologically, one sees mucus-filled cysts in the submucosa, muscularis propria, and serosa. These are lined by cuboidal to columnar epithelium containing goblet cells, enterocytes, and Paneth cells, all supported by a normal lamina propria. The major differential diagnosis in such lesion is between

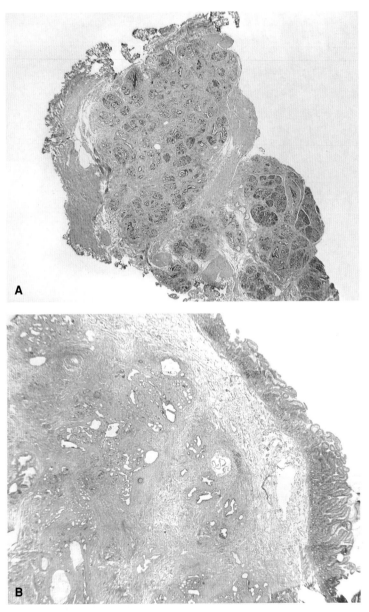

FIGURE 10.16 Heterotopic pancreas. **A.** Heterotopic pancreas typically demonstrates a prominent lobular architecture similar to that of the native pancreas. **B.** In some cases, there is scant acinar tissue present, and the lesion is comprised mainly of ducts. The lobular architecture remains however. **C.** At higher power, there is no cytologic atypia present. (*continued*)

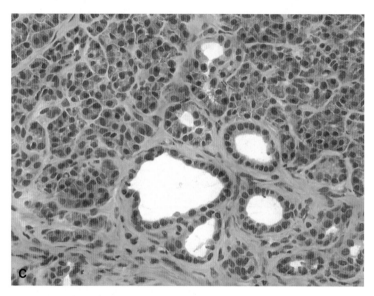

FIGURE 10.16 (Continued)

displaced epithelium and invasive adenocarcinoma. Features that help rule out malignancy include the absence of desmoplasia around the glands and the presence of surrounding lamina propria, and an absence of cytologic atypia within the displaced glands. In some cases, it may be impossible to determine whether one is dealing with displaced epithelium or an invasive cancer. Careful sampling and examination of the surface epithelium may help resolve the diagnostic dilemma as the presence of dysplasia in the overlying epithelium increases the probability that the lesion is invasive.

Occasionally, the pathologist may be called upon to determine whether a neoplasm involving the small bowel is primary or a metastasis. This determination may be difficult when the lesion is an adenocarcinoma. It is important to remember first that metastatic tumors are more common than primary small bowel malignancies. Features that suggest that the lesion is primary include identification of a precursor lesion (adenoma) and the presence of the majority of the lesion in the superficial layers of the bowel wall. The presence of multiple lesions, or the appearance that the bulk of the lesion is present in the outer layers of the bowel wall, is more suggestive of metastasis (Fig. 10.17).

Appendix: Major Intraoperative Questions

Surgical removal of the appendix is rarely performed for neoplasia diagnosed preoperatively. Instead, most appendices are removed for symptoms of appendicitis, and neoplasms are sometimes discovered incidentally in these circumstances. As a result, an appendix that appears enlarged, or involved by a mass lesion, may be sent for frozen section evaluation.

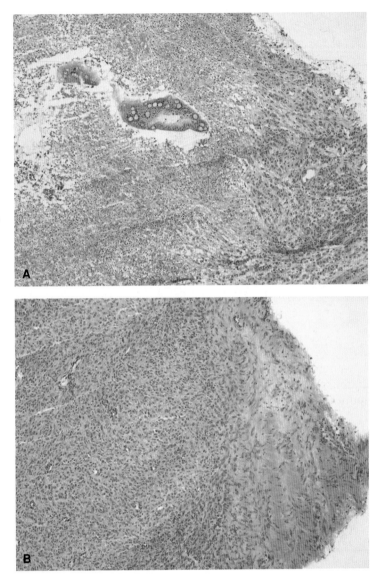

FIGURE 10.17 Small bowel metastasis. **A.** The tumor involves the full thickness of the small bowel wall. There is evidence of surface ulceration with only small fragments of residual mucosa. **B.** The bulk of the tumor, however, is located in the deeper layers of the intestinal wall. A small amount of smooth muscle of the muscularis propria is seen in the lower right of the photograph. **C.** High power shows an undifferentiated neoplasm, which on permanent sections was diagnosed as metastatic melanoma. (*continued*)

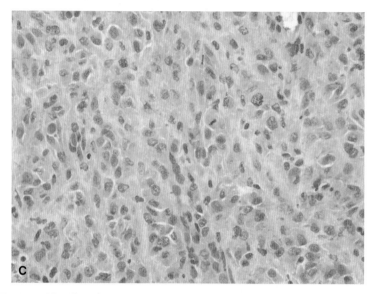

FIGURE 10.17 (*Continued*)

Appendix: Interpretation of the Frozen Section

Appendiceal neoplasms may obstruct the lumen of the appendix, resulting in superimposed acute appendicitis. As a result, frozen sections obtained for evaluation of preoperatively unsuspected appendiceal mass lesions often show features of acute inflammation. Primary appendiceal adenocarcinomas are rare, but may be diagnosed at frozen section. The margin of resection of appendectomy specimens with primary adenocarcinoma do not need to be frozen, since this diagnosis results in a right hemicolectomy regardless of the status of the margin. If the mass lesion is a carcinoid tumor, however, the margin should be evaluated by frozen section, since appendectomy with a negative margin of resection is sufficient treatment for these tumors. Other lesions that may be encountered on frozen sections from the appendix include mucinous cystadenomas, mucoceles, endometriosis, diverticula, and metastatic carcinomas (Figs. 10.18 and 10.19).

Colon and Rectum: Major Intraoperative Questions

The most common reason for requesting frozen section evaluation of a colectomy specimen is for establishing the diagnosis of deep mural or serosal lesions, or distinction of inflammatory from neoplastic masses. Frozen sections are rarely performed for assessment of resection margins in patients undergoing colectomy for primary colonic neoplasms. In most cases, the margins are sufficiently far away from the main tumor mass that they do not need to be examined intraoperatively. Occasionally, gross evaluation and measurement of the distance of the tumor from the distal

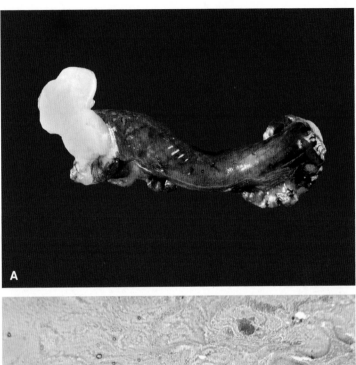

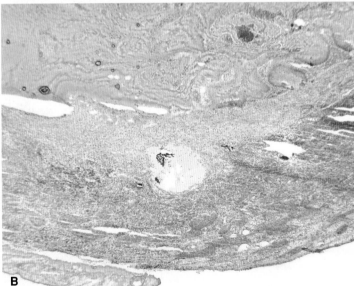

FIGURE 10.18 Mucocele of the appendix. **A.** Gross photograph of the appendectomy specimen demonstrating abundant mucin extravasating from the lumen. **B.** Low-power view of the frozen section from this same specimen. The lumen contains a large mucin collection, but obvious invasive neoplasia is not identifiable. **C.** Higher-power view of the appendiceal wall showing a bland, nonneoplastic-appearing epithelial lining, and no evidence of invasive carcinoma in the deeper layers. (*continued*)

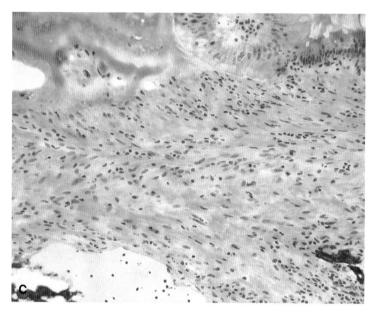

FIGURE 10.18 (*Continued*)

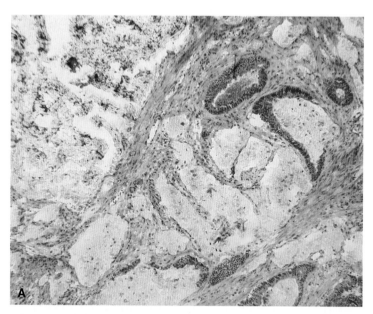

FIGURE 10.19 Appendiceal adenocarcinoma. **A.** Low-power view showing neoplastic glands invading the wall of the appendix. **B.** Higher-power view demonstrating infiltrating signet ring cells. It is not uncommon for appendiceal adenocarcinomas to show signet ring cell features. The major differential diagnosis in such a case is with adenocarcinoid. However, the intraoperative diagnosis of either entity results in similar surgical therapy, right hemi-colectomy; therefore, differentiating between these two entities on frozen section is not necessary. (*continued*)

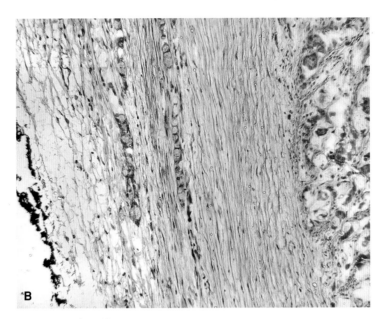

FIGURE 10.19 (*Continued*)

resection margin may be requested in cases of extremely low-lying rectal adenocarcinomas.

Colon and Rectum: Interpretation of the Frozen Section

EVALUATION OF RESECTION MARGINS. Evaluation of the adequacy of resection of a primary colorectal neoplasm can always be done grossly, and does not require frozen section. For primary colorectal adenocarcinomas, the distal edge of the tumor should be at least 2.5 cm from the distal resection margin (43,44). Some studies, however, suggest that local recurrence, at least in cases of rectal adenocarcinoma where a total mesorectal excision has been performed, is unrelated to the distance of the tumor from the distal resection margin (45,46). The proximal resection margin should be at least 5 cm from the primary tumor, but this is almost never a difficulty for the surgeon to accomplish, and therefore, the pathologist is almost never called upon to assess the proximal margin in a colectomy specimen.

EVALUATION OF MASS LESIONS. As discussed in the section on small bowel frozen section evaluation, distinction between inflammatory and neoplastic mass lesions may sometimes be difficult. Inflammatory masses or strictures occur in patients with diverticular disease, inflammatory bowel disease, or those with colonic perforation occurring for other reasons.

REFERENCES

1. Manner H, May A, Pech O, et al. Early Barrett's carcinoma with "low-risk" submucosal invasion: long-term results of endoscopic resection with a curative intent. *Am J Gastroenterol.* 2008;103:2589–2597.
2. Larghi A, Lightdale CJ, Ross AS, et al. Long-term follow-up of complete Barrett's eradication endoscopic mucosal resection (CBE-EMR) for the treatment of high grade dysplasia and intramucosal carcinoma. *Endoscopy.* 2007;39:1986–1091.
3. Ell C, May A, Pech O, et al. Curative endoscopic resection of early esophageal adenocarcinomas (Barrett's cancer). *Gastrointest Endosc.* 2007;65:3–10.
4. Casson AG, Darnton SJ, Subramanian S, et al. What is the optimal distal resection margin for esophageal carcinoma? *Ann Thorac Surg.* 2000;69:205–209.
5. Tsutsui S, Kuwano H, Watanabe M, et al. Resection margin for squamous cell carcinoma of the esophagus. *Ann Surg.* 1995;222:193–202.
6. Yuasa N, Miyachi M, Yasui A, et al. Clinicopathological features of superficial spreading and nonspreading squamous cell carcinoma of the esophagus. *Am J Gastroenterol.* 2001;96:315–321.
7. Younes M. Frozen section of the gastrointestinal tract, appendix, and peritoneum. *Arch Pathol Lab Med.* 2005;129:1558–1564.
8. Barbour AP, Rizk NP, Gonen M, et al. Adenocarcinoma of the gastroesophageal junction. Influence of esophageal resection margin and operative approach on outcome. *Ann Surg.* 2007;246:1–8.
9. Mariette C, Castel B, Balon JM, et al. Extent of oesophageal resection for adenocarcinoma of the oesophagogastric junction. *Eur J Surg Oncol.* 2003;29:588–593.
10. Ikeda Y, Kurihara H, Niimi M, et al. Esophageal intramural spreading from an adenocarcinoma of the esophagogastric junction. *Hepatogastroenterology.* 2004;51: 1382–1383.
11. Shen JG, Cheong JH, Hyung WJ, et al. Intraoperative frozen section margin evaluation in gastric cancer of the cardia surgery. *Hepatogastroenterology.* 2006;53:976–978.
12. Nigro JJ, Hagen JA, DeMeester TR, et al. Prevalence and location of nodal metastases in distal esophageal adenocarcinoma confined to the wall: implications for therapy. *J Thorac Cardiovasc Surg.* 1999;117:16–23.
13. Kodama M, Kakegawa T. Treatment of superficial cancer of the esophagus: a summary of responses to a questionnaire on superficial cancer of the esophagus in Japan. *Surgery.* 1998;123:432–439.
14. Georgakoudi I, Jacobson BC, Van Dam J, et al. Fluorescence, reflectance, and light-scattering spectroscopy for evaluating dysplasia in patients with Barrett's esophagus. *Gastroenterology.* 2001;120:1620–1629.
15. Guelrud M, Ehrlich EE. Endoscopic classification of Barrett's esophagus. *Gastrointest Endosc.* 2004;59:58–65.
16. DeWitt J, Kesler K, Brooks JA, et al. Endoscopic ultrasound for esophageal and gastroesophageal junction cancer: impact of increased use of primary neoadjuvant therapy on preoperative locoregional staging accuracy. *Dis Esophagus.* 2005;18:21–27.
17. Zuccaro G Jr, Rice TW, Vargo JJ, et al. Endoscopic ultrasound errors in esophageal cancer. *Am J Gastroenterol.* 2005;100:601–606.
18. Prasad GA, Wang KK, Lutzke LS, et al. Frozen section analysis of esophageal endoscopic mucosal resection specimens in the real-time management of Barrett's esophagus. *Clin Gastroenterol Hepatol.* 2006;4:173–178.
19. O'Donovan DG, Kell P. Malignant granular cell tumour with intraperitoneal dissemination. *Histopathology.* 1989;14:417–419.
20. Prematilleke V, Sujendran V, Warren BF, et al. Granular cell tumour of the oesophagus mimicking a gastrointestinal stromal tumour on frozen section. *Histopathology.* 2004;44:502–514.
21. Ichikura T, Chochi K, Sugasawa H, et al. Individualized surgery for early gastric cancer guided by sentinel node biopsy. *Surgery.* 2006;139:501–507.
22. Tanaka K, Tonouchi H, Kobayashi M, et al. Laparoscopically assisted total gastrectomy with sentinel node biopsy for early gastric cancer: preliminary results. *Am Surg.* 2004;70:976–981.

23. Lee YJ, Moon HG, Park ST, et al. The value of intraoperative imprint cytology in the assessment of lymph node status in gastric cancer surgery. *Gastric Cancer.* 2005;8:245–248.

24. Matsusaka S, Nagareda T, Yamasaki H, et al. Immunohistochemical evaluation for intraoperative rapid pathological assessment of the gastric margin. *World J Surg.* 2003;27:715–718.

25. Dworak O, Wittekind C. A 30-s PAS stain for frozen sections. *Am J Surg Pathol.* 1992;16:87–88.

26. Soans S, Galindo LM, Garcia FU. Mucin stain on frozen sections: a rapid 3-minute method. *Arch Pathol Lab Med.* 1999;123:378–380.

27. Monig SP, Luebke T, Soheili A, et al. Rapid immunohistochemical detection of tumor cells in gastric carcinoma. *Oncol Rep.* 2006;16:1143–1147.

28. Rindi G, Bordi C, Rappel S, et al. Gastric carcinoids and neuroendocrine carcinomas: pathogenesis, pathology, and behavior. *World J Surg.* 1996;20:168–172.

29. Gough DB, Thompson GB, Crotty TB, et al. Diverse clinical and pathologic features of gastric carcinoid and the relevance of hypergastrinemia. *World J Surg.* 1994;18:473–479.

30. Modlin IM, Gilligan CJ, Lawton GP, et al. Gastric carcinoids. The Yale experience. *Arch Surg.* 1995;130:250–255.

31. Thomas RM, Baybick JH, Elsayed AM, et al. Gastric carcinoids. An immunohistochemical and clinicopathologic study of 104 patients. *Cancer.* 1994;73:2053–2058.

32. Dakin GF, Warner RRP, Pomp A, et al. Presentation, treatment, and outcome of type 1 gastric carcinoid tumors. *J Surg Oncol.* 2006;93:368–372.

33. Hou W, Schubert ML. Treatment of gastric carcinoids. *Curr Treat Option Gastroenterol.* 2007;10:123–133.

34. Hirschowitz BI, Griffith J, Pellegrin D, et al. Rapid regression of enterochromaffinlike cell gastric carcinoids in pernicious anemia after antrectomy. *Gastroenterology.* 1992;102:1409–1418.

35. Kern SE, Yardley JH, Lazenby AJ, et al. Reversal by antrectomy of endocrine cell hyperplasia in the gastric body in pernicious anemia: a morphometric study. *Mod Pathol.* 1990;3:561–566.

36. Higham AD, Dimaline R, Varro A, et al. Octreotide suppression test predicts beneficial outcome from antrectomy in a patient with gastric carcinoid tumor. *Gastroenterology.* 1998;114:817–822.

37. Pennington L, Hamilton SR, Bayless TM, et al. Surgical management of Crohn's disease. Influence of disease at margin of resection. *Ann Surg.* 1980;192:311–318.

38. Hamilton SR, Reese J, Pennington L, et al. The role of resection margin frozen section in the surgical management of Crohn's disease. *Surg Gynecol Obstet.* 1985;160:57–62.

39. McLeod RS. Resection margins and recurrent Crohn's disease. *Hepatogastroenterology.* 1990;37:63–66.

40. Katanagi H, Kramer K, Fazio VW, et al. Do microscopic abnormalities at resection margins correlate with increased anastomotic recurrence in Crohn's disease? Retrospective analysis of 100 cases. *Dis Colon Rectum.* 1991;34:909–916.

41. Cooper JC, Williams NS. The influence of microscopic disease at the margin of resection on recurrence rates in Crohn's disease. *Ann R Coll Surg Engl.* 1986;68:23–26.

42. Fazio VW, Marchetti F, Church JM, et al. Effect of resection margins on the recurrence of Crohn's disease in the small bowel. A randomized controlled trial. *Ann Surg.* 1996;224:563–573.

43. Hughes TG, Jenevein EP, Poulos E. Intramural spread of colon carcinoma: a pathologic study. *Am J Surg.* 1983;146:697–699.

44. Weese JL, O'Grady MG, Ottery FD. How long is the five centimeter margin? *Surg Gynecol Obstet.* 1986;163:101–103.

45. Karanjia ND, Schache DJ, North NR, et al. "Close shave" in anterior resection. *Br J Surg.* 1990;77:510–512.

46. Thompson WHF, Foy CJW, Longman RJ. The nature of local recurrence after colorectal cancer resection. *Colorectal Dis.* 2007;10:69–74.

11

LIVER, EXTRAHEPATIC BILIARY TREE, GALLBLADDER, AND PANCREAS

RISH K. PAI, REBECCA WILCOX, AMY NOFFSINGER, AND JOHN HART

LIVER

Liver: Major Intraoperative Questions

Frozen sections of the liver are usually performed to evaluate a mass lesion. In general, frozen sections for the diagnosis of a medical liver condition, such as chronic hepatitis, steatohepatitis, metabolic disorders, or chronic cholestatic conditions, should be strongly discouraged. The diagnosis of these entities requires excellent slide quality, clinicopathologic correlation, and the use of special stains. Since this is usually not practical in the frozen section suite, the likelihood of diagnostic error is too high to make frozen section evaluation worthwhile in these settings. Moreover, artifactual distortion of the biopsy specimens utilized for frozen section makes this tissue unsuitable for optimal permanent section diagnosis. In any case, the widespread availability of same-day processing of biopsy specimens makes it unnecessary to perform frozen sections on liver biopsies for diagnosis of medical conditions. Of course, there are rare exceptions to this rule of thumb. For instance, frozen sections are required to evaluate for the presence of microvesicular steatosis by oil-red-O or Sudan Black stain. Also, frozen section analysis of potential donor livers can be essential in predicting the function of the allograft posttransplant.

In contrast, there are many situations in which frozen section evaluation of a mass lesion in the liver is indicated. Surgeons routinely examine the surface of the liver for lesions during abdominal surgery, and, in many cases, an intraoperative ultrasound is performed for suspected deeper lesions. These lesions are commonly submitted for frozen section diagnosis. Occasionally, primary liver tumors are submitted for frozen section diagnosis for histologic confirmation as well as for assessment of the surgical margin. During surgical resections of pancreatic, gastric, and esophageal tumors, the presence of a liver metastasis is a contraindication to resection for cure; thus the intraoperative consultation directly guides surgical

TABLE 11.1 Differential Diagnosis of Mass Lesion in Cirrhotic and Noncirrhotic Livers	
Cirrhotic Liver	Noncirrhotic Liver
Macroregenerative nodule (large regenerative nodule)	Metastatic carcinoma
Dysplastic nodule	Cholangiocarcinoma
Hepatocellular carcinoma	Bile duct adenoma
Cavernous hemangioma	Bile duct hamartoma
Focal scarring (parenchymal extinction)	Vascular tumors
	Cavernous hemangioma
	Epithelioid hemangioendothelioma
Bile duct adenoma	Focal fatty change
Bile duct hamartoma	Hepatic adenoma
Cholangiocarcinoma	Focal nodular hyperplasia
Metastatic adenocarcinoma[a]	Hepatocellular carcinoma
	Fibrolamellar carcinoma
	Sclerosing hepatic carcinoma
	Cystic biliary lesions
	Hepatobiliary cystadenoma
	Benign biliary cyst
	Parasitic cysts

[a]Very rare.

therapy. For colorectal and gynecologic malignancies, finding a small metastatic tumor deposit in the liver will guide postoperative therapy and does not usually guide intraoperative decision making; nevertheless, surgeons routinely ask for an intraoperative consultation in these cases.

When reviewing a frozen section on a liver mass, it is essential to know whether the liver is cirrhotic or not, since the differential diagnosis is quite different in these two settings (Table 11.1). For instance, in a noncirrhotic liver metastatic tumor is always a leading diagnostic consideration while metastatic tumor in cirrhosis is distinctly uncommon. Also, by convention, the diagnosis of hepatic adenoma is not rendered in the setting of cirrhosis.

When performing a frozen section on a small hepatic lesion, it is important to first grossly identify the lesion either visually or with gentle palpation. If no gross lesion is identified, bisecting the tissue may be helpful. When interpreting the frozen section, it is important to keep in mind that the surgeon visualized a lesion; thus, if no mass lesion is evident in the slide, deeper sections should be cut in order to avoid the unpleasant finding of a worrisome lesion on the permanent sections. Larger lesions should be weighed and the resection margin inked. Since the hepatic capsule does not represent a true oncologic margin, it is not necessary to ink this surface. Serial sections of the specimen should then be performed before selecting the portion of tissue to be frozen.

If a metabolic disorder is suspected, tissue can be snap frozen for possible future enzymatic or genetic testing. However, the first responsibility of the pathologist is to be sure that adequate tissue is reserved for routine H&E examination. If all of the tissue is submitted to rule out a metabolic disorder and the test is negative, then no diagnosis can be rendered. Tissue for enzymatic or genetic testing should be wrapped in aluminium foil (without OTC) and snap frozen, and then stored at −70°C. It should not be sent for testing until the H&E sections of the other tissue has been examined. Electron microscopy is sometimes helpful in the evaluation of mass lesions, metabolic disorders, and infectious diseases. If a needle core sample is provided, then 1-mm portions from each end of the biopsy can be fixed in glutaraldehyde.

Liver: Frozen Section Interpretation

METASTATIC TUMORS. By far the most common frozen section diagnosis on liver lesions is for metastatic tumor, as the liver is an extremely common site for metastases. Thankfully, the diagnosis of metastatic tumor on a frozen section is usually not difficult. As with other sites of metastasis, desmoplasia is usually very helpful along with the other cytomorphologic features of malignancy (nuclear enlargement, hyperchromasia, irregular nuclear membranes, atypical mitotic figures, and architectural complexity). Suggesting a source of the primary tumor is not necessary unless asked specifically by the operating surgeon. If the patient has a previous history of a malignancy, review of the prior slides can be extremely helpful.

It is not possible to distinguish between primary hepatic cholangiocarcinoma and metastatic adenocarcinoma unless an in situ component can be documented. Colon cancer is the most common metastatic adenocarcinoma, and the presence of tall columnar cells with dirty necrosis is highly suggestive of a colorectal primary (Fig. 11.1). Metastatic pancreatic cancer often induces an exuberant desmoplastic response (Fig. 11.2), although many other tumors such as lung carcinoma can also do this. Gynecologic malignancies have a wide morphologic spectrum, and they can be very difficult to distinguish on a frozen section. A sinusoidal pattern of infiltration by a malignant tumor should suggest the possibility of lymphoma, melanoma, or breast carcinoma. In all cases, if uncertainty exists, it is best to convey that uncertainty to the surgeon and defer a definitive diagnosis until the permanent sections are available.

Bile duct hamartoma/von Meyenburg complex. Bile duct hamartomas are the most common diagnoses rendered during frozen section of a liver nodule sampled during abdominal surgery at the University of Chicago. They are often present just beneath the capsule, and thus are noted by the

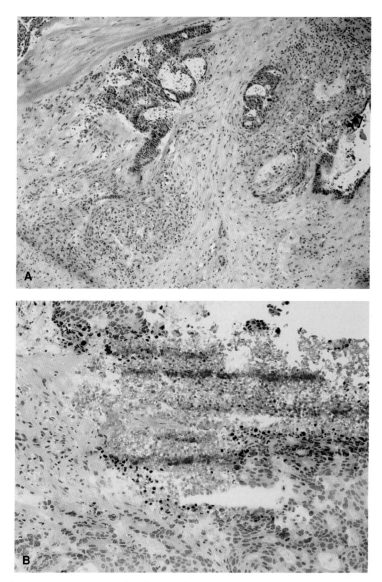

FIGURE 11.1 Metastatic colonic adenocarcinoma. **A.** Note the presence of columnar cells with pencillate nuclei. **B.** In other areas, there was extensive necrosis.

surgeon. In one autopsy series, bile duct hamartomas were found in 5.6% of individuals (1). Most are less than 5 mm in size. In the majority of cases, distinction between metastatic carcinoma and bile duct hamartoma is straightforward; however, in one study, bile duct hamartomas were the most common lesion mistaken for metastatic tumor (2). Bile duct hamartomas are well circumscribed, unlike metastatic tumors (Fig. 11.3, e-Fig. 11.1). Moreover, the glandular structures in bile duct hamartomas are

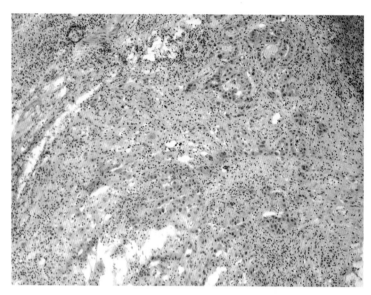

FIGURE 11.2 Metastatic pancreatic adenocarcinoma. The desmoplastic stroma is characteristic, but it is not possible to distinguish from a primary intrahepatic cholangiocarcinoma.

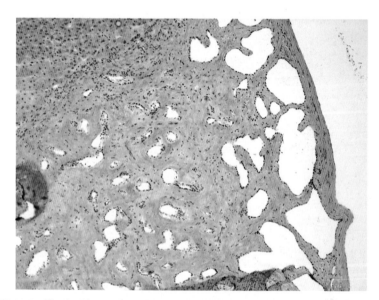

FIGURE 11.3 Bile duct hamartoma (von Meyenburg complex). The frozen section from the same case as Figure 11.2 also contained a bile duct hamartoma adjacent to the metastatic pancreatic carcinoma. The ectatically dilated glandular profiles with bland cytologic features is characteristic.

lined by cuboidal cells with dilated lumens and rounded contours. Bile or inspissated proteinaceous material can sometimes be present within these lesions. Additionally, the stroma surrounding the glands in a bile duct hamartoma is fibrous and quite unlike the desmoplastic stroma seen in metastatic tumors. Distinction between bile duct hamartoma and bile duct adenoma can be difficult at times, but this distinction is of no practical consequence since both lesions are benign and of no clinical significance.

Bile duct adenoma. Differentiating between bile duct adenomas and metastatic carcinomas can be more challenging. Bile duct adenomas are also fairly small (<1 cm) but can occasionally be quite large (up to 4 cm). They are discovered incidentally during abdominal surgery and are typically subcapsular, circumscribed white-gray firm masses (e-Fig. 11.2). Histologically, they are composed of tightly packed small tubules with scant intervening fibrous stroma (Fig. 11.4, e-Fig. 11.3). At low-power magnification, a bile duct adenoma can closely resemble a metastatic tumor deposit especially when inflamed; however, close inspection reveals glands lined by low-cuboidal epithelium without the histologic features of malignancy (3).

Hepatic granulomas. On occasion, a frozen section consultation is requested to evaluate a tiny subcapsular nodule to exclude metastatic adenocarcinoma at the time of resection of a gastrointestinal or pancreatic primary. Often the sections reveal a bile duct adenoma or bile duct hamartoma, but not infrequently a hyalinized nodule consistent with an old granuloma is identified (e-Figs. 11.4, 11.5). These granulomas are generally of no

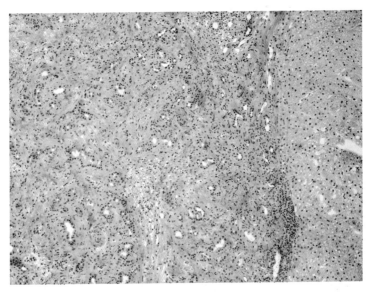

FIGURE 11.4   Bile duct adenoma. Note the closely packed bland-appearing glandular profiles with a sharp demarcation with the surrounding liver.

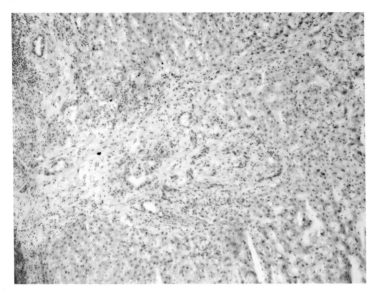

FIGURE 11.5 Mechanical extrahepatic biliary obstruction. The proliferating bile ducts exhibit architectural and cytologic atypia. However, the presence of surrounding normal portal structures, portal edema, bile, and intense acute inflammatory cell infiltrate argues against a malignant diagnosis.

clinical consequence, even when there is a small area of central necrosis. If a GMS stain is performed on a permanent section, *Histoplasma* organisms are sometimes identified, particularly in patients from the midwestern United States. Nonetheless, this finding has no bearing on the surgical management of the patient.

Biliary obstruction. In biliary obstruction caused by pancreatic and common bile duct tumors, numerous small white spots dot the surface of the liver giving the impression to the surgeon of multiple metastatic tumor deposits. A frozen section from these lesions can be quite difficult without complete knowledge of the clinical history particularly when the ductular reaction is florid. The proliferating ductules appear infiltrative and angulated, and a fibrous stromal reaction mimicking a desmoplastic response is also a feature (Fig. 11.5). Recognizing that the proliferating ductules are centered on portal tracts containing portal veins and hepatic artery branches is essential to making this diagnosis.

Focal nodular hyperplasia. Focal nodular hyperplasia (FNH), a benign lesion with no risk of malignant degeneration, is sometimes resected to alleviate symptoms. Although FNH occurs in both sexes, these lesions are more common in adult women. Usually such lesions are more than 10 cm in diameter, and a well-developed central scar containing an anomalous vessel is evident grossly. FNH is usually circumscribed and paler than the surrounding hepatic parenchyma (Fig. 11.6).

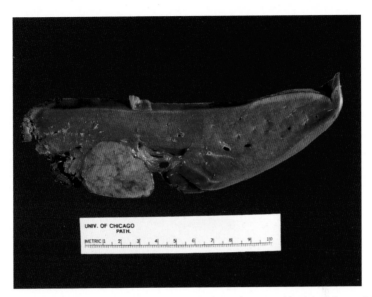

FIGURE 11.6 Focal nodular hyperplasia. A central scar is not evident in this small lesion. However, note the nodular cut surface of the lesion compared to the smooth surface of the surrounding parenchyma.

FNH can also present as an incidental mass lesion discovered during abdominal surgery. In this setting, the lesion is usually smaller and the central scar may not be grossly evident. In fact, lesions less than 3 cm in diameter usually lack a central scar with a large anomalous vessel. Whether small or large, FNH classically demonstrate three characteristic histologic findings: abnormal lobular architecture, abnormal arteries, and bile ductular proliferation (4). The usual lobular architecture of the liver is disrupted by the presence of thin fibrous septa, which can produce a cirrhosis-like pattern within the lesion. In fact, a clue to the diagnosis of FNH in a needle biopsy is the presence of apparent "cirrhosis," when in fact the surrounding parenchyma is noncirrhotic. It may even be worthwhile to ask the surgeon to procure a biopsy of the surrounding parenchyma for comparison. The second element of the diagnosis is the presence of abnormal large arteries with intimal proliferation and muscular hypertrophy and a disrupted elastic lamina. The third important component for the diagnosis of FNH is the presence of bile ductules at the periphery of the fibrous septa (Fig. 11.7). Although at first glance, the fibrous septa may appear to represent normal portal tracts, in fact no true native bile ducts are present. Native bile ducts are recognized by their location within the substance of the portal tract (rather than at the interface with the parenchyma), the presence of a normal arteriole of the same caliber nearby (so-called parallelism), and the presence of a well-formed lumen and surrounding basement membrane. The hepatocytes that make up an FNH are morphologically normal appearing and are arranged in a normal

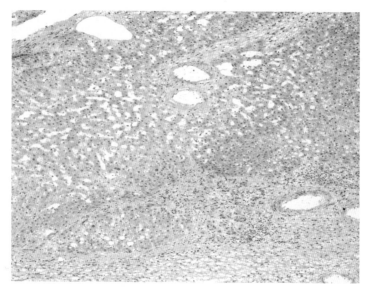

FIGURE 11.7   Focal nodular hyperplasia. The presence of proliferating bile ductules at the periphery of fibrous septa is characteristic (bottom right).

trabecular cord pattern. The hepatocytes near the fibrous septa usually show some evidence of cholate stasis with feathery degeneration, Mallory hyaline, and copper deposition. Steatosis is not uncommon within an FNH. A mild mononuclear cell inflammatory infiltrate is commonly present at the periphery of the fibrous septa along with the proliferating ductules. Needle biopsy frozen section diagnosis of FNH can be challenging, especially without knowledge of clinical impression and radiological features.

As the surgeon usually asks for a frozen section consultation to exclude metastatic tumor, rendering a descriptive frozen section diagnosis stating no evidence of metastatic tumor and deferring further classification of the benign hepatic lesion until the permanent sections is appropriate. Specifically, distinction between FNH and a hepatic adenoma is usually not critical at the time of frozen section consultation. Because FNH is benign, resection is not necessary for asymptomatic lesions if a confident frozen section diagnosis is made on a needle biopsy specimen. Likewise, a negative surgical margin is not critical (5).

Hepatic adenoma. Hepatic adenomas occur only in noncirrhotic livers and never cause an elevation in serum alpha-fetoprotein, two facts that the surgical pathologist should always keep in mind when evaluating a frozen section of a hepatic mass lesion. Large adenomas may cause abdominal pain, while smaller lesions are usually discovered incidentally. Adenomas are much more common in females than males. In fact, the diagnosis of a hepatic adenoma in a male patient who is not taking anabolic steroids should not be made without serious consideration of the possibility of well-differentiated hepatocellular carcinoma (6).

Symptomatic tumors are usually larger than 10 cm in diameter and can be quite a bit larger than that. Adenomas are not encapsulated and are often not well demarcated from the surrounding normal parenchyma. Large adenomas may have large areas of recent and organizing hemorrhage, resulting in a variegated cut surface. Rupture of a very large adenoma through the hepatic capsule can result in catastrophic bleeding, necessitating emergency surgery and a request for a diagnostic frozen section consultation. This dramatic clinical presentation and gross appearance can lead the surgical pathologist to an unwarranted bias toward a malignant diagnosis. Rupture of an adenoma usually occurs in women on oral contraceptives.

Microscopically, adenomas can be difficult to distinguish from normal liver and from well-differentiated hepatocellular carcinoma (6). The key to the distinction from normal liver is the lack of portal tracts within the tumor. Adenomas are composed of cytologically bland hepatocytes arranged in the usual pattern of two-cell-thick trabecular cords. Macrovesicular steatosis is common within the tumor. Characteristically, there are scattered thin-walled vessels dispersed through the lesion. The fibrous septa with proliferating bile ductules characteristic of FNH are absent in hepatic adenoma. Although there may be extensive hemorrhage, necrosis and fibrosis are quite unusual. Mitotic figures should be very rare to absent, but scattered hepatocytes with enlarged hyperchromatic nuclei are not uncommon (Fig. 11.8), and should not raise suspicion of hepatocellular carcinoma. Features that do raise the possibility of well-differentiated hepatocellular carcinoma include mitotic figures, tumor necrosis, significant increase in nuclear cytoplasmic ratio, and trabecular cords that are more than two to three cells thick. In some cases, it may not be possible to definitely exclude HCC; in such cases, a diagnosis of hepatocellular neoplasm may be rendered. In most such cases, the surgeon can proceed with the same operation, complete surgical resection of the tumor.

The hepatocytes of an adenoma tend to merge imperceptibly with those of the surrounding parenchyma, making it difficult to evaluate the adequacy of surgical resection (Fig. 11.8, e-Fig. 11.6). The best way to determine the limits of the lesion is to search for portal tracts, which only occur outside the tumor. Although the surgical aim is always to completely excise the lesion, it is not absolutely critical to do so, since the risk of malignant degeneration is extremely low (7). In rare instances, very large tumors may abut important vascular or biliary structures that make it impossible to completely resect without removal of an unacceptably large portion of the liver.

Hepatocellular carcinoma. The diagnosis of hepatocellular carcinoma by frozen section can be quite challenging. These tumors can develop in either a cirrhotic or noncirrhotic setting, but knowledge of the condition

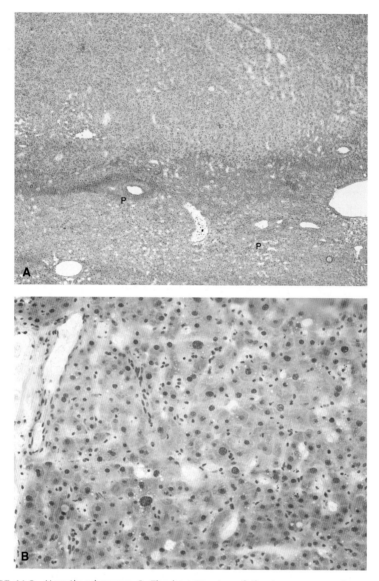

FIGURE 11.8   Hepatic adenoma. **A.** The hepatocytes of the tumor merge imperceptibly with the surrounding normal parenchyma. The presence of a portal tract *(P)* marks the boundary of the tumor. **B.** Note the presence of thin-walled vessels unaccompanied by bile duct as well as the random nuclear atypia.

of the surrounding parenchyma is still valuable as it influences the differential diagnosis. In a noncirrhotic liver, the distinction between well-differentiated hepatocellular carcinoma and hepatic adenoma can be extremely problematic. In some cases, only a diagnosis of hepatocellular neoplasm will be possible, as described aforementioned. Fortunately, this is usually sufficient information for the surgeon to make a decision regarding resection of the mass. On the other hand, in a cirrhotic liver, the problematic distinction is between a well-differentiated hepatocellular carcinoma and a dysplastic nodule. Again, however, narrowing the differential to these two alternatives is usually adequate for the purposes of surgical management. If the surrounding parenchyma is sampled, the presence or absence of cirrhosis and the degree of macrovesicular steatosis should be made known to the surgeon, since this will influence the decision as to how much of the liver can be resected without threat of postoperative liver failure. The presence of cirrhosis and/or significance macrovesicular steatosis adversely affects the synthetic capacity of the liver, and large resections in the face of these two features can be life threatening, particularly in the elderly or very sick patients. If cirrhosis and/or significant steatosis is present, the surgeon may opt to perform an ablative procedure rather than a resection of the tumor.

The microscopic diagnosis of hepatocellular carcinoma rests first upon the recognition of hepatocellular origin of the tumor. Most hepatocellular carcinomas are composed of large polygonal cells with abundant cytoplasm and a large nucleus containing a single prominent nucleolus. Only hepatocytes make bile, so if cytoplasmic bile pigment can be identified the diagnosis of a hepatocellular lesion is ensured. However, care must be taken when assessing for this feature, since inconspicuous isolated normal hepatocytes can be trapped within a metastatic tumor deposit. Better-differentiated examples of HCC typically maintain a trabecular growth pattern, albeit with abnormally thickened cords. The presence of endothelial cells lining the trabecular cords of tumor cells is also characteristic of hepatocellular neoplasms. However, other richly vascular tumors may have arborizing vascular channels that are difficult to distinguish from the endothelial lining of HCC.

Once a tumor has been determined to be of hepatocellular origin, the differential diagnosis is narrowed considerably. As discussed, possibilities in a noncirrhotic liver include FNH, hepatic adenoma, and HCC, while in a cirrhotic liver the differential diagnosis includes a large regenerative nodule, dysplastic nodule, and HCC. This is usually little confusion between FNH and HCC, since FNH is composed of normal-appearing hepatocytes in the usual trabecular arrangement. Distinction between a dysplastic nodule and well-differentiated HCC in the setting of cirrhosis can be very difficult, and rests upon the complete absence of portal tracts in the lesion and the presence of high-grade cytologic features, such as increased cell density and significant nuclear pleomorphism. Fortunately, in most patients the surgical management of these two lesions will be similar. Higher-grade HCCs usually also exhibit thickening of the trabecular cords (Fig. 11.9), numerous mitotic figures, invasion of surrounding portal tracts, tumor necrosis, and/or production of a desmoplastic stroma (8,9). In HCC, the malignant hepatocytes may exhibit macrovesicular steatosis, or contain Mallory bodies or alpha-1-antitrypsin globules. Clear

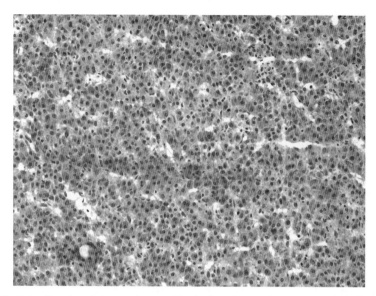

FIGURE 11.9 Hepatocellular carcinoma. The trabecular cords are more than three cells thick, which is diagnostic of malignancy.

cell change is occasionally evident, raising the possibility of metastatic renal cell carcinoma. However, the rich vascular network typical of renal cell carcinoma is not characteristic of HCC. Some HCCs exhibit prominent pseudoglandular arrangement of tumor cells reminiscent of metastatic adenocarcinoma. However, the basal arrangement of nuclei usually evident in adenocarcinoma is not present in HCC.

Liver Biopsy Obtained at the Time of Bariatric Surgery

In many centers, intraoperative liver biopsies are routinely obtained at the time of bariatric surgery for morbid obesity. However, most surgeons agree that frozen section assessment of these biopsies is not usually necessary (10). Steatosis and steatohepatitis are highly prevalent in this patient population, but the presence of these disorders does not influence the surgical management. If there is gross suspicion of cirrhosis, the surgeon may ask for a frozen section specifically to assess the degree of fibrosis (Fig. 11.10). The presence of cirrhosis could result in an unacceptably high risk of postoperative morbidity or death in this patient population, and therefore the surgeon may elect to abort the planned procedure. The surgical pathologist in this situation does not have to worry about the grade of steatohepatitis but rather simply report how much fibrosis is present. Overestimation of fibrosis is common when shallow wedge biopsies are provided, and therefore a needle biopsy might be preferable in this situation (11).

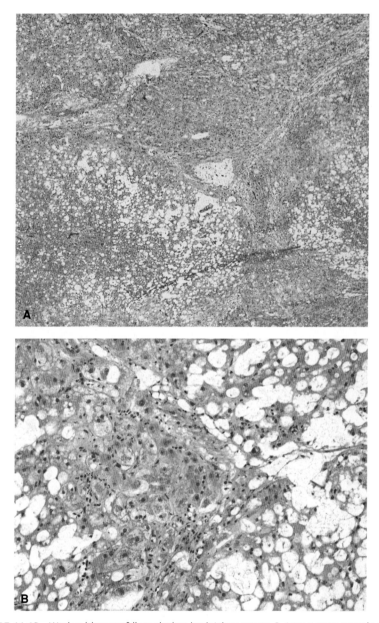

FIGURE 11.10   Wedge biopsy of liver during bariatric surgery. **A.** Low power reveals extensive macrovesicular steatosis and fibrous bands linking portal tracts and central veins. **B.** This
is most likely a central vein with ballooning degeneration of hepatocytes and sinusoidal fibrosis.

TABLE 11.2 Guidelines for Evaluation of Donor Livers
• There is no universally accepted threshold for the degree of macrovesicular steatosis that makes a cadaveric donor organ unusable
• Microvesicular steatosis cannot be reliably recognized in routine frozen sections and there are no convincing data to suggest that its presence adversely affects donor organ function
• A needle biopsy is best to evaluate the degree of macrovesicular steatosis but a wedge biopsy is suitable as long as it is deep (not just a subcapsular sample)
• Biopsies should be transported on saline moistened gauze, *not* submerged in saline
• Other histologic features that should be assessed include the degree of hepatocyte necrosis and fibrosis
• The presence of mild nonspecific chronic portal inflammation is acceptable for transplantation

Cadaveric Donor Biopsy Evaluation

INTRODUCTION. The evaluation of the suitability of a cadaveric liver for use as an allograft is not standardized, but rather varies according to the practice of individual transplant centers, and in many cases, individual transplant surgeons (Table 11.2). The degree of hepatic steatosis is the primary factor that the surgical pathologist is asked to assess at the time of frozen section of a donor liver. Although there is evidence that suggests that gross inspection of the organ by the surgeon as a means to estimate degree of steatosis is not accurate, this practice widely persists (Fig. 11.11) (12). In one study, the positive predictive value of gross inspection was reported to be 71% for severe, 46% for moderate, and 17% for mild steatosis (13). In practice, the gross estimation of the degree of steatosis is only one aspect of the surgeon's decision-making process. The appearance of the organ in regard to color, texture, sharpness of the liver edges, and size all play a part in the evaluation of organ suitability for transplantation. Moreover, the gross appearance is only a small part of the overall evaluation. Clinical features such as the serum transaminase levels, metabolic panel results, donor history (e.g., duration of ICU stay), and the projected total cold ischemia time are all factored in as well. Thus, in U.S. centers, only approximately 30% of potential donor organs are biopsied for frozen section evaluation of suitability (OPTN database).

FROZEN SECTION ASSESSMENT OF DONOR LIVERS. Either wedge or needle biopsy specimen may be submitted for evaluation. Wedge biopsies should be deep rather than broad, such that more than the subcapsular region is sampled. Needle biopsies should be approximately 2 cm in length for

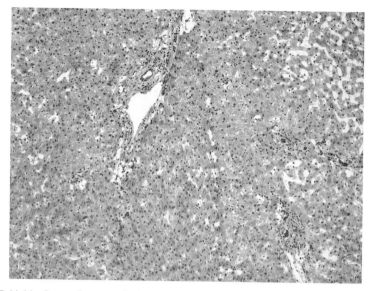

FIGURE 11.11 Donor liver needle biopsy. This liver was turned down by a transplant surgeon because the organ was felt to be too steatotic by gross inspection. However, this biopsy in fact reveals no steatosis, and the liver was utilized successfully for transplantation.

adequate evaluation. The decision to perform a needle or wedge biopsy may depend on the availability of a needle biopsy instrument in the operating room. Also, some pathologists are more comfortable performing and reading a frozen section on a wedge biopsy specimen. The biopsy should be submitted on saline moistened gauze but not submerged in saline, as this causes hepatocyte swelling that makes evaluation for steatosis difficult (Fig. 11.12). The biopsy should be blotted dry before freezing to reduce ice crystal artifact. Standard 4- to 5-μm sections and H&E staining are all that are required. Oil red stains are not necessary and in fact are often misleading, leading to overestimation of degree of steatosis (14). In most centers, only the degree of macrovesicular steatosis is graded. Microvesicular steatosis is quite difficult to recognize on frozen section, and there are data to suggest that surgical pathologists overestimate its severity (15). Several studies have indicated that the degree of microvesicular steatosis has no significant impact on posttransplant graft function (12,16,17).

The degree of macrovesicular steatosis is estimated by the pathologist as the percentage of hepatocytes throughout the biopsy that contain a large lipid droplet (Figs. 11.13–11.15). Ice crystal artifact can produce uniform medium-sized vacuoles within hepatocytes that resemble fat vacuoles (Fig. 11.16). One clue to the recognition of this artifact is the uniformity of this change through the biopsy (or a part of the biopsy). Although a variety of ancillary techniques have been proposed to increase the accuracy of the recognition and grading of steatosis in donor biopsies,

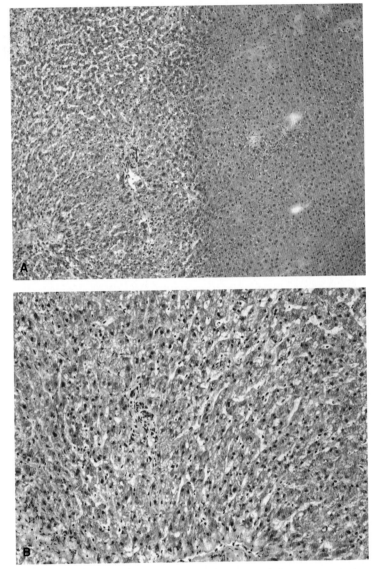

FIGURE 11.12 **A.** This wedge biopsy was partially submerged in saline, producing the artifactual hepatocyte swelling evident in the left side of the photograph. **B.** The artifactual distortion caused by submersion of the tissue in saline makes it difficult to assess for steatosis.

at present routine H&E stains and visual estimation remain the standard of care (18).

The surgical pathologist should be aware that the there is no rigid threshold for the degree of steatosis that precludes use of the organ. In the literature, steatosis more than 60% is usually reported as causing a significant increased risk of primary nonfunction (PNF). In the

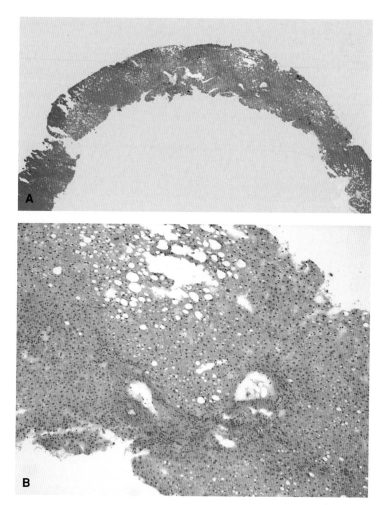

FIGURE 11.13 **A&B** Donor needle biopsy. There is 10% macrovesicular steatosis in this biopsy.

early-transplant era, PNF rates of up to 80% were reported when severely steatotic donor organs were used. When these organs were excluded the overall rate of PNF dropped dramatically. The risk of PNF is regarded as the primary reason to avoid heavily steatotic donor organs (13,19). It is thought that lipid metabolites escape from hepatocytes during the period of cold ischemia and cause damage to sinusoidal endothelial cells. During the immediate posttransplant period, there is resultant patchy hepatocyte ischemic necrosis, which ultimately cascades to produce graft infarction.

The significance of a diagnosis of steatohepatitis in a donor biopsy has not been addressed in the liver transplant literature to date. It would

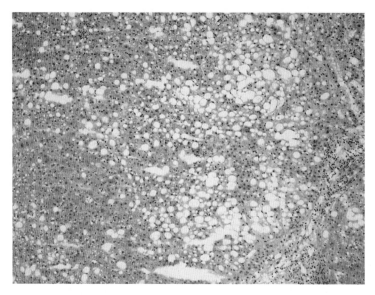

FIGURE 11.14   Donor liver wedge biopsy. There is 50% macrovesicular steatosis. This liver was not utilized for transplantation.

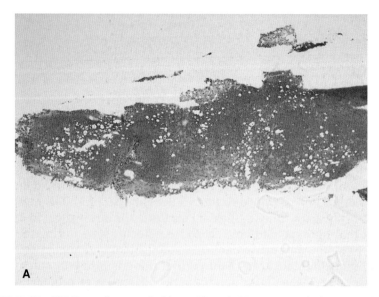

FIGURE 11.15   **A&B** Donor liver needle biopsy. There is 25% macrovesicular steatosis in this biopsy. This liver was successfully utilized for transplantation. (*continued*)

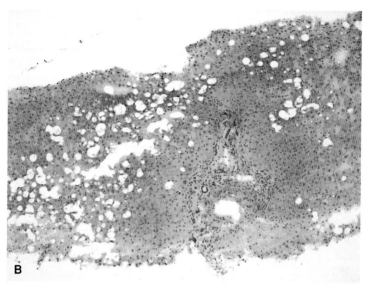

FIGURE 11.15 (*Continued*)

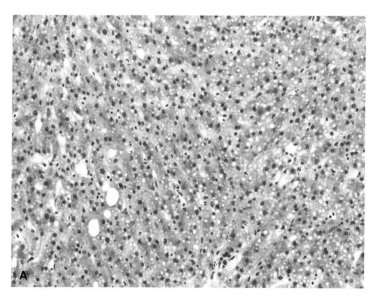

FIGURE 11.16 **A&B** Donor liver wedge biopsy. The tissue was wet when it was frozen, resulting in artifactual medium-sized vacuoles in each hepatocyte. This artifact should not be mistaken for steatosis. (*continued*)

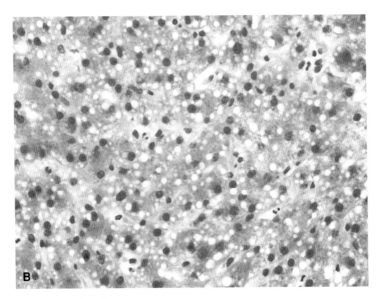

FIGURE 11.16 *(Continued)*

seem reasonable that the presence of significant hepatocyte injury, in the form of prominent hepatocyte ballooning, Mallory bodies, centrilobular fibrosis, and/or lobular inflammation, might increase the risk of posttransplant allograft dysfunction (even if the degree of steatosis was not great), but this scenario has not yet been studied. It is also true that recognizing these histologic features of steatohepatitis in a frozen section is not trivial (Fig. 11.17).

Lesser degrees of donor organ steatosis may not significantly increase the risk of PNF but there are data to suggest an increased risk of poor graft function in the immediate posttransplant period (20,21). While the graft damage is usually transient, poor initial function may result in significant risk of acute renal failure and mortality, particularly in high-risk recipients (those of older age with multiorgan failure at the time of transplant). Thus, a surgeon may be happy to use a donor organ with 40% macrovesicular steatosis for a young, otherwise healthy patient with fulminant hepatic failure because of acetaminophen toxicity, but turn down the same organ for use in a 65-year-old male patient with alcoholic cirrhosis and severe cardiovascular disease. The pathologist should recognize that there is no "magic cutoff" for the degree of steatosis that makes a particular organ usable or not. Rather, the degree of steatosis is merely one of a complex mix of factors involving the donor, recipient, and a large number of other graft factors (including the presence of anomalous vascular or biliary anatomy).

OTHER DONOR BIOPSY PATHOLOGY. Macrovesicular steatosis is not the only pathologic process that should be assessed in the frozen section

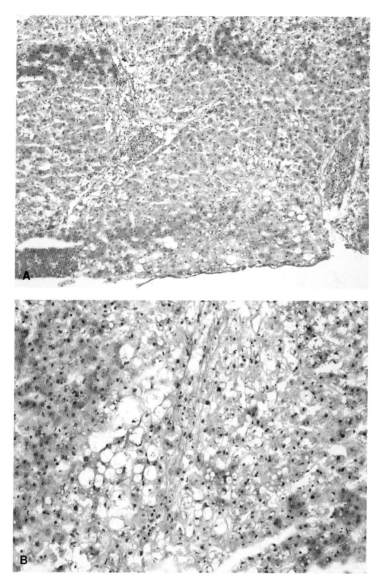

FIGURE 11.17 **A&B** Donor liver needle biopsy. This biopsy exhibits features of nonalcoholic steatohepatitis, with ballooned hepatocytes and lobular inflammation in addition to the 30% macrovesicular steatosis. This liver was not utilized for transplantation. The permanent sections confirmed the diagnosis of non-alcoholic steatohepatitis (NASH).

evaluation of donor biopsies. The presence of hepatocyte necrosis should be reported if present. Centrilobular necrosis may be subtle if it is recent. It causes slight shrinkage and smudginess of hepatocytes with condensation of the cytoplasm and mild nuclear hyperchromasia (Fig. 11.18). It most often occurs as a consequence of hepatic ischemia related to the use

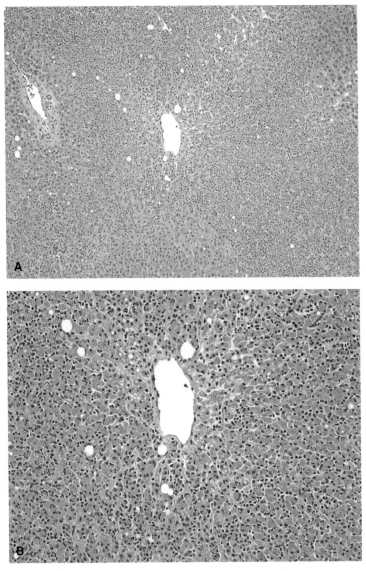

FIGURE 11.18 Donor liver wedge biopsy. **A.** At low power, this biopsy appears relatively normal. **B.** Higher power reveals extensive recent hepatocyte necrosis because of the use of high doses or pressor agents.

of high dose of pressor agents and/or the development of hypernatremia and other metabolic derangements preceding the development of brain death. At an earlier stage, there may be random individual apoptotic hepatocytes (acidophil bodies), but this degree of hepatocyte injury probably will not cause significant posttransplant graft dysfunction (Fig. 11.19). Although not yet a common practice in the United States, the use of organs

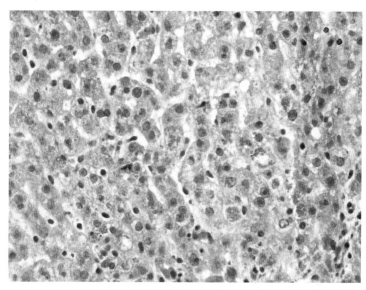

FIGURE 11.19 Donor liver wedge biopsy. There are randomly scattered acidophil bodies because of the use of high doses of pressor agents. This liver was utilized for transplantation for a patient with fulminant hepatic failure. Although graft function was poor initially, the recipient ultimately did well.

donated after cardiac death has been explored in regions where there is a particular shortage of cadaveric grafts or where the concept of donation after brain death is not accepted. Careful assessment of the degree of centrilobular hepatocyte necrosis is particularly important in this situation (22).

A mild degree of portal mononuclear cell infiltration is acceptable, and the cause is generally never learned (donors are screened for HBV and HCV hepatitis). It is possible that chronic intermittent biliary obstruction, celiac disease, or prior resolved episodes of HBV or HCV hepatitis are responsible for these infiltrates in some donor organs (Fig. 11.20). The degree of portal inflammation is often overestimated in donor biopsies (13). Unexplained heavy portal or lobular inflammatory cell infiltrates should be mentioned to the surgeon and likely will lead to rejection of the organ. Likewise significant fibrosis (stage 2 or worse) is generally unacceptable, except for recipients with fulminant hepatic failure.

Recently the practice of utilizing HCV positive grafts for recipients with cirrhosis because of chronic HCV hepatitis has been explored. This strategy has been utilized particularly in patients with cirrhosis and hepatocellular carcinoma, and in patients undergoing retransplantation for recurrent HCV cirrhosis. Donor organ biopsies are often obtained for frozen section evaluation in this situation. The pathologist should report the degree of necroinflammatory activity (interface activity and lobular inflammation) and fibrosis. There are no agreed upon guidelines for what grade

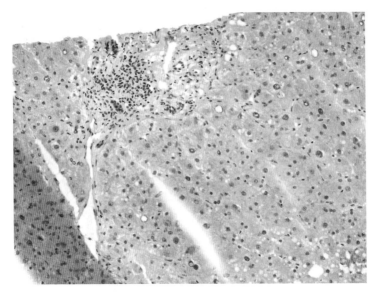

FIGURE 11.20 Donor liver needle biopsy. This mild degree of portal inflammation does not preclude use of this liver for transplantation. The cause of the inflammation is usually never determined.

and stage of chronic hepatitis is acceptable for use as an allograft, and the decision is individualized based on recipient factors and individual transplant center practice.

Available data indicate that the use of donor organs from patients with hereditary hemochromatosis or secondary iron overload does not cause posttransplant allograft dysfunction (provided that significant fibrosis had not developed). Likewise, undetected alpha-1-antitypsin disease in an allograft does not appear to lead to increased posttransplant morbidity or mortality (23,24).

MASS LESIONS IN DONOR ORGANS. On rare occasions, small mass lesions may be identified by the transplant surgeon at the time of organ harvest. Bile duct hamartomas (von Meyenburg complexes), even if numerous, are not a contraindication to the use of an organ (25). Likewise, bile duct adenomas are regarded as benign lesions that pose no risk to the recipient. These two lesions are often recognized by the surgeon as small well-circumscribed subcapsular nodules and are often ignored. Walled-off hyalinized granulomas are also regarded as innocuous lesions, but the presence of numerous caseating or necrotizing granulomas should probably lead to rejection of the donor organ. Small cavernous hemangiomas are common incidental findings (~1% of livers at autopsy), and are usually easily recognized by both surgeons and surgical pathologists (26).

The presence of FNH is also not a contraindication to the use of a donor organ, as these lesions have no malignant potential. Small lesions often do not exhibit a central scar with an obvious abnormal vessel, so the diagnosis rests upon recognition of the "focal cirrhosis" pattern of fibrous septa containing proliferating bile ductules. Although not well studied, organs containing hepatic adenomas have also been utilized after complete excision of the mass. Naturally, confident exclusion of a well-differentiated hepatocellular carcinoma must be ensured, and this can be problematic by frozen section examination. Thus, many of these organs end up not being used.

FROZEN SECTIONS ON LIVER ALLOGRAFTS. In general, frozen sections should not be performed on percutaneous needle biopsy specimens from allograft livers. Diagnosis and grading of acute cellular rejection are not reliable on frozen section slides, and many other processes can be missed or misinterpreted. For instance, a low-grade posttransplant lymphoproliferative disorder may be mistaken for acute cellular rejection or recurrent HCV hepatitis. Also, the permanent sections of a biopsy specimen utilized for frozen section are almost always small and of poor quality, precluding full assessment. On rare occasions, a frozen section may be indicated to assess for widespread parenchymal necrosis and the need to list the patient for retransplantation. Even in this situation the recognition of very recent hepatocyte necrosis can be problematic. Since rapid same-day processing is available in most pathology departments, the need for frozen section consultation is not necessary.

GALLBLADDER AND EXTRAHEPATIC BILIARY TREE

Gallbladder and Extrahepatic Biliart Tree: Major Intraoperative Question

The major intraoperative question involves the margins as they are most likely to be submitted for frozen section diagnosis. The margin should be entirely frozen and both dysplasia and invasive carcinoma should be carefully sought.

Gallbladder and Extrahepatic Biliary Tree: Frozen Section Interpretation

CHOLANGIOCARCINOMA. Proper surgical management of these tumors can be quite complex, sometimes necessitating a pancreaticoduodenectomy for ampullary carcinomas and cholangiocarcinoma arising from the distal common bile duct, resection of the proximal extrahepatic bile ducts for extrahepatic cholangiocarcinoma arising from the more proximal extrahepatic biliary tree, or partial hepatectomy for intrahepatic and hilar cholangiocarcinomas. Frozen section diagnosis is usually not performed on the main tumor mass; rather the surgical margins are likely to be submitted. As the bile duct has numerous peribiliary glands, the histologic evaluation of bile duct margins for invasive carcinoma can be extremely difficult. In one recent study of 90 patients who initially had negative margins by frozen section, 8 (9%) had invasive carcinoma on the permanent sections. Those with wide true-negative margins had a disease-specific survival of 56 months compared with 36 months for those with narrow negative margins and 32 months for those with positive margins (27). Thus, frozen section analysis is important in predicting survival postoperatively. In another study specifically of the intrahepatic bile duct margin of hilar cholangiocarcinoma, the accuracy, sensitivity, and specificity of the frozen section diagnosis of invasive tumor was 56.5%, 75.0%, and 46.7% respectively (28). The high error rate is largely because of the marked reactive changes produced by mucosal erosion and intense acute inflammation, which is often a consequence of stent placement.

When faced with a bile duct margin, it is important to receive an oriented specimen with the margin side indicated by the surgeon. The margin side is placed up on the chuck and frozen sections are cut. Beside the usually cytomorphologic features, the malignancy, the presence of perineural invasion can be extremely helpful in differentiating benign from malignant glands (Fig. 11.21). Nuclei four times the size of clearly benign nuclei is usually indicative of malignancy. Finally, benign peribiliary glands are not located near large vessels in contrast to invasive cancer.

The interobserver agreement in the diagnosis of dysplasia throughout the GI and biliary tract on routine H&E sections among expert GI pathologists is only fair to moderate, thus the diagnosis of dysplasia in frozen sections is fraught with difficulty. However, in contrast to invasive carcinoma, the presence of dysplasia at the margin does not seem

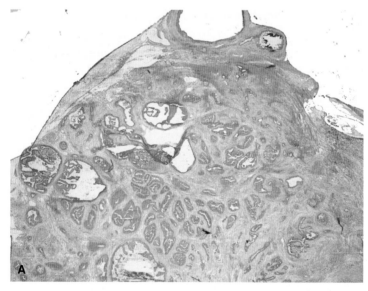

FIGURE 11.21 Cholangiocarcinoma. **A.** The common bile duct margin is involved by adenocarcinoma with malignant glands extending to the serosal surface. **B.** Note the presence of perineural invasion. (*continued*)

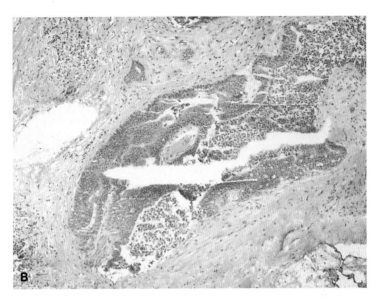

FIGURE 11.21 *(Continued)*

to affect disease-specific survival (29). Nevertheless, if unequivocal dysplasia is found, it should be reported as the surgeon may attempt to resect and additional margin is possible. Low-grade dysplastic biliary epithelium has enlarged hyperchromatic nuclei with nuclear overlap and increased mitotic figures. In contrast, high-grade dysplasia is architecturally complex with cribriforming and gland fusion. In addition, the nuclei lose polarity and have irregular membranes (Fig. 11.22). However, caution should be given when interpreting specimens taken from areas in which a stent was placed as inflamed biliary epithelium can closely mimic dysplasia. Because of the difficulty in interpretation of these biopsies, the opinions of multiple pathologists are often required to render a diagnosis.

GALLBLADDER ADENOCARCINOMA. The gallbladder is rarely submitted for frozen section diagnosis. The risk of adenocarcinoma is much higher in gallbladders removed for cholecystitis in patients older than 50 years. During an elective cholecystectomy, a gallbladder with unusual gross features is occasionally submitted for intraoperative consultation. Close analysis of the gallbladder specimen is important to indentify the suspicious lesion. Induration or wall thickening may be the only gross evidence of malignancy.

When analyzing the frozen section, care must be made to not interpret dysplasia extending into Rokitansky-Aschoff sinuses as invasive carcinoma. Gallbladder adenomyoma can also be mistaken for invasive adenocarcinoma. The bland cytology of this glandular component of the

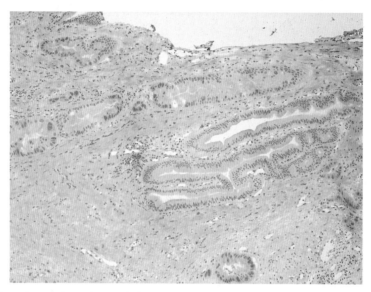

FIGURE 11.22 High-grade dysplasia. The common bile duct margin demonstrates high-grade dysplasia. The nuclei are enlarged and irregular and clearly different from the unremarkable adjacent biliary epithelium.

lesion and the surrounding bundles of smooth muscles are the keys for proper diagnosis.

PANCREAS

Pancreas: Introduction

Frozen section evaluation of pancreatic malignancies, like those of the biliary tree, is notoriously difficult. Malignancies involving the head of the pancreas are often small, diffuse infiltrative lesions, and may be difficult to diagnose preoperatively. Interpretation of the frozen section of such lesions is complicated by the frequent presence of coexistent chronic pancreatitis, atrophy, and reactive changes in the native pancreas, and the often minor degree of cytologic atypia displayed by infiltrating pancreatic adenocarcinomas. These features make primary diagnosis of such tumors, or evaluation of resection margins for such pancreatic cancers among the most difficult frozen sections to interpret. It is critical that the submitting surgeon be aware of these factors, since discrepancies between frozen section and permanent section diagnosis are almost certain to occur at some time in this area. Although some studies suggest that frozen section is a reliable mechanism for establishing the initial diagnosis of pancreatic neoplasms (30), it is our strong feeling that the surgeon should be strongly discouraged from taking a patient with a pancreatic head mass to surgery without a primary tissue diagnosis, since establishing a definitive diagnosis at the time of surgery by frozen section may be extremely difficult. In many cases, the mass lesion must be removed surgically regardless of the diagnosis, and therefore the surgeon may be willing to wait until permanent section for the final answer.

Pancreas: Major Intraoperative Questions

The types of specimens that may be received for intraoperative examination during surgery involving the pancreas include needle biopsies from mass lesions undiagnosed preoperatively, lymph nodes or peritoneal biopsies to exclude metastatic disease, enucleated intrapancreatic mass lesions, distal pancreatectomy specimens (with or without splenectomy), pancreaticoduodenectomies (Whipple resections), and total pancreatectomies.

In some cases, a patient with a pancreatic mass lesion identified radiographically may be taken to surgery without a tissue diagnosis, and the pathologist may be called upon to make a diagnosis intraoperatively by frozen section of a needle core or wedge biopsy. This scenario is becoming increasingly uncommon, however, as endoscopic techniques such as endoscopic ultrasound continue to improve, and allow sampling of an increasing number of previously inaccessible sites.

Once a diagnosis of pancreatic malignancy is established, the surgeon will generally explore the abdomen searching for sites of possible metastatic disease (liver, lymph nodes, and peritoneum). Suspicious lesions are often sent for frozen section because the presence of metastatic disease will stop any attempt at curative resection, and will result in the surgeon performing at most a palliative procedure. An exception to this rule is the finding of a metastatic well-differentiated endocrine neoplasm. Metastatic islet cell tumors do not preclude surgical procedures aimed at resecting as much tumor as possible.

When curative resection for a pancreatic malignancy is being performed, the resection margin(s) may be sent for frozen section evaluation. The most commonly evaluated specimens are the pancreatic parenchymal and bile duct margins. The uncinate or retroperitoneal margin, though important from a staging and prognostication standpoint, is generally not sent for frozen section evaluation because the surgeon usually cannot resect additional tissue from this area even if the margin is positive.

Frozen sections are also sometimes performed to guide the extent of pancreatectomy in infants undergoing surgery for correction of congenital hyperinsulinism. In these patients, frozen section has been used to distinguish between focal and diffuse forms of hyperinsulinism, and thereby guide the extent of surgery, possibly preventing postoperative diabetes mellitus (31). This procedure is generally only carried out in a few specialized centers, and is not one that will be encountered by the pathologist in general surgical pathology practice.

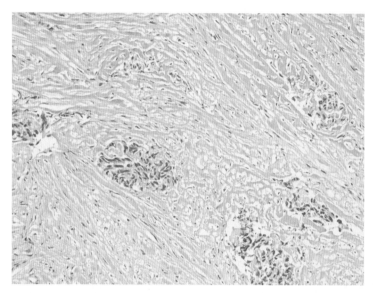

FIGURE 11.23 Severe electrocautery artifact is sometimes present at the pancreatic parenchymal margin. In cases such as this, it is impossible to determine whether the ductal structures that are present are malignant or not. If additional noncauterized tissue in unavailable, the diagnosis in such cases must be deferred to permanent sections.

Frozen Section Interpretation

A diagnosis of pancreatic adenocarcinoma, as mentioned earlier in the chapter, can sometimes be quite difficult to establish on frozen section. The reason for this is pancreatic ductal carcinomas, in particular, are often associated with extensive chronic pancreatitis, atrophy, fibrosis, and reactive changes. The result is the presence of ductal structures of varying type within the microscopic field. These are frequently artifactually distorted either as a result of crushing or electrocautery artifact, making their characterization that much more difficult (Fig. 11.23). This problem applies to both surgical resection margins as well as biopsies to establish a primary diagnosis.

There are a number of histologic features, however, that when carefully applied, may be used to assist in differentiating neoplastic and non-neoplastic ductal structures in frozen material. Most of these criteria were established in the now classic paper published by Hyland and coworkers in 1981 (32). In this study, Hyland et al. prospectively reviewed 64 frozen sections and their associated permanent sections, and established three major and five minor criteria for the diagnosis of pancreatic carcinoma. The major criteria were (i) nuclear size variation of 4:1 of greater in ductal epithelial cells, (ii) incomplete ductal lumens, and (iii) disorganized duct distribution (Fig. 11.24). Minor criteria are as follows: (i) large irregular nucleoli in epithelial cells, (ii) necrotic glandular debris, (iii) glandular mitoses, (iv) glands unaccompanied by connective tissue stroma within

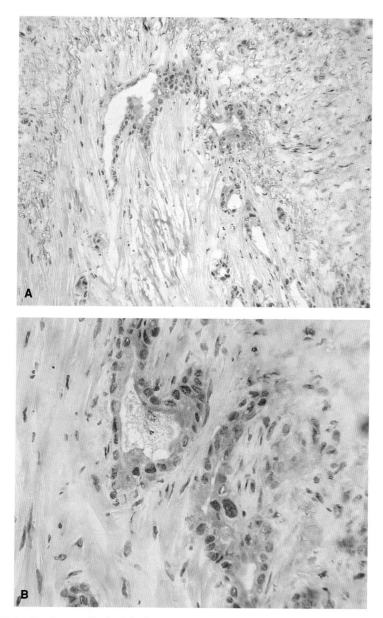

FIGURE 11.24 Pancreatic ductal adenocarcinoma. **A.** Low-power view of this frozen section taken from a resection margin positive for ductal adenocarcinoma demonstrates ducts with variably sized nuclei and incomplete glands. **B.** Higher-power view of a duct in which the largest epithelial nucleus exceeds four times the area of the smallest nucleus. **C.** Another group of ducts shows a ductal cell with a nucleus at least four times larger than that of the adjacent cells. **D.** An incomplete gland is present in which the glandular lumen contacts the periglandular stroma. (*continued*)

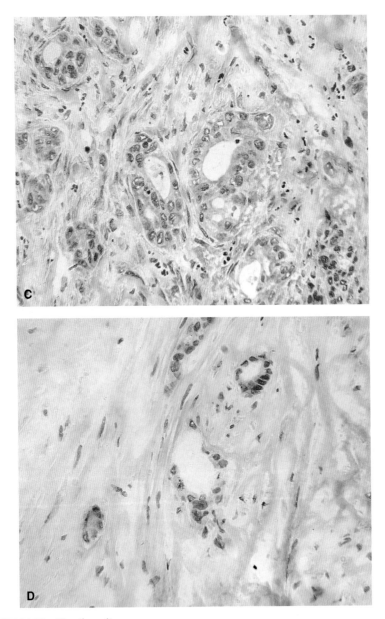

FIGURE 11.24 (*Continued*)

smooth muscle bundles (in periampullary biopsies), and (v) perineural invasion (Fig. 11.25).

Other useful features for establishing the diagnosis of pancreatic adenocarcinoma in areas of chronic pancreatitis include the presence of ductal structures in areas where they should not normally be found. The normal pancreatic architecture is lobular, and this anatomy is maintained

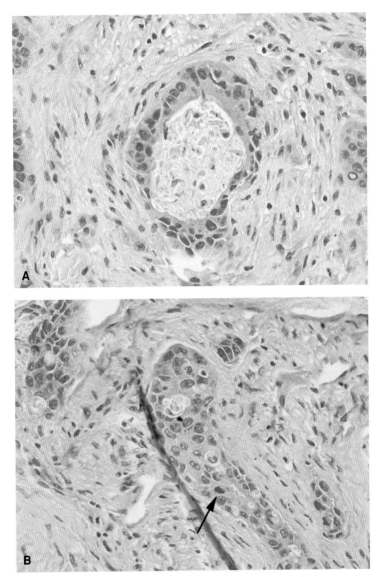

FIGURE 11.25 Pancreatic ductal adenocarcinoma. **A.** Malignant gland containing luminal debris. **B.** Mitotic figures can sometimes be seen in adenocarcinomas (arrow), and when identified may be helpful in establishing the diagnosis since they are rarely seen otherwise. **C.** Ductal adenocarcinomas sometimes demonstrate large irregular nucleoli. Luminal debris is also present in the gland in this photograph. (*continued*)

even in the face of atrophy in chronic pancreatitis (Fig. 11.26). In particular, the larger muscular vessels are located in the interlobular connective tissue, an area normally devoid of glandular structures. The presence of glands in close proximity to such vessels is an indication of invasion and malignancy (Fig. 11.27).

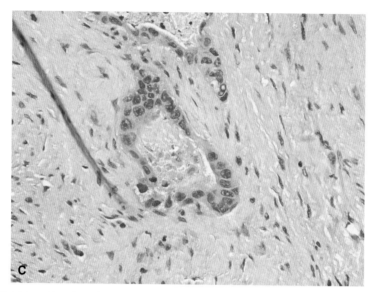

FIGURE 11.25 *(Continued)*

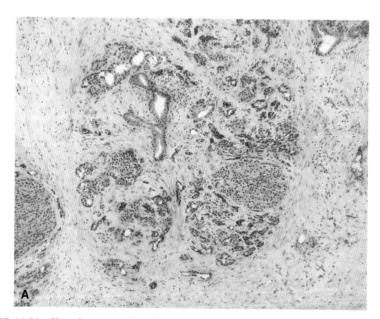

FIGURE 11.26 Chronic pancreatitis. **A.** Low-power photomicrograph demonstrating the lobular architecture of the pancreas, even when there is atrophy secondary to chronic pancreatitis. **B.** A muscular vessel is present in the interlobular septum. **C.** Higher-power view of another vessel between the pancreatic lobules. Note that there are no ductal structures adjacent to the vessel. *(continued)*

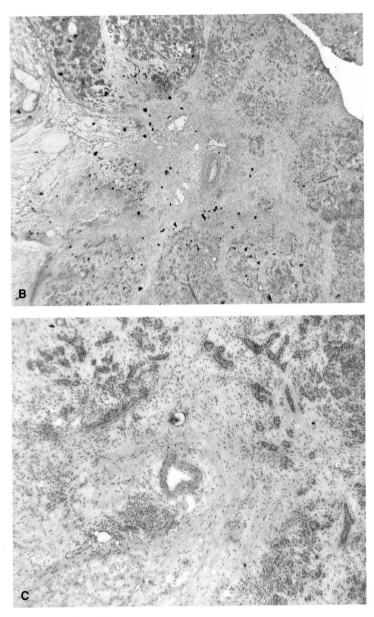

FIGURE 11.26 (*Continued*)

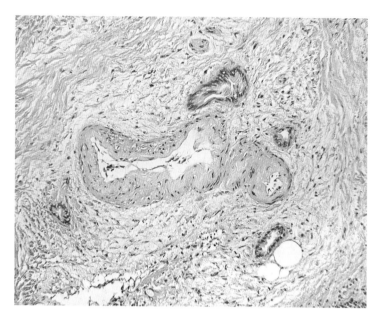

FIGURE 11.27 Invasive pancreatic adenocarcinoma. Neoplastic ducts are present next to this muscular vessel in the pancreas. There is cautery artifact present, making evaluation of the cytologic features of the epithelial cells difficult. A diagnosis of adenocarcinoma can be made despite this fact since these glands are present in a location where normal ducts should not be.

It is important to remember, however, that some forms of chronic pancreatitis (e.g., autoimmune or lymphoplasmacytic sclerosing pancreatitis) may themselves produce pancreatic mass lesions. Up to 2.5% of pancreaticoduodenectomies performed for presumed pancreatic cancer, in fact, turn out at final diagnosis to represent autoimmune pancreatitis (33–35). The morphologic hallmarks of autoimmune pancreatitis include periductal infiltration by a dense population of lymphocytes and plasma cells, neutrophilic destruction of duct epithelium, venulitis, and periductal fibrosis. These features may sometimes be appreciated on frozen section (Fig. 11.28).

Margins of resection may also be evaluated in patients undergoing surgical resection for mucinous cystic neoplasms. Intraductal papillary mucinous neoplasms, in particular, demonstrate differing patterns of ductal involvement, which may determine the extent of surgical resection necessary for their removal. As a result, frozen section of resection margins may be performed to determine the need for further resection. Current evidence suggests that the presence of nondysplastic or borderline intraductal papillary mucinous neoplasms in a duct at the resection margin does not warrant resection of additional pancreas (36) (Fig. 11.29). However, high-grade dysplasia or invasive carcinoma involving the

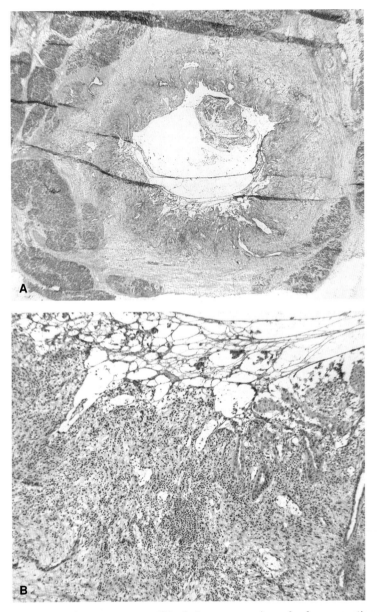

FIGURE 11.28   Autoimmune pancreatitis. **A.** Low-power view of a frozen section taken from the pancreatic parenchymal margin of a pancreas resected for presumed carcinoma. The main pancreatic duct is surrounded by a dense inflammatory infiltrate. **B.** On higher power, this infiltrate is composed of lymphocytes and plasma cells. **C.** There is also neutrophilic infiltration of the ductal epithelium. The diagnosis of autoimmune pancreatitis was suggested at the time of frozen section, and was confirmed by elevated serum IgG4 levels and characteristic features on permanent sections. (*continued*)

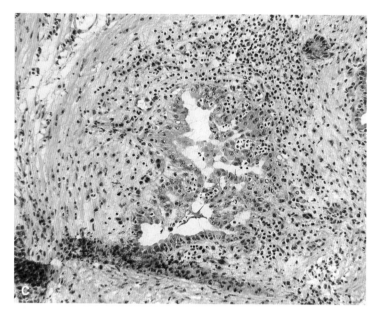

FIGURE 11.28 (*Continued*)

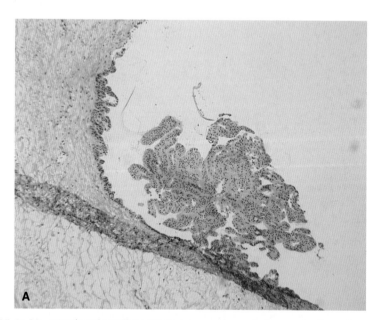

FIGURE 11.29 Intraductal papillary mucinous neoplasm. **A.** Frozen section of a resection margin in a patient with a cystic lesion of the pancreas. A papillary structure is present in a dilated pancreatic duct. **B.** On higher power, no features of high-grade dysplasia are present. **C.** In the surrounding tissue, scattered ductal structures were present, which showed severe cautery artifact. It was unclear at the time of frozen section whether these represented atrophic ducts or infiltrating carcinoma, and the diagnosis with regard to invasive carcinoma was deferred. On permanent sections, invasive ductal carcinoma was present in the pancreatectomy specimen, but did not involve the margin of resection. (*continued*)

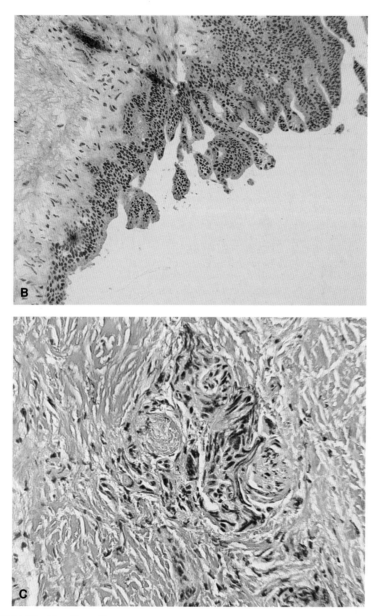

FIGURE 11.29 (*Continued*)

margin of resection should prompt the surgeon to remove additional tissue or perform a completion pancreatectomy. Therefore, resection margins from patients with cystic neoplasms should be evaluated for the presence of cystic ductal dilation, degree of dysplasia, and the presence of absence of invasive carcinoma. The invasive carcinomas arising in association with intraductal papillary mucinous neoplasms may be of two types, typical pancreatic ductal adenocarcinoma, with the features described earlier in the chapter, and mucinous adenocarcinoma, similar to that occurring in the colon or appendix.

REFERENCES

1. Brunt EM. Benign tumors of the liver. *Clin Liv Dis.* 2001;5:1–15.
2. Rakha E et al. Accuracy of frozen section diagnosis of liver mass lesions. *J Clin Pathol.* 2006;59:352–354.
3. Allaire GS et al. Bile duct adenoma: a study of 152 cases. *Amer J Surg Pathol.* 1988; 12:708–715.
4. Makhlouf HR et al. Diagnosis of focal nodular hyperplasia of the liver by needle biopsy. *Hum Pathol.* 2005;36:1210–1216.
5. Cherqui D et al. Management of focal nodular hyperplasia and hepatocellular adenoma in young women: a series of 41 patients with clinical, radiological, and pathological correlations. *Hepatology.* 1995;22:1674–1681.
6. Bioulac-Sage P et al. Pathological diagnosis of liver cell adenoma and focal nodular hyperplasia: Bordeaux update. *J Hepatol.* 2007;46:521–527.
7. Micchelli STL et al. Malignant transformation of hepatic adenomas. *Mod Pathol.* 2008;21:491–497.
8. Kondo F et al. Biopsy diagnosis of well differentiated hepatocellular carcinoma based on new morphologic criteria. *Hepatology.* 1989;9:751–755.
9. Wanless IR. Liver biopsy in the diagnosis of hepatocellular carcinoma. *Clin Liver Dis.* 2005;9(2):281–285.
10. Guarrera JV et al. Discovery of diffuse biliary microhamartomas during liver procurement. *Liver Transpl.* 2007;13:1470–1471.
11. Markin RS et al. Frozen section evaluation of donor livers before transplantation *Transplantation.* 1993;56:1403–1409.
12. Fernandez ED et al. Intraoperative assessment of liver organ condition by the procurement surgeon. *Transplant Proc.* 2007;39:1485–1487.
13. Adams R et al. The outcome of steatotic grafts in liver transplantation. *Transplant Proc.* 1991;23:1538.
14. Nocito A et al. When is steatosis too much for transplantation. *J Hepatol.* 2006; 45:494–498.
15. Lo IJ et al. Utility of liver allograft biopsy obtained at procurement. *Liver Transpl.* 2008;14:639–646.
16. Fishbein TM et al. Use of livers with microvesicular fat safely expands the donor pool. *Transplantation.* 1997;64:248–251.
17. Crowley H et al. Steatosis in donor and transplant liver biopsies. *Hum Pathol.* 2000;31:1209–1213.
18. Fiorini RN et al. Development of an unbiased method for the estimation of liver steatosis. *Clin Transplant.* 2004;18:700–706.
19. D'Alessandro AM et al. The predictive value of donor liver biopsies for the development of primary non-function after orthotopic liver transplantation. *Transplantation.* 1991; 51:157–163.
20. Rerez-Dega JA et al. Influence of degree of hepatic steatosis on graft function and postoperative complications of liver transplantation. *Transplant Proc.* 2006;38:2468–2470.
21. Nikeghbalain S. Does donor's fatty liver change impact on early mortality and outcome of liver transplantation. *Transplant Proc.* 2007;39:1181–1183.
22. Deshpande R, Heaton N. Can non-heart-beating donors replace cadaveric heart-beating liver donors? *J Hepatol.* 2006;45:499–502.

23. Pungpapong S et al. Clinicopathologic findings and outcomes of liver transplantation using grafts from donors with unrecognized and unusual diseases. *Liver Transpl.* 2006; 12:310–315.

24. Dabkowski PL et al. Site of principal metabolic defect in idiopathic hemochromatosis: insights from transplantation of an affected organ. *Br Med J.* 1993;306:1726–1728.

25. Shalhub S et al. The importance of routine liver biopsy in diagnosing nonalcoholic steatohepatitis in bariatric patients. *Obesity Surg.* 2004;14:54–59.

26. Padoin AV et al. A comparison of wedge and needle biopsies in open bariatric surgery. *Obesity Surg.* 2006;16:178–182.

27. Endo I et al. Clinical significance of intraoperative bile duct margin assessment for hilar cholangiocarcinoma. *Ann Surg Oncol.* 2008;15:2104–2012.

28. Horimi OY et al. Study of the intrahepatic surgical margin of hilar bile duct carcinoma. *Hepatogastroenterology.* 2002;49:625–627.

29. Wakai T et al. Impact of ductal resection margin status on long-term survival in patients undergoing resection for extrahepatic cholangiocarcinoma. *Cancer.* 2005;103:1210–1216.

30. Doucas H, Neal CP, O'Reilly K, et al. Frozen section diagnosis of pancreatic malignancy: a sensitive diagnostic technique. *Pancreatology.* 2006;6:210–214.

31. Suchi M, Thornton PS, Adzick NS, et al. Congenital hyperinsulinism. Intraoperative biopsy interpretation can direct the extent of pancreatectomy. *Am J Surg Pathol.* 2004;28:1326–1335.

32. Hyland C, Kheir SM, Kashlan MB. Frozen section diagnosis of pancreatic carcinoma. A prospective study of 64 biopsies. *Am J Surg Pathol.* 1981;5:179–191.

33. Wakabayashi T, Kawaura Y, Satomura Y, et al. Clinical study of chronic pancreatitis with focal irregular narrowing of the main pancreatic duct and mass formation comparison with chronic pancreatitis showing diffuse irregular narrowing of the main pancreatic duct. *Pancreas.* 2002;25:283–289.

34. Yadav D, Notohara K, Smyrk TC, et al. Idiopathic tumefactive chronic pancreatitis: clinical profile, histology, and natural history after resection. *Clin Gastroenterol Hepatol.* 2003;1:129–135.

35. Abraham SC, Wilentz RE, Yeo CJ, et al. Pancreaticoduodenectomy (Whipple resections) in patients without malignancy: are they all "chronic pancreatitis"? *Am J Surg Pathol.* 2003;27:110–120.

36. Tanaka M, Chari S, Adsay V, et al. International consensus guidelines for management of intraductal papillary mucinous neoplasms and mucinous cystic neoplasms of the pancreas. *Pancreatology.* 2006;6:17–31.

12

THE SKIN

CHRISTOPHER KINONEN AND VIJAYA B. REDDY

INTRODUCTION

Skin cancer is the most common form of cancer in the United States, with basal cell carcinoma (BCC) and squamous cell carcinoma (SCC) being the two most frequent types of dermatologic malignancies. Melanoma is the third most common type of skin cancer. In 2004, melanomas and other nonepithelial skin cancers accounted for 50,039 new cancer diagnoses and 7,952 deaths (1). Surgical resection is the mainstay of treatment for these lesions, and many can be resected without frozen section analysis. In fact, routine frozen section analysis on all skin specimens is not clinically indicated, can be very time and resource intensive, and in many cases is not cost effective (2). A portion of skin lesions, however, requires frozen section margin assessment and potentially primary diagnosis if it is unclear if the lesion is benign versus malignant or primary versus metastatic. Overall, accuracy of frozen section analysis of skin specimens has been reported to range from 71% to 99% (3,4). Literature evaluating the usage of frozen section for specific skin cancers primarily focuses on BCC, SCC, melanoma, and Mohs micrographic surgery.

For BCC, complete excision results in 99% cure rate while recurrence rates for incompletely excised tumors have been reported to be between 19% and 67% (5). Incompletely excised SCC has similar recurrence rates ranging from 30% to 60% (6); thus, accurate assessment of resection margins is critically important. In a study of 450 patients, Cataldo et al. reported complete excision, without the aid of frozen section, in 90% of patients with primary tumors having clinically distinct borders. However in recurrent tumors, where microscopic foci can extend beyond clinically detectable margins, 24% of patients had incomplete excisions when frozen section analysis was not performed. The authors concluded that routine frozen section examination of primary lesions with clinically distinct borders was of little benefit. For recurrent lesions, when margins were clinically indistinct, or when tissue preservation was deemed important however, frozen section may be of value (2). Similar conclusions regarding frozen section usage for skin specimens have been documented in other literature as well (3,4,7).

Thus for nonmelanoma skin cancers, there are several general indications for frozen section. Appropriate lesions for frozen section include those that are large, clinically ill defined, recurrent, or have an infiltrating growth pattern. Other indications include lesions located in areas where wide margin excision is not possible or tissue sparing is desirable, such as the eye, forehead, cheek, nose, and ears. Eyelid tumors, in particular, have shown benefit from frozen section margin assessment (2). Additionally, frozen section diagnoses may be indicated if reconstructive surgery is to be performed immediately following resection or if there is a question as to whether the lesion is benign or malignant. Although metastatic disease to the skin is uncommon, it has been reported to occur in 5% to 10% of internal malignancies (8) where it can occur as the initial manifestation of an undiscovered malignancy or potentially as the first indication of metastasis of a previously diagnosed and treated tumor. These lesions may also require frozen section as a means of primary diagnosis.

Malignant melanoma represents a different type of skin cancer, and frozen section analysis should be discouraged for suspected melanocytic lesions. Depth of invasion, presence of ulceration, and margin assessment are critically important factors for diagnosis, prognostication, and treatment of melanoma. Freezing causes tissue distortion, which can preclude accurate measurement of depth of invasion on the permanent sections. Similarly, the ability to determine cytologic atypia is compromised with freezing. This can be especially problematic when assessing intraepidermal spread of single atypical melanocytes or on sun-damaged skin that frequently contains melanocytic hyperplasia. Determining the degree of atypia in these specimens can be difficult enough on permanent sections, and hence freezing artifact should not be added as an additional pitfall. Rare cases when freezing may be appropriate include when the lesion is in a cosmetically important area, such as the face, or in a difficult-to-heal surgical site (e.g., acral sites such as the heel). In general, however, frozen section evaluation of melanocytic lesions should be discouraged and if performed, the surgeon should be made aware of the pitfalls and limitations. The use of frozen section in Mohs micrographic surgery to evaluate melanomas is discussed in the chapter.

Literature evaluating the role of frozen section in nonneoplastic lesions such as necrotizing fasciitis, toxic epidermal necrolysis/erythema multiforme (TEN/EM), calciphylaxis, vasculitis, and infections is less extensive. Nevertheless, skin biopsies to evaluate for these life-threatening conditions are frequently requested in a tertiary care setting. Early, accurate diagnosis in these cases is essential to implement potentially life-saving therapies. In a study by Majeski et al., 43 patients had bedside biopsies to evaluate for necrotizing fasciitis by frozen section. Twelve of the forty-three patients were diagnosed with necrotizing fasciitis. Each patient had immediate surgical debridement and supportive therapy, and all patients survived (9).

Mohs Micrographic Surgery

Mohs micrographic surgery is a procedure for select skin cancers intended to resect tumors with complete assessment of surgical margins and minimal wound size. It involves removing the tumor in stages and microscopically examining the entire resection margin. Since tissue sparing is a primary goal of the surgery, it can be useful in anatomically and cosmetically important sites, such as the eyes, ears, nose, and lips. It can also be used for recurrent tumors or lesions, which have a high likelihood of recurrence (10,11). Mohs surgeons are trained to histologically evaluate their resections so general surgical pathologists are typically not involved with frozen section examination. This is not the case at all medical centers however, so it is important for the surgical pathologists to be aware of this procedure as an alternative to traditional dermatologic resections. The exact procedure and method of cutting the tissue for frozen section is primarily dependent on the specific Mohs surgeon as well as the lesion itself; thus, the following information is intended to provide a general overview of the process. The procedure is typically done as an outpatient procedure using local anesthesia. The surgeon begins by removing visible cancer along with a thin rim of surrounding tissue extending peripherally and deep to the lesion. The specimen is then oriented, sectioned, and inked before standard frozen section processing. The specimen is cut such that 100% of the surgical margin is evaluated. The location of each positive margin is then carefully mapped so that the procedure can be repeated in those areas as many times as necessary to completely excise the tumor. A final margin can then be taken from around the tumor and sent for permanent sections to confirm the initial frozen section margin assessment (12).

Extensive literature exists pertaining to the indications and therapeutic success of Mohs surgery. It has been reported to be superior to standard resection for nonmelanoma malignancies that display features that increase the risk of recurrence (11). Success is probably largely dependent on the experience and skill of the Mohs surgeon as well as associated histotechnologists who prepare and process the tissue. As stated previously, it is commonly performed in sites where cosmesis is of concern. In addition, it can be used for recurrent tumors or tumors with increased risk of recurrence. The procedure has been utilized with multiple types of nonmelanoma malignancies including, but not limited to, BCC, SCC, dermatofibrosarcoma protuberans (DFSP), atypical fibroxanthoma, microcystic adnexal carcinoma, and leiomyosarcoma (13).

Mohs micrographic surgery is also increasingly performed on certain lower-risk subtypes of melanoma, such as lentigo maligna melanoma and melanoma in situ, and in melanomas that are clinically ill defined. However its usage with melanocytic lesions remains controversial primarily because of the questionable accuracy of detecting atypical melanocytes on the frozen section (11). This can be especially difficult on chronically sun-damaged skin, which frequently contains prominent melanocytes with pleomorphic hyperchromatic nuclei (14).

Other areas of controversy also exist with regard to Mohs surgery. Critics cite the lack of prospective randomized trials to evaluate the Mohs technique, potential overestimation of cure rates, and the effectiveness of alternative therapies (e.g., cryosurgery, excision, and electrosurgery) (13). Nevertheless, Mohs surgery remains a widely utilized technique and frozen section examination is an integral part of the process.

Specimen Types and Biopsy Techniques

Common skin biopsy techniques that may be submitted for frozen section analysis include punch biopsies, superficial and deep shave biopsies, curettage, and excisions. There are specific clinical indications for each biopsy type, which can assist with the differential diagnosis. Additional factors that influence biopsy technique include anatomic site, size and shape of the lesion, cosmesis, and general health of the patient (8).

A punch biopsy is often performed to evaluate for inflammatory dermatoses, but may also be used to completely excise small lesions or sample large lesions. Punch biopsies can be 2 to 8 mm in diameter. The first step, as with any skin specimen, is to orient, measure, and describe the specimen, including skin color and presence or absence of lesions. If lesions are present, describe the size, type (e.g., papular, vesicular, or macular), color, borders (irregular vs well-circumscribed), and distance to the closest margin. Ink the margin of resection, a single color is adequate. For 3-mm punch biopsies, the entire lesion can be submitted without sectioning. Larger biopsies require bisecting or trisecting, so as to have sections no larger than 3 mm in thickness. Maintain vertical orientation when sectioning. Ideally, at least two levels should be obtained for permanent sections.

Shave biopsies can either be superficial or deep, and are used primarily for nonmalignant lesions in which the key histologic changes are expected to be present in the epidermis or superficial dermis, such as seborrheic keratoses, solar keratoses, and benign nevi. Shave biopsies can also be used to diagnose BCCs, since this technique will leave the lower portion of the dermis intact and amenable to subsequent complete resection. First, orient, measure, describe, and ink resection margins of the specimen. If the specimen is more than 3 mm in diameter, bisect or trisect so that vertical orientation is maintained. Generally, the entire specimen should be submitted for frozen section. Order two levels on the permanent block of the frozen section.

Curettage specimens are meant to be diagnostic, usually for seborrheic keratosis, actinic keratosis, or BCC, and may consist of multiple variably sized tissue fragments. These specimens may be difficult or impossible to orient as they are usually superficial and without architectural landmarks. Note the number of fragments (or an estimate of the number), aggregate measurement, and color. Inking is not necessary since tissue fragmentation precludes margin evaluation. Order two levels on the permanent block of the frozen section.

Excisions are generally received as skin ellipses, although they may be round or irregularly shaped. These procedures are most commonly performed to remove malignant tumors such as BCC, SCC, melanoma, or atypical melanocytic nevi. They may also be used for nonmalignant lesions such as panniculitis. Excisions are usually oriented in some manner (e.g., with suture) and the purpose of frozen section in most instances is to assess margins. Less frequently, a primary diagnosis will be requested. Although excisions can be very large, most of the ones that are sent for frozen section evaluation are small enough so that the entire specimen can be submitted.

The initial steps to process an excision are to orient, measure (in three dimensions), and describe the specimen including skin color. Also note the presence of lesions, their size, type (e.g., papular, vesicular, or macular), color, and borders (irregular vs well-circumscribed). There is typically a suture, or another identifying mark, that is designated 12 o'-clock. If no orientation is provided, speak with the surgeon to clarify if orientation is needed. Next, ink the resection margins so as to maintain orientation. If no orientation is provided, the entire margin can be inked one color, otherwise, ink so that margins in four quadrants can be identified microscopically. Inking is a crucial step because the location of involved margins must be correctly identified, as well as the distance of the tumor from the margin. Next, serially section the entire specimen along the short axis, in 3-mm intervals, to evaluate the relationship of the lesion(s) to the margins as well as to identify any additional deep lesions. In most cases, the entire specimen should be submitted for frozen section. If the specimen is larger and cannot be processed in four blocks, a cross-section through the center and perpendicular margins of the tips can be submitted for frozen sections. The closest margin should always be evaluated with either an en face or perpendicular cut. The remainder of the specimen can be processed for permanent sections (8,15).

If any of the margins are positive for tumor, an additional strip of skin will often be reexcised and also sent for frozen section. It is important that the true resection margin be identified, either by the surgeon directly or by some other indication (e.g., suture), so that ink may be properly applied. The additional material may then be submitted enface or horizontally sectioned (7).

Generally, sections should be no larger than 0.3 cm in thickness, and are placed on a thin layer of media that is prefrozen on a chuck. Length and width are dependent on chuck size but should probably not be larger than 1 cm × 1 cm. If multiple pieces are submitted, they should each be placed in the same plane (7).

Cytologic preparations are not necessary for margin evaluation but may be required in cases of primary diagnoses. If performed, a touch preparation as well as a smear are recommended on separate slides. These are particularly useful in diagnosis of small blue cell tumors involving the skin, such as Merkel cell carcinoma and lymphoma.

The standard stain for frozen section processing in general surgical pathology laboratories is hematoxylin-eosin (H&E). Toluidine blue is an alternate stain used by some Mohs surgeons, particularly for BCC, because it is more rapid (7). Toluidine blue metachromatically stains the mucopolysaccharides and hyaluronic acid in the stroma present around BCC tumor cells. This yields a characteristic magenta color that contrasts with the dark blue stain of the actual tumor cells. This staining is said to help differentiate BCC from tangentially cut hair follicles and benign follicular tumors (16). It can also be helpful if there is obscuring inflammation. For cytologic preparations, a Romanowsky stain is the standard.

Basal Cell Carcinoma

BCC typically affects older individuals, most often occurring as single lesions on sun-exposed hair-bearing skin, particularly the face. BCC may appear as small well-circumscribed pearly tan-gray papules devoid of scale. Over time, the lesions enlarge and tend to ulcerate giving the characteristic "rodent ulcers" (8). Most often, these lesions have been previously biopsied, and a specimen will be sent for frozen section to assess excisional margins. Less frequently, a primary diagnosis may be requested.

The general histopathology of BCC shows prominent nests and islands of basaloid cells attached to the undersurface of the epidermis, invading to varying degrees into the dermis. These nests will show characteristic palisading of basaloid cells at the periphery. The tumor cells tend to be uniform with frequent mitoses. Other important features include the presence of clefting artifact between the epithelium and stroma as well as the connective tissue stroma itself that proliferates around the tumor. This stroma tends to be composed of parallel bundles of young fibroblasts, occasionally in a mucinous background. There are multiple variants of BCC including superficial, nodular, sclerosing (morphea-like), keratotic, adenoid, and fibroepithelial (8). The most common subtype evaluated for frozen section at Rush University Medical Center is the nodular subtype and less commonly the superficial and sclerosing variants.

The nodular subtype of BCC shows a nodular proliferation of uniform basophilic tumor cells with characteristic peripheral palisading. The nodules are larger and typically extend deeper into the dermis than with the superficial variant (Fig. 12.1).

Superficial BCC shows buds and irregular proliferations of tumor cells, with peripherally palisading nuclei, attached to the undersurface of the epidermis with minimal penetration into the dermis (Fig.12.2). There can be fibroblasts arranged around the tumor cells as well as a mild to moderate inflammatory cell infiltrate in the upper dermis. The overlying epidermis is often atrophic. In contrast to most subtypes of BCC, the superficial subtype occurs predominantly on the trunk rather than the face (8).

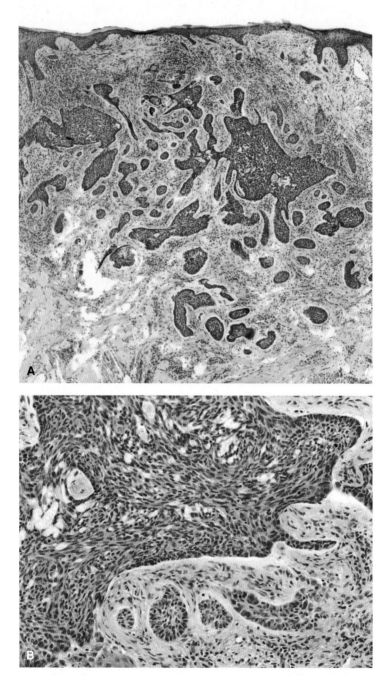

FIGURE 12.1   Basal cell carcinoma, nodular type. **A.** Deeply infiltrative nodules of basaloid cells. **B.** On higher power, peripheral palisading and beginning of stromal retraction artefacts can be seen.

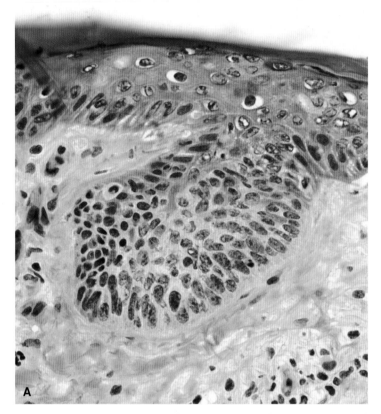

FIGURE 12.2 Basal cell carcinoma, superficial type. **A.** A single elongated nest of basaloid cells emanating from the undersurface of the epidermis. **B.** The presence of characteristic retraction artifact around this focus of superficial basal cell carcinoma is more diagnostic. (*continued*)

Sclerosing (morphea-like) BCC demonstrates irregular thin branching strands of basaloid cells infiltrating into a dense fibrotic stroma (Fig. 12.3).

DIAGNOSTIC PITFALLS. As previously stated, margin assessment is the most common intraoperative question addressed with frozen section analysis of BCC. A primary diagnostic pitfall can be distinguishing BCC from tangentially cut hair follicles, which can appear as nests of basaloid cells. Clues to the presence of BCC include stromal changes and cleft formation around the tumor nests. Hair follicles are surrounded by a dense fibrous sheath, in contrast to the looser parallel bundles of young fibroblasts surrounding BCC (Fig. 12.4).

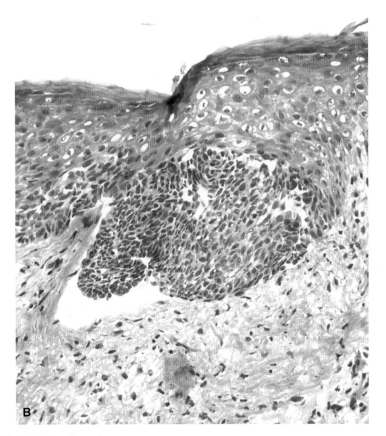

FIGURE 12.2 (*Continued*)

On specimens from sun-damaged skin submitted for frozen section, a potential diagnostic pitfall is mistaking the buds of atypical keratinocytes of actinic keratosis for BCC. However, the cells of actinic keratosis have more abundant eosinophilic cytoplasm and the buds lack typical peripheral lacking and retraction artifacts (Fig. 12.4).

Squamous Cell Carcinoma

SCC commonly affects men older than 60 years, favoring sun-exposed areas including the upper face, ears, lower lip, and the dorsum of hands. In addition to sun exposure, risk factors include x-ray therapy, local carcinogens such as tars and oils, and hereditary diseases such as xeroderma pigmentosa (17). SCC also arises in scars from burns and in stasis ulcers. Clinically, lesions generally present as a slow-growing indurated nodule that may develop central ulceration (8). As with BCC, many of these lesions have been previously diagnosed with biopsy, and the frozen section question will involve margin assessment of an excision.

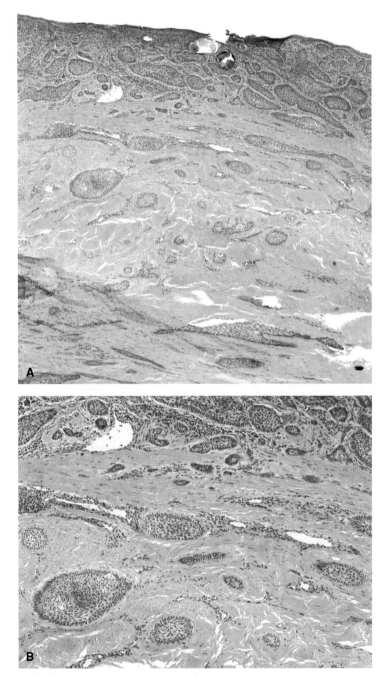

FIGURE 12.3 Basal cell carcinoma, sclerosing (morphea) type. **A.** Nests and cords of basaloid cells infiltrating in collagenous stroma. **B.** Higher power shows basaloid cells with peripheral palisading.

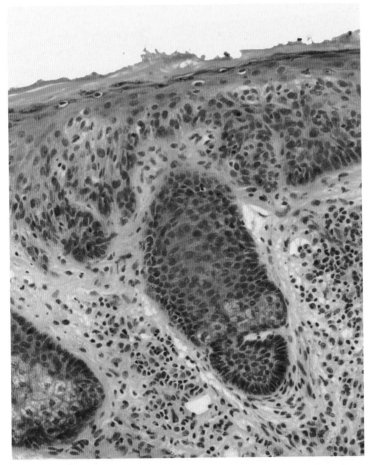

FIGURE 12.4 Actinic keratosis. This image shows a proliferation of keratinocytes of the lower part of the epidermis. In contrast to basal cell carcinoma, these cells have more abundant eosinophilic cytoplasm. Notice the follicular germ that can also mimic a nest of basal cell carcinoma. However, the relationship to a sebaceous lobule and the cellular stroma (papilla) surrounding the nest helps in identifying the follicular unit.

There are classic morphologic features of SCC in situ and invasive SCC. In situ lesions show downward epidermal proliferation of squamous epithelial cells with full-thickness cellular atypia. The atypical cells are large with a moderate amount of eosinophilic cytoplasm, nuclear enlargement, hyperchromasia, and presence of intercellular bridges (Fig. 12.5). Invasive lesions can have the same features plus infiltration into at least the reticular dermis (Fig. 12.6). The degree of differentiation is determined by the degree of keratin pearl formation (8,17).

DIAGNOSTIC PITFALLS. Variants of SCC can present diagnostic pitfalls. Spindle cell SCC closely resembles atypical fibroxanthoma. A differentiating

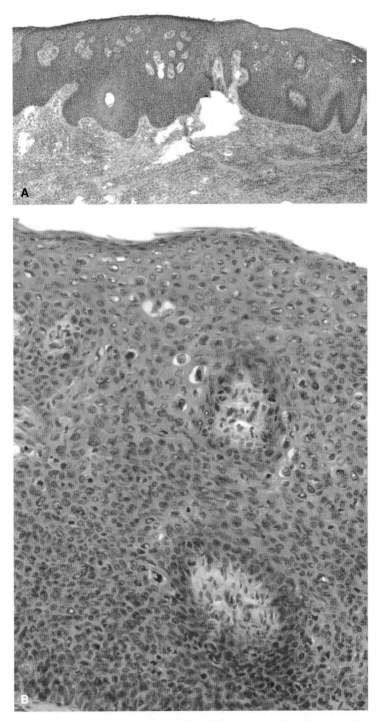

FIGURE 12.5 Squamous cell carcinoma in situ. **A.** Low-power view demonstrates marked increase in the thickness of the epidermis, which shows no maturation of the keratinocytes. **B.** High-power view highlights the keratinocytic atypia, dyskeratosis, and mitotic figures.

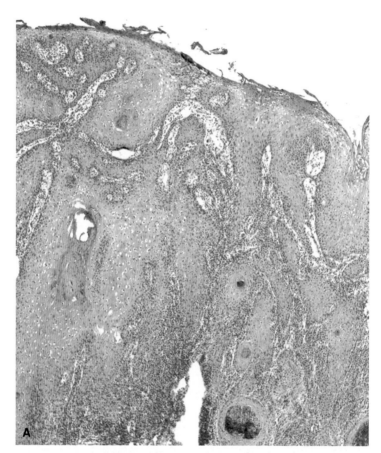

FIGURE 12.6 Squamous cell carcinoma, invasive. **A.** Low-power view shows an irregular proliferation of squamous epithelium. **B.** High-power view shows keratin pearls characteristic of squamous cell carcinoma. (*continued*)

histologic feature is the presence of intercellular bridges in SCC, which are lacking in atypical fibroxanthomas. These two lesions may be indistinguishable on frozen section however, and immunohistochemistry may be required on permanent sections (17). More importantly, the margin requirements at the time of frozen section are identical for both the entities, and the distinction is not critical as long as spindle cell melanoma is not a consideration.

Poorly differentiated SCC can also be a diagnostic challenge, since these lesions often lack keratinization and so the site of origin may be difficult to ascertain. This is not an issue with margin analysis but rather when a primary diagnosis is requested.

Pseudoepitheliomatous hyperplasia (pseudocarcinomatous hyperplasia) occurs at the edges of ulcers, in burns, deep fungal infections,

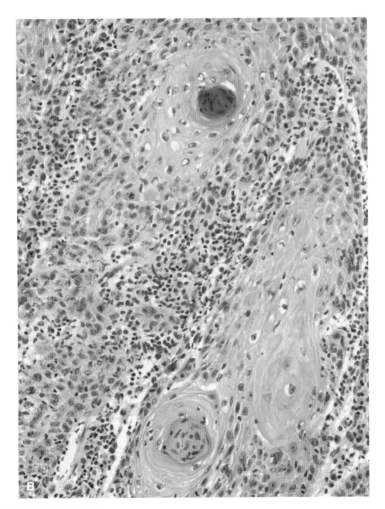

FIGURE 12.6 (*Continued*)

pyodermias, hidradenitis suppurativa, and other chronic proliferative in-flammatory processes (8). The lesion produces epithelial hyperplasia that closely resembles well to moderately differentiated SCC; however cellular atypia is usually minimal with less nuclear hyperchromasia and individual cell keratinization than in SCC. An added key differentiating feature is the presence of an inflammatory infiltrate such as neutrophilic microabscesses and granulomas, which are suggestive of an inflammatory process instead of SCC. Similar difficulty may be encountered by prior biopsy sites, which may show inflammatory features, despite the presence of SCC. Differenti-ating the two lesions can be difficult, and multiple biopsies may be re-quired in addition to clinical correlation (8).

Finally, cautery artifact can present a diagnostic pitfall by obscuring atypical epithelial cells, particularly with in situ lesions. A tangentially cut

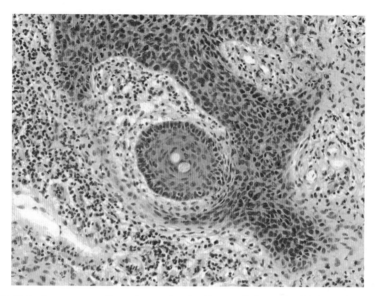

FIGURE 12.7 Squamous cell carcinoma in situ. Tangentially embedded section showing atypical squamous epithelial cells extending into the dermis in a pseudoinvasive pattern.

section of in situ SCC can show areas that can be mistaken for invasion (Fig. 12.7).

Melanoma

Melanomas present as asymmetric irregularly pigmented lesions with ill-defined borders. Up to 20% originate in association with nevi, including congenital nevi and Clark's dysplastic nevi. Histopathology shows broad, poorly circumscribed, asymmetric proliferations of large atypical melanocytes. These occur as single atypical cells and nests, which may be distributed unevenly, at the dermoepidermal junction. Single melanocytes can extend into the overlying epidermis in a pagetoid pattern (Fig. 12.8). Superficial spreading melanoma refers to the histologic pattern where a prominent pagetoid spread is present. Nodular melanoma refers to a thick, more advanced melanoma involving the dermis (17).

As discussed previously, frozen section evaluation of melanoma specimens, particularly for primary diagnoses, is difficult and should generally be discouraged. Margin assessment is occasionally requested, particularly in cosmetically sensitive areas and with narrow margins.

DIAGNOSTIC PITFALLS. The primary diagnostic pitfall involves differentiating melanoma in situ from junctional melanocytic hyperplasia on sun-damaged skin. This differentiation can be difficult even on permanent sections, and freezing artifact further complicates the process. Architectural and cytologic features should be evaluated in conjunction with the

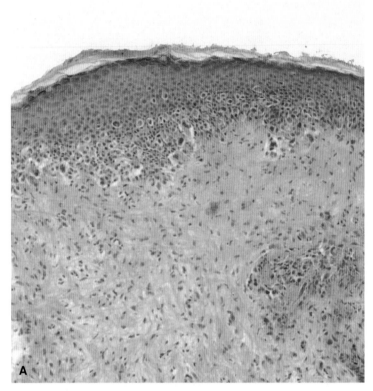

FIGURE 12.8 Malignant melanoma: **A.** Irregular nests and solitary units of large melanocytes at the dermoepidermal junction. Extension around the adnexal epithelium may give a false impression of dermal invasion. **B.** On high magnification, the melanocytes have pale cytoplasm (pagetoid) and atypical nuclei and extend above the junction in a pagetoid pattern. (*continued*)

clinical history. In frozen section evaluation for margins, clues to the diagnosis of melanoma in situ include a contiguous proliferation of uniformly atypical melanocytes that are larger than normal melanocytes. It is helpful if the sections contain part of the melanoma so that the lateral progression and the point of changes to normal skin can be assessed.

Other Cutaneous Neoplasms

Although BCC and SCC are the most common lesions evaluated by frozen section, other less common cutaneous neoplasms seen at the University of Chicago Hospitals and Rush University Medical Center include angiosarcoma, DFSP, and Merkel cell carcinoma.

Angiosarcoma commonly affects males in the sixth to seventh decade of life with a predilection for the face, scalp, and neck. Angiosarcoma can also occur secondary to chronic lymphedema (Stewart-Treves syndrome)

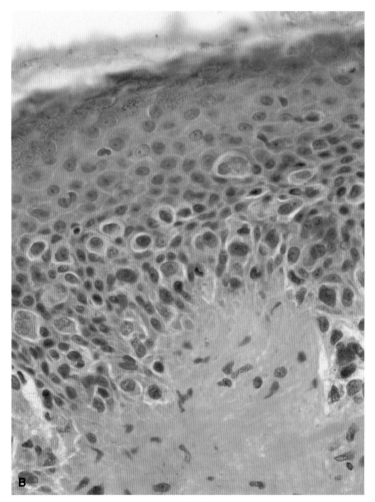

FIGURE 12.8 (*Continued*)

and as a complication of radiodermatitis or arising from the effects of skin trauma or ulceration (8). There are rare occurrences in postmastectomy patients. Clinically, patients present with dusky irregular erythematous plaques. The lesions tend to progress rapidly leading to ulceration and hemorrhage. Histopathology shows a tumor consisting of a proliferation of malignant epithelial cells that appear as an asymmetric collection of angulated, irregular vascular spaces infiltrating between collagen bundles. The endothelial cells lining the vascular spaces have hyperchromatic, irregular nuclei; prominent nucleoli; and a high mitotic rate. Commonly, there is also a lymphocytic infiltrate and adjacent dilated vascular channels (Fig. 12.9). Frozen sections may be requested for margin assessment, especially for lesions from the head and neck area. Again, the ability to

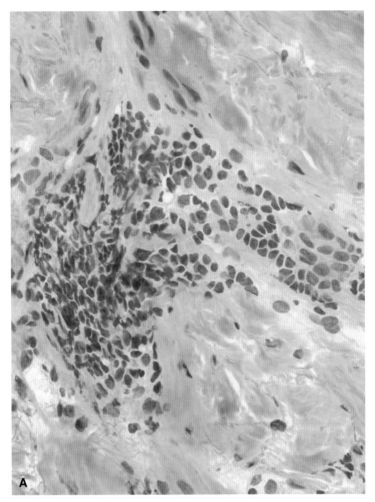

FIGURE 12.9 Angiosarcoma. **A.** Frozen section for evaluation of margins in a case of angiosarcoma shows an infiltrate of cells with hyperchromatic nuclei. In the absence of vascular lumina, the diagnosis of angiosarcoma requires a high degree of suspicion. **B.** In other areas, irregular vascular channels lined by atypical endothelial cells can be seen, which aids in the diagnosis. (*continued*)

compare areas of unequivocal angiosarcoma with the changes closer to the margins would be most helpful. Differential diagnoses to consider include epithelioid hemangioma, Kaposi sarcoma, and intravascular papillary endothelial hyperplasia (17).

DFSP can occur at any age, but young adults are most commonly affected, males more often than females. DFSP presents as an indurated plaque or subcutaneous mass on which multiple congested, firm nodules arise, occasionally with ulceration (8). It most frequently involves the

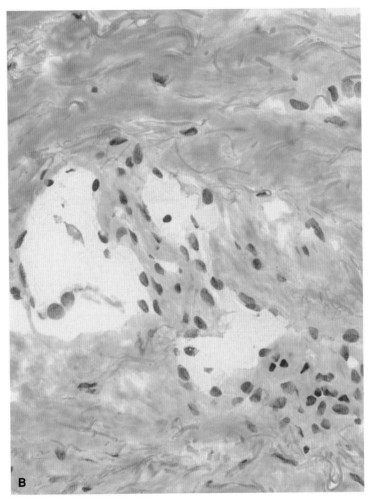

B

FIGURE 12.9 *(Continued)*

trunk and extremities, less commonly the head and neck. It is a locally aggressive tumor with destruction of surrounding tissue. The neoplasm originates in the subcutis or dermis, and is composed of relatively bland, homogenous spindle cells arranged in monotonous sheets or a storiform pattern (Fig. 12.10). The tumor cells may be arranged around small blood vessels, and areas of myxoid degeneration are common. Mitoses may or may not be prominent. Multinucleated giant cells, xanthoma cells, and foci of inflammation may also be seen. On frozen sections, the spindle cell proliferation of DFSP can be subtle, and the presence of transition from tumor to the uninvolved areas can be helpful in assessing the surgical margins. Differential diagnoses to consider include fibrous histiocytoma (dermatofibroma), fibrosarcoma, and malignant fibrous histiocytoma (17).

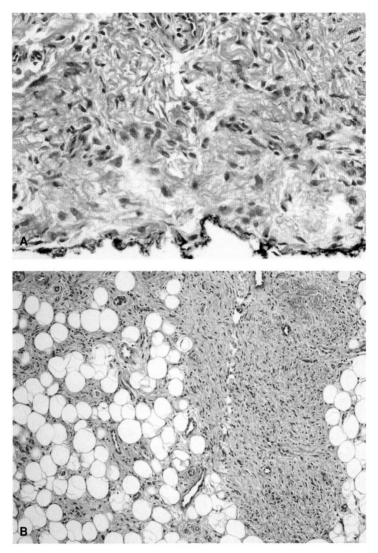

FIGURE 12.10 Dermatofibrosarcoma protuberans. **A.** Frozen section shows rather bland spindle-shaped cells close to the inked margin. **B.** Permanent section of the tumor shows spindle-shaped cells infiltrating the subcutaneous fat in a lacelike pattern, characteristic of dermatofibrosarcoma protuberans.

Merkel cell carcinoma is an uncommon neoplasm with neuroendocrine differentiation. Cutaneous involvement is usually on the head or extremities where it presents as a solitary nodule or rarely as multiple nodules. Skin ulceration is uncommon. Histopathology shows a dermal nodule composed of small round blue cells with scant cytoplasm and irregular nuclei with uniformly distributed chromatin (Fig. 12.11). Tumor cells

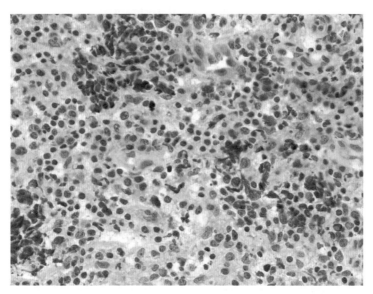

FIGURE 12.11   Merkel cell carcinoma. Frozen section shows a small blue cell proliferation some of which show crush artifact. Preserved cells show minimal cytoplasm and hyperchromatic nuclei with coarse chromatin typical of neuroendocrine differentiation.

are arranged in sheets or trabeculae and may form pseudorosettes. Nucleoli are inconspicuous and nuclear molding may be present. Mitotic figures and individually necrotic tumor cells are common. Stroma between the nests of tumor cells is scant. The overlying epidermis may show varying degrees of atypia and occasionally SCC. Frozen sections may be requirement in the assessment of surgical margins and occasionally for diagnosis. Differential diagnoses to consider include metastatic small cell carcinoma, malignant lymphoma, and other primitive neuroectodermal tumors such as Ewing sarcoma and neuroblastoma.

Metastatic Malignancies

Various cutaneous metastases occur in different proportions in women and men. For women, 69% of cutaneous metastases originate from the breast, 9% from the large intestine, and 4% from the lungs and ovaries. In men, lung carcinomas represent 24% of skin metastases, 19% are from the large intestine, 12% from the oral cavity, and 6% from the kidney and stomach (8).

Suspected metastatic lesions may be sent for frozen section for primary diagnosis or possibly margin assessment. Obviously the histologic pattern of the lesion is dependent on the site of origin (Figs. 12.12, 12.13). Certain primary carcinomas of the skin are difficult to distinguish from metastatic lesions, especially ones that are solitary. Examples of primary skin lesions that can closely mimic metastatic tumors include primary

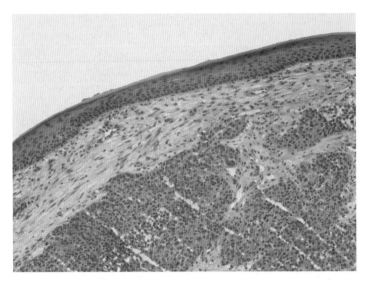

FIGURE 12.12 Metastatic poorly differentiated carcinoma. Section shows unremarkable epidermis and a poorly differentiated carcinoma in the dermis consistent with metastasis.

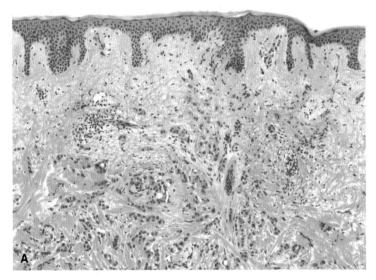

FIGURE 12.13 Metastatic breast carcinoma. **A.** Low-power view shows unremarkable epidermis and a diffuse infiltrate of atypical cells in the dermis. **B.** High-power view of atypical cells in a single cell pattern, which can be difficult to discern as epithelial in nature. **C.** In other areas, there is gland formation, which is helpful in making the correct diagnosis. (*continued*)

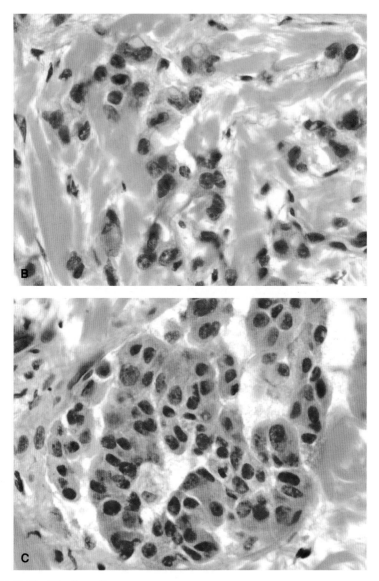

FIGURE 12.13   (*Continued*)

mucinous adenocarcinoma of the skin, adenocarcinoma of the mammary-like glands of the vulva, primary carcinoids, cutaneous signet ring carcinoma, and adnexal carcinomas (8). Close clinical correlation is required in these instances and in some cases, distinguishing between primary and metastatic lesions may not always be possible on frozen section.

Potentially Life-Threatening Inflammatory Conditions

Occasionally, skin biopsies from hospitalized patients are sent for frozen section diagnosis for inflammatory diseases. This occurs most often in tertiary care centers with relatively busy oncologic services where even a preliminary diagnosis may be most helpful in the immediate management of a seriously ill patient.

ERYTHEMA MULTIFORME/TOXIC EPIDERMAL NECROLYSIS. The distinction and classification of EM, TEN, and Stevens-Johnson syndrome (SJS) has been controversial. These three entities have been thought to represent a spectrum of disease with overlapping histopathologic features; however there are clinical differences between the entities. In EM, patients develop target lesions or raised atypical target lesions involving less than 10% of the body surface area. TEN shows flat, atypical targets that progress to diffuse, generalized detachment of the epidermis, involving more than 30% of the body surface area. SJS has flat atypical targets and confluent purpuric macules on the face and trunk as well as severe mucosal ulcerations involving less than 10% of the body surface area (18).

The etiology is believed to be a cell-mediated hypersensitivity immune reaction to infections agents (e.g., herpes simplex virus, *Mycoplasma pneumoniae*, and fungal infections) or medications (18).

Patients with infections or on multiple medications for systemic diseases develop rapidly progressive cutaneous eruption. Although there are typical lesions as described previously, the eruption can take on many different morphologic expressions (multiform), and consists of macules, papules, or vesicles. In some patients, the rash may progress rapidly into large flaccid bullae with detachment of the epidermis (TEN) and/or involvement of the mucosal surfaces (SJS). A biopsy for frozen section should ideally be taken from the area of erythema or periphery of a vesicle when present.

Histopathologic features of EM/TEN/SJS include vacuolar alteration of the basal cell layer above which there are necrotic keratinocytes. Full-thickness epidermal necrosis may be seen in advanced lesions of EM and TEN (Fig. 12.14).

Acute graft versus host disease remains in the differential diagnosis in all expressions of EM and cannot be distinguished on morphologic basis alone. In some patients, more commonly in the pediatric age group, staphylococcal scalded skin syndrome (SSSS) is in the clinical differential diagnosis. On frozen section, histopathologic distinction can be relatively easy since staphylococcal scalded skin syndrome is characterized by a split in the granular layer and more significantly by the absence of necrotic keratinocytes that is so characteristic of EM/TEN.

INFECTIONS: VIRAL: HERPES. In suspected cases of herpes infection, perhaps a much easier method of diagnosis is by preparing a smear from the

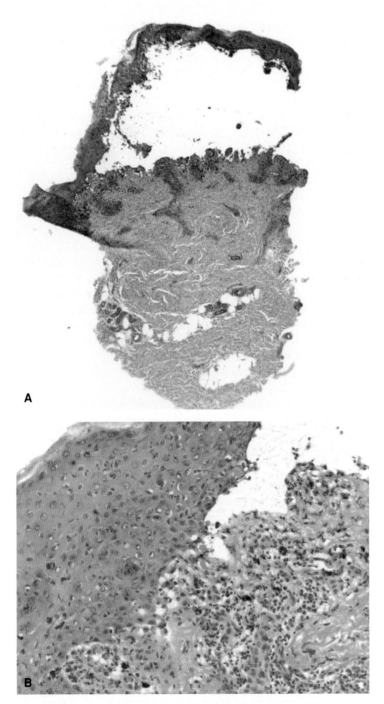

FIGURE 12.14 Erythema multiforme/toxic epidermal necrolysis. **A.** Low-power view shows a subepidermal blister. **B.** High-power view shows cause of the blister to be an interface dermatitis above which there is full-thickness necrosis of the epidermis.

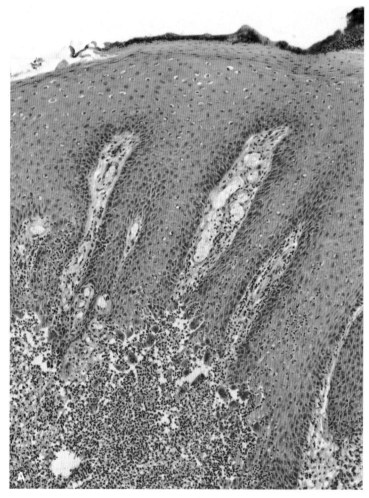

FIGURE 12.15 Herpes virus infection. **A.** Low-power view shows acantholysis in the lower part of the epidermis. **B.** High-power view shows multinucleated cells with nuclear changes characteristic of herpesvirus infection. (*continued*)

roof of a blister (Tzanck smear). A frozen section diagnosis may be requested in clinically challenging situations or when the differential diagnosis is EM. The histologic changes of herpes virus infection include necrosis of the epidermal keratinocytes and acantholysis. Classic multinucleated giant cells with viral cytopathic effect are required for a definite diagnosis (Fig. 12.15). Differential diagnostic considerations include primary bullous disease with acantholysis, such as pemphigus vulgaris in addition to EM.

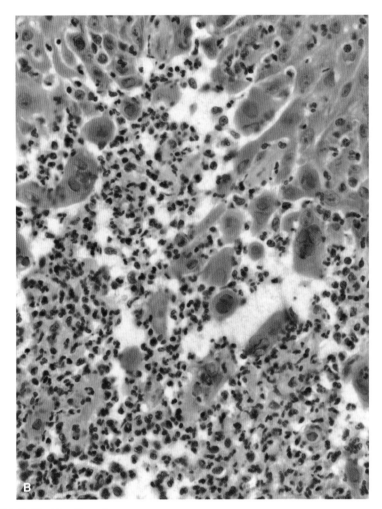

FIGURE 12.15 (*Continued*)

INFECTIONS: BACTERIAL

Necrotizing fasciitis. Necrotizing fasciitis is a rapidly progressive life-threatening disease that requires prompt diagnosis and aggressive medical and surgical treatment. Necrotizing fasciitis can develop either from an injury to the skin or from systemic spread of an infection. In some instances, the initial trauma is minor, such as needle puncture, insect bite, or other forms of trauma that disrupt the integrity of the skin surface. Group A beta-hemolytic streptococcus is most often associated with necrotizing fasciitis, although other serotypes and a wide range of other bacteria are also implicated. Erythema and edema of the skin may be the initial manifestation that may lead to an initial diagnosis of cellulitis.

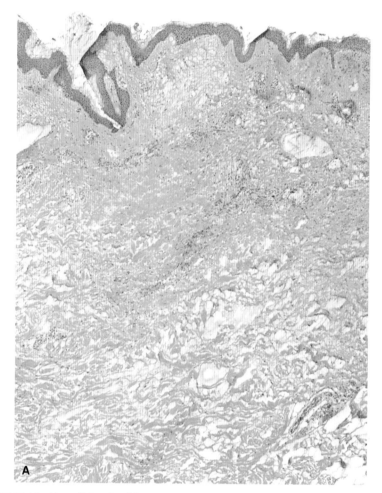

FIGURE 12.16 Necrotizing fasciitis. **A.** Low-power view of skin shows inflammation in the mid-dermis. **B.** Deeper tissue shows necrosis and numerous bacterial colonies. **C.** Neutrophilic inflammation of the fascial tissue. (*continued*)

However, the erythema rapidly progresses to painful, patchy discoloration of the skin without clear borders with subsequent vesiculation or bullae formation (19).

Frozen sections are requested not only for primary diagnosis but also in evaluating the margins for viability as the surgeon proceeds to debride the affected tissue. The specimen received for initial frozen section typically is a deep incisional biopsy from the blotchy erythematous skin and underlying soft tissue. On frozen section examination, the epidermis may be necrotic. Necrosis of the underlying soft tissue and superficial fascia with varying numbers of neutrophils and blood vessels occluded by fibrin thrombi are noted (Fig. 12.16). In most instances, bacterial organisms can

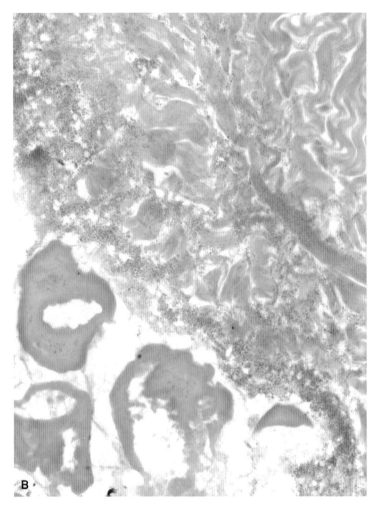

FIGURE 12.16 (*Continued*)

be seen. Advanced lesions show necrosis of all layers of skin and under-lying soft tissue and may include the sweat glands (19). A potential pitfall may be the paucity of neutrophils on frozen section, which should not de-ter one from looking for the organisms. Once the diagnosis of necrotizing fasciitis is confirmed, additional frozen sections from the advancing bor-ders of the lesion are sent for assessment of viability.

An early diagnosis, aggressive surgical management with debride-ment of dead tissues, and antibiotics are the mainstay of management of necrotizing fasciitis.

Vasculitis. Cutaneous vasculitis encompasses a wide range of primary and secondary vasculitic syndromes. Clinical symptoms range from benign,

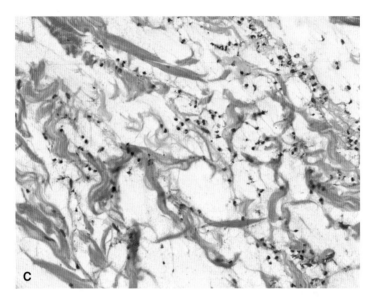

FIGURE 12.16 (*Continued*)

self-limiting cutaneous eruptions to severe systemic disease with multisystem organ failure. Commonly, primary vasculitis is classified according to size of the vessels involved and then further delineated based on histopathologic features, such as the composition of the inflammatory infiltrate, as well as clinical and serologic data. In many cases, final diagnosis is dependent on close clinical and histopathologic correlation (20). Cutaneous vasculitis is most often a manifestation of underlying systemic disease and because of the ease of access, a punch biopsy of skin may be sent for frozen section diagnosis.

The most common form of vasculitis encountered is leukocytoclastic vasculitis, which involves the small blood vessels of the superficial dermis. Characteristic histologic features include superficial perivascular inflammatory cell infiltrates with neutrophils and neutrophilic nuclear dust. Extravasated red cells in significant numbers may be present. In well-established lesions, fibrin deposits are present around the affected blood vessels (Fig. 12.17).

In the differential diagnosis, thrombotic vasculopathies such as those seen in disseminated intravascular coagulation and Coumadin/heparin thrombosis may be considered. These disorders typically lack the prominent inflammatory component seen in leukocytoclastic vasculitis and contain fibrin thrombi that occlude the vascular lumina rather than as deposits in the walls only.

When a diagnosis of small vessel vasculitis is fairly certain on frozen section evaluation, the frozen section remnant can be submitted for immunofluorescence studies. This is particularly of value in pediatric

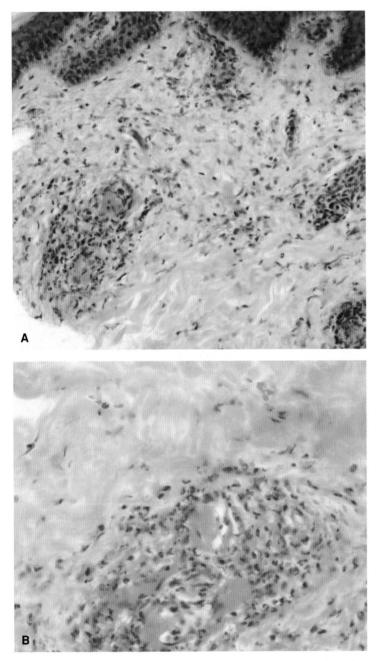

FIGURE 12.17 Leukocytoclastic vasculitis. **A.** Low-power view of skin with perivascular in-flammation. **B.** On higher power, there is perivascular infiltrate of neutrophils and fibrin thrombi in the lumen.

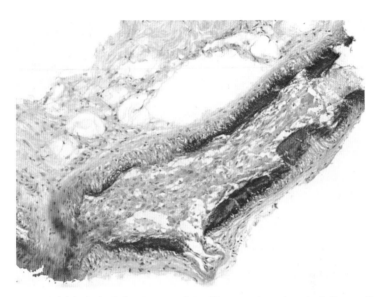

FIGURE 12.18 Calciphylaxis. Subcutaneous fat with necrosis and acute inflammation and an arteriole with calcific deposits in the wall and marked endothelial proliferation.

patients or severely ill patients where a second biopsy for fluorescence studies is not plausible. Positive immunofluorescence for immunoglobulin A versus IgM or IgG differentiates Henoch-Schönlein purpura from other forms of leukocytoclastic vasculitis.

The overlying epidermis may be necrotic in all forms of vasculitis as well as vasculopathies because of resulting ischemia and differentiating from erythema multiforme-type disorders requires a high degree of suspicion in addition to the clinical context.

Calciphylaxis (calcific uremic arteriolopathy). Calciphylaxis is an uncommon but a potentially life-threatening complication in patients with chronic renal disease. Hyperparathyroidism and elevated increased levels of serum phosphate are consistent findings in most patients (21). Calciphylaxis is increasingly recognized as the contributing factor to death in dialysis patients. Most patients present with skin manifestations ranging from solitary to multiple lesions, which often evolve rapidly into painful ulcerating lesions of the skin associated with necrosis and inflammation of the underlying subcutaneous fat. Calcification with intimal arterial hypertrophy and superimposed small vessel thrombosis is pathognomic of calciphylaxis (Fig. 12.18). In early lesions, granules of calcium may be seen in the walls and lumina of the small blood vessels as well as in the interstitium, in association with thrombosis and necrosis of the overlying skin secondary to ischemia.

Differential diagnostic considerations of specimens received for frozen section include other forms of vasculitis and vasculopathies, necrotizing fasciitis, and panniculitis. The histologic findings should be interpreted in the clinical context of renal disease, hyperparathyroidism, and elevated concentrations of serum phosphate. Potential benefits from parathyroidectomy in these patients are under consideration (21).

REFERENCES

1. Center for Disease Control and Prevention. 2008/2009 Skin cancer prevention and education initiative fact sheet. www.cdc.gov/Cancer/Skin

2. Cataldo PA, Stoddard PB, Reed WP. Use of frozen section analysis in the treatment of basal cell carcinoma. *Am J Surg.* 1990;159:561–563.

3. Ghauri RR, Gunter AA, Weber RA. Frozen section analysis in the management of skin cancers. *Ann Plast Surg.* 1999;43(2):156–160.

4. Manstein ME, Manstein CH, Smith R. How accurate is frozen section for skin cancers? *Ann Plast Surg.* 2003;50(6):607–609.

5. De Silva SP, Dellon L. Recurrence rate of positive margin basal cell carcinoma: results of a five-year prospective study. *J Surg Oncol.* 1985;28:72–74.

6. Fleming ID, Amonette R, Monaghan T, et al. Principles and management of basal and squamous cell carcinoma of the skin. *Cancer.* 1995;75(2):699–704.

7. Smith-Zagone MJ, Schwartz MR. Frozen section of skin specimens. *Arch Pathol Lab Med.* 2005;129:1536–1543.

8. Elder DE ed. *Lever's Histopathology of the Skin.* Philadelphia: Lippincott Williams & Wilkins; 2009.

9. Majeski J, Majeski E. Necrotizing fasciitis: improved survival with early recognition by tissue biopsy and aggressive surgical treatment. *South Med J.* 1997;90(11):1065–1068.

10. American Society for Mohs Surgery. Important patient information regarding Mohs micrographic surgery in the treatment of skin cancer. www.mohssurgery.org/pdfs/patient_information_brochure.pdf

11. Minton TJ. Contemporary Mohs surgery applications. *Curr Opin Otolaryngol & Head Neck Surg.* 2008;16:376–380.

12. Dawn ME, Dawn AG, Miller SJ. Mohs surgery for the treatment of melanoma in situ: a review. *Dermatol Surg.* 2007;33:395–402.

13. Garcia C, Holman J, Poletti E. Mohs surgery: commentaries and controversies. *Int J Dermatol.* 2005;44:893–905.

14. Barlow RJ, White CR, Swanson NA. Mohs' micrographic surgery using frozen sections alone may be unsuitable for detecting single atypical melanocytes at the margins of melanoma in situ. *Br J Dermatol.* 2002;146:290–294.

15. Lester SC. *Manual of Surgical Pathology.* Philadelphia: Elsevier Inc; 2006.

16. Goldberg LH, Wang SQ, Kimyai-Asadi A. The setting sun sign: visualizing the margins of a basal cell carcinoma on serial frozen sections stained with toluidine blue. *Dermatol Surg.* 2007;33:761–763.

17. Reddy VB, Hsu J. Skin and adnexal structures. In: Haber MH, Gattuso P, Spitz DJ, eds. *Differential Diagnosis in Surgical Pathology.* Philadelphia: W.B. Saunders Company; 2002.

18. Lamoreux MR, Sternbach MA, Hsu WT. Erythema multiforme. *Am Fam Physician.* 2006;74(11):1883–1888.

19. Kihiczak GG, Schwartz RA, Kapila R. Necrotizing fasciitis: a deadly infection. *J Eur Acad Dermatol Venereol.* 2006;20:365–369.

20. Carlson JA, Chen KR. Cutaneous vasculitis update: small vessel neutrophilic vasculitis syndromes. *Am J Dermatopathol.* 2006;28(6):486–506.

21. Rogers NM, Teubner DJ, Coates TH. Calcific uremic arteriolopathy: advances in pathogenesis and treatment. *Sem Dial.* 2007;20(2):150–157.

13

CENTRAL NERVOUS SYSTEM

JACK RAISANEN, KIMMO J. HATANPAA, AND CHARLES L. WHITE III

INTRAOPERATIVE DIAGNOSIS IN NEUROPATHOLOGY

Intraoperative diagnosis often plays a role in the care of the patient with an intracranial or intraspinal mass. The reason for intraoperative diagnosis is to help the surgeon determine the endpoint of the operation. In some cases, because of the clinical presentation and preoperative imaging, a mass is widely exposed and the extent of the operation is based, in part, on the intraoperative diagnosis. Specifically, for surgeons operating to resect a mass, the extent of the procedure is based on the intraoperative diagnosis and the surgeon's ability to identify an interface between the lesion and adjacent normal tissue. An intraoperative diagnosis may also hasten the postoperative care of a patient by leading to immediate body scans in cases of metastatic disease or, in unusual instances, immediate treatment of a life-threatening mass. Intraoperative diagnosis also helps to determine the need to set aside tissue for additional studies to characterize a neoplasm or for culture to identify microorganisms.

In other cases, again because of the patient's presentation and the characteristics of a lesion on preoperative images, a limited procedure is used to sample it, and the intraoperative consultation is used to confirm that tissue has been obtained that will lead to a diagnosis upon which care of the patient can be based. It is during these biopsies that surgeons sometimes request an intraoperative diagnosis inappropriately. For example, a surgeon who has decided to stop the procedure, perhaps because of bleeding, may request an intraoperative diagnosis using tissue that has already been obtained. Although, as above, treatment of a patient may be based on intraoperative preparations, it is usually based, more confidently, on formalin-fixed, paraffin-embedded sections, and in these instances it is necessary to discuss the importance of conserving the tissue.

There are a variety of diseases, including many types of neoplasms, that affect the central nervous system (CNS) and cause mass effect that is symptomatic and possibly life-threatening. Because of this variety, it is best to render a specific intraoperative diagnosis in the context of the patient's clinical presentation. The patient's age and history and the location of the lesion and its radiographic features are pieces of information that are key to diagnosis. Radiographs, particularly magnetic resonance images, indicate the location of a lesion and may indicate its demarcation as well as whether it is cystic, surrounded by edema, causes mass effect, or exhibits contrast enhancement.

A number of excellent references are available to the pathologist who consults intraoperatively in neuropathology (1–15); we have drawn some of the information for this chapter from those references.

Intraoperative Diagnosis during Resection

A neurosurgeon who is operating on a lesion using wide exposure and with an intent to potentially resect the entire lesion will often submit a small fragment of the lesion for intraoperative diagnosis. The lesion may be contained in, or be submitted along with, normal CNS parenchyma. Unfixed normal CNS gray matter is reddish brown and normal white matter is white or near white. Lesional tissue often can be identified in normal parenchyma by finding areas of hemorrhage or necrosis or, sometimes, in cases of diffusely infiltrating gliomas, by finding areas that are yellowish or gray, or softer than the surrounding parenchyma. It is also possible to locate a diffusely infiltrating glioma by identifying areas where the normally sharp gray/white matter junction is effaced.

It is best to divide the lesion into at least three fragments: one for frozen section and a second for a cytologic preparation, both of these for intraoperative diagnosis, and a third for formalin fixation for final diagnosis. In some cases, depending upon the intraoperative diagnosis, it is helpful to further divide the tissue for final diagnosis and to put fragments in glutaraldehyde for electron microscopy or in media for flow cytometric or cytogenetic studies. If cultures are indicated, it is preferable that they be obtained within the sterile environment of the operative suite rather than at the surgical pathology bench.

For intraoperative cytology, we prefer smear preparations instead of touch preparations because of the increased cellularity obtained. We use approximately 1 mm^3 of tissue and simultaneously crush and smear it between two glass slides. We fix the smear in 100% methanol and stain it with hematoxylin and eosin.

Intraoperative Diagnosis during Biopsy

A neurosurgeon who is operating to biopsy a lesion wants to know if he or she has submitted tissue that will lead to a diagnosis upon which appropriate treatment can be based. Usually the biopsy is done with a needle with a hollow core, and small, cylindrical fragments are submitted. Once again, the lesion may be submitted in or along with normal CNS parenchyma, and it may be necessary to identify areas that are necrotic, hemorrhagic, yellowish gray, or gelatinous.

Intraoperative diagnosis of a neoplasm, an infection, or, possibly, an infarct or focus of demyelination indicates to the surgeon that he or she has sampled the lesion. It is best, however, if the neurosurgeon stops the procedure only if sufficient tissue has been or will be obtained for formalin fixation, culture, or other studies necessary to confirm the intraoperative impression.

NONNEOPLASTIC LESIONS

Some of the most important intraoperative diagnoses in neurosurgery are the diagnoses of nonneoplastic lesions, because patients with such lesions often do not benefit from resection. Thus, the first thing to consider when examining a CNS lesion during a planned resection is whether the pathologic findings represent a reaction to a destructive, but nonneoplastic process; for example, does the presence of increased cellularity represent hyperplasia and not neoplasia? The most common destructive, but nonneoplastic, lesions that mimic neoplasms clinically and radiologically are (i) infections/abscesses, (ii) infarcts, and (iii) plaques of demyelinating diseases like multiple sclerosis.

At the time that they are most likely to mimic neoplasms, infarcts are usually organizing and the parenchyma contains inflammatory cells, especially abundant foamy macrophages, and reactive astrocytes. Similarly, at the time demyelination mimics a neoplasm, there is ongoing destruction and the plaque contains lymphocytes, many foamy macrophages, and reactive astrocytes. Thus, the key to identification of these two lesions intraoperatively is recognition of foamy macrophages and reactive astrocytes (16) (Fig. 13.1). Frozen sections of parenchyma infiltrated by foamy macrophages can be particularly confusing because the cell borders of macrophages are often difficult to distinguish, their nuclei are monomorphic and resemble those of oligodendrocytes, and their clear cytoplasm

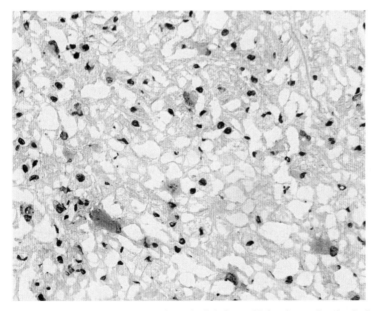

FIGURE 13.1   Intraoperative frozen section of a left frontal lobe demyelinating lesion. Sections that show reactive astrocytes and infiltrates of foamy macrophages should raise the possibilities of infarct or demyelination.

resembles ice crystal artifact. In these cases, cytologic preparations that reveal individual cells are very useful. They show cells with monomorphic nuclei with diameters that are approximately 1.5 to 2 times that of normal oligodendrocytes, abundant foamy or granular cytoplasm, and low nuclear-to-cytoplasmic (N/C) ratios (Fig. 13.2, e-Fig. 13.1). Sections and smears show reactive astrocytes with low N/C ratios; abundant perinuclear cytoplasm; and multiple long, highly fibrillar processes (e-Fig. 13.2). In both organizing infarcts and active plaques of demyelination, reactive astrocytes are greatly outnumbered by foamy macrophages.

The observation of necrotic neuronal cell bodies suggests infarct instead of demyelination, but they are often not identifiable on intraoperative preparations, and the distinction must be made using formalin-fixed, paraffin-embedded sections and special stains.

It is ultimately up to the surgeon to correlate the intraoperative diagnosis of inflammation and astrocytosis with his or her impression of the lesion. As neurosurgeons reach an organizing infarct or a plaque of demyelination, they often suspect that the lesion is nonneoplastic and, in these cases, an intraoperative diagnosis of inflammation with abundant foamy macrophages and reactive astrocytosis will usually lead them to abandon a plan for complete resection. However, the presence of reactive astrocytes and infiltrates of inflammatory cells alone merely indicates tissue injury and may be observed in the parenchyma adjacent to a neoplasm; thus, the surgeon who suspects a neoplasm may persist in obtaining additional samples for microscopic examination.

Infection of the CNS parenchyma by bacteria, fungi, or parasites often leads to an infiltrate composed of combinations of neutrophils, lymphocytes, plasma cells, and macrophages. Macrophages may be foamy, epithelioid, or multinucleated, and there are usually nearby reactive astrocytes. As with infarcts and demyelinating plaques, neurosurgeons often recognize an abscess as they approach it during the surgical procedure, and intraoperative diagnosis is used to confirm their impression. Surgeons may then turn their attention to draining or resecting an abscess and sending tissue to the microbiology laboratory for identification of microorganisms. Sometimes it is possible to identify organisms intraoperatively on sections or smears, for instance, fungi or *Toxoplasma*.

NEOPLASMS

Many types of neoplasms arise in the CNS, impinge on it, or are metastatic to it, and, as in other systems, specific types occur most frequently in specific locations in specific age groups. Because of this, it is best to make the diagnosis of a specific type of neoplasm in the context of the patient's age and history, the location of the neoplasm, and its radiographic features. With regard to location, it is useful to divide the CNS into supratentorial, infratentorial, and spinal compartments, and to consider whether a supratentorial or infratentorial neoplasm is intraventricular,

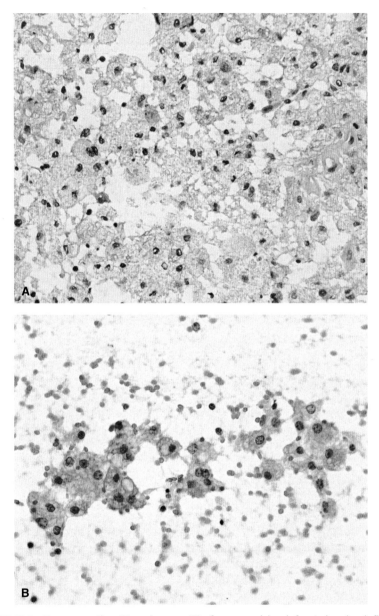

FIGURE 13.2 Frozen section (A) and smear (B) of an organizing infarct showing infiltrates of foamy macrophages. Intraoperatively, smears are invaluable for identifying macrophages in infarcts and demyelinating lesions.

intraparenchymal (intraaxial), or extraparenchymal (extraaxial), and whether a spinal neoplasm is intraparenchymal (intramedullary), extra-parenchymal but intradural, or epidural. Supratentorial neoplasms may be localized further to the sellar or pineal regions. In addition, some cerebral

TABLE 13.1 Most Common CNS Neoplasms in Adults

Cerebral hemispheres
Intraaxial
- Diffusely infiltrating astrocytoma
- Oligodendroglioma
- Metastatic carcinoma
- Metastatic melanoma
- Lymphoma

Extraaxial, intradural
- Meningioma

Lateral ventricles
- Ependymoma
- Neurocytoma
- Subependymoma

Sellar region
- Pituitary adenoma
- Meningioma
- Craniopharyngioma

Pineal region
- Germinoma
- Pineal cell tumor
- Astrocytoma

Posterior fossa
Intraaxial/intraventricular
- Metastatic carcinoma
- Metastatic melanoma
- Ependymoma
- Pilocytic astrocytoma
- Hemangioblastoma
- Choroid plexus tumor

Extraaxial, intradural (cerebellopontine angle)
- Schwannoma
- Meningioma
- Epidermoid cyst
- Ependymoma
- Choroid plexus tumor

Spinal canal
Intramedullary
- Ependymoma
- Pilocytic astrocytoma
- Diffusely infiltrating astrocytoma
- Hemangioblastoma

Extramedullary, intradural
- Schwannoma
- Meningioma
- Neurofibroma

Epidural
- Metastatic carcinoma
- Lymphoma
- Plasmacytoma
- Schwannoma
- Neurofibroma

parenchymal neoplasms extend into the lateral or third ventricle and some sellar or pineal region neoplasms are found mostly in the third ventricle. Tables 13.1 and 13.2 list the most common neoplasms in these specific CNS locations in adults and children.

The intraoperative diagnosis of a specific neoplasm helps the neurosurgeon determine the extent of the resection, a decision based in part on the known, usual biologic behavior of the neoplasm. For instance, individual cells of some CNS neoplasms are able to infiltrate normal parenchyma diffusely, while other neoplasms are composed of cells that do not infiltrate aggressively and are relatively well-circumscribed. Metastatic neoplasms may be relatively well-circumscribed, but are often multifocal.

Sometimes, even with clinical and radiographic information, is not possible to make a specific diagnosis of neoplasm type intraoperatively

TABLE 13.2 Most Common CNS Neoplasms in Children

Cerebral hemispheres
- Pilocytic astrocytoma
- Diffusely infiltrating astrocytoma
- Ganglion cell tumor
- Pleomorphic xanthoastrocytoma
- Dysembryoplastic neuroepithelial tumor
- Primitive neuroectodermal tumor

Lateral ventricles
- Ependymoma
- Choroid plexus tumor
- Subependymal giant cell astrocytoma

Sellar region
- Craniopharyngioma
- Pilocytic astrocytoma
- Germinoma

Pineal region
- Germinoma
- Pineal cell tumor
- Astrocytoma

Posterior fossa
- Medulloblastoma
- Pilocytic astrocytoma
- Ependymoma
- Hemangioblastoma

Spinal canal

Intramedullary
- Ependymoma
- Pilocytic astrocytoma
- Diffusely infiltrating astrocytoma
- Hemangioblastoma

Extramedullary, intradural
- Schwannoma
- Neurofibroma

either because of artifact, because the amount of tissue is too small, or because immunohistochemistry or other studies are necessary. In these instances, the most helpful intraoperative diagnosis describes the likely biologic behavior of the neoplasm. Thus, the intraoperative diagnosis of "low-grade diffusely infiltrating glioma" states that the specific differentiation of the neoplastic cells is uncertain but indicates their likely behavior. Sometimes, when it is not possible to be this specific, it is helpful to clarify a prediction of likely biologic behavior with a differential diagnosis. For instance, an intraoperative diagnosis for a posterior fossa neoplasm in an adult may be "low-grade neoplasm: schwannoma versus fibrous meningioma."

Supratentorial Neoplasms of the Cerebrum and Associated Meninges: Adults

In adults, the most common primary neoplasms of the cerebral parenchyma are diffusely infiltrating gliomas, and the most common metastatic neoplasms are carcinomas. Melanomas, usually metastatic, and lymphomas, either primary or metastatic, are also encountered intraoperatively, but less frequently. The most common supratentorial, extraaxial, but intradural neoplasms are meningiomas.

DIFFUSELY INFILTRATING ASTROCYTOMA. Diffusely infiltrating astrocytomas are neoplasms composed of incompletely differentiated astrocytic cells. According to the 2007 World Health Organization (WHO) *Classification of Tumours of the Central Nervous System* (15), diffusely infiltrating astrocytomas are graded as 2, 3, or 4, with grade 3 synonymous with anaplastic astrocytoma and grade 4 with glioblastoma. The peak incidence of grade 2 neoplasms is between age 30 and 40 and of grade 4 neoplasms between age 45 and 75. Individual cells of diffusely infiltrating astrocytomas invade surrounding normal CNS parenchyma and, therefore, the intraoperative diagnosis of an infiltrating glioma indicates to the surgeon that all of the neoplastic cells probably cannot be resected.

The nuclei of grade 2 neoplasms are more consistently round to oval or elliptical and are not as atypical or pleomorphic as those of higher-grade gliomas. Chromatin is more finely granular, usually with one or several slightly larger chromocenters and discernible parachromatin spaces. Few mitotic figures may be observed in grade 2 neoplasms. The cells have scant perinuclear cytoplasm and at least some have well-differentiated fibrillar processes. The cellularity of grade 2 diffusely infiltrating astrocytomas is often low, but the neoplastic cells almost always occur among axons with associated normal glial cells, and comparison of normal nuclei with neoplastic nuclei is often the key to intraoperative diagnosis. In normal cerebral white matter, most glial nuclei are oligodendrocyte nuclei that are round or almost round with diameters of approximately 8 μm. Nuclear membranes are smooth and chromatin is often densely packed. Normal astrocytes are less frequent and have round to oval or elliptical nuclei with diameter of approximately 10 μm and smooth membranes. Nuclei of grade 2 diffusely infiltrating astrocytomas are generally bean-shaped or elliptical, but some have diameters that are approximately 1.5 to 2.5 times that of normal oligodendrocytes, are pleomorphic, and have atypical membranes. Because of edema, frozen sections of low-grade diffusely infiltrating astrocytomas almost always exhibit severe artifact, and it is often difficult to be certain of nuclear size, atypia, and pleomorphism (Fig. 13.3, e-Fig. 13.3). It is often easier to observe these features on cytologic preparations. Smears usually show neoplastic cells mixed with normal cells on a background of crushed granular cytoplasm, crushed axons and fibrillar processes (Fig. 13.4).

Low-grade oligodendrogliomas are usually composed of cells with uniformly round or almost round nuclei that are neither as atypical nor as pleomorphic as those of low-grade diffusely infiltrating astrocytomas. However, it is sometimes difficult, even with excellent smears, to distinguish a low-grade diffusely infiltrating astrocytoma from a low-grade oligodendroglioma or a low-grade oligoastrocytoma intraoperatively, and in those cases, "low-grade infiltrating glioma" is an appropriate diagnosis.

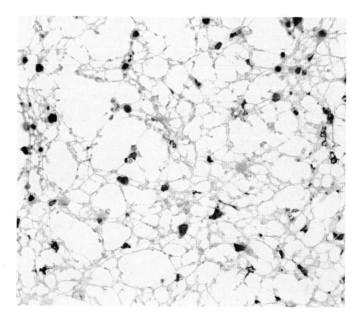

FIGURE 13.3 Intraoperative frozen section of a grade 2 diffusely infiltrating glioma. Cells of low-grade diffusely infiltrating gliomas may be difficult to distinguish from normal or reactive cells that are distorted by freezing and cutting.

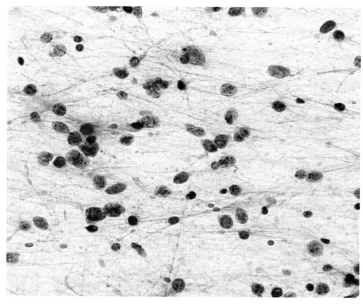

FIGURE 13.4 Smear of a low-grade diffusely infiltrating glioma. Neoplastic nuclei are larger than those of normal glia (compare their sizes with those of normal oligodendrocytes); the oval or elliptical shapes and the degree of atypia and pleomorphism suggest astrocytic differentiation.

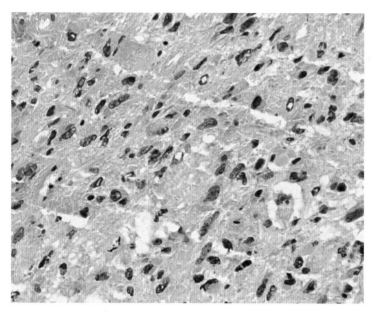

FIGURE 13.5 Frozen section of a high-grade diffusely infiltrating astrocytoma. The small, round nuclei with densely packed chromatin are the nuclei of normal oligodendrocytes.

The cells of high-grade diffusely infiltrating astrocytomas have atypical and pleomorphic nuclei usually with coarsely granular, irregularly dispersed chromatin; sometimes, the chromatin appears clumped or smudged. Some cells contain mitotic figures. Usually some of the cells have relatively abundant perinuclear cytoplasm and many have long, stellate processes characteristic of glial differentiation. Glioblastomas have tumor cell necrosis or contain microvascular proliferation or both. Frozen sections of high-grade diffusely infiltrating astrocytomas often show individual infiltrating neoplastic cells surrounded by normal parenchyma (Fig. 13.5). Sometimes, though, the central portion of a high-grade astrocytoma is submitted and, on frozen sections, it may be difficult to discern the cytoplasmic processes that indicate glial differentiation. In these cases, cytologic preparations are key to distinguishing a glioma from a carcinoma, lymphoma, or melanoma (Fig. 13.6, e-Fig. 13.4).

OLIGODENDROGLIOMA. Oligodendrogliomas are diffusely infiltrating gliomas composed of cells that resemble normal oligodendrocytes. As with diffusely infiltrating astrocytomas, individual cells invade surrounding normal parenchyma and, therefore, an intraoperative diagnosis of oligodendroglioma indicates to the surgeon that all of the neoplastic cells probably cannot be resected.

According to WHO (15), oligodendrogliomas are grade 2 or 3; peak incidence of grade 2 neoplasms is between age 40 and 45 years. Grade 3

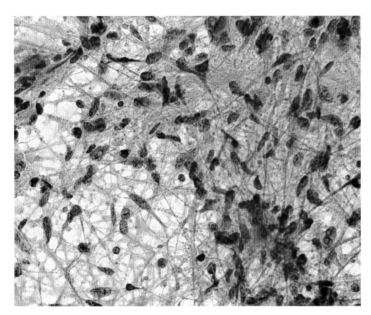

FIGURE 13.6 Intraoperative smear of glioblastoma. The overlapping, intersecting cytoplasmic processes indicate glial differentiation.

neoplasms have relatively abundant mitotic figures and/or microvascular proliferation or tumor cell necrosis, or both. Grade 2 neoplasms are usually composed mostly of round to oval cells, though in some neoplasms, some of the neoplastic cells have short cytoplasmic processes. Nuclei are consistently round or nearly round, usually with diameters that are approximately 1.5 to 2.5 times that of normal oligodendrocytes. Chromatin is finely granular, often with one or several larger chromocenters. Sometimes parachromatin spaces are relatively wide, creating a salt and pepper appearance. Like low-grade infiltrating astrocytomas, the cells are often arranged diffusely among normal parenchyma. Sometimes, they occur in sheets or nodules.

In formalin-fixed, paraffin-embedded sections, the cytoplasm of the neoplastic cells of low-grade oligodendrogliomas often appears clear, but on frozen sections, this is difficult to discern (Fig. 13.7, e-Fig. 13.5). Therefore, as with low-grade diffusely infiltrating astrocytomas, intraoperative diagnosis often depends on comparison of oligodendroglial nuclei and identification of separate normal and neoplastic populations, and this is often easiest on smear preparations (Fig. 13.8, e-Fig. 13.6).

Again, it is often difficult to distinguish low-grade oligodendrogliomas from low-grade diffusely infiltrating astrocytomas or low-grade oligoastrocytomas intraoperatively, because of the degree of overlap of nuclear and cytoplasmic features. Findings that suggest oligodendroglioma or a component of oligodendroglial differentiation include uniformly

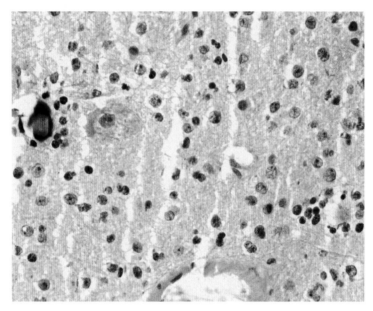

FIGURE 13.7 The neoplastic cells of grade 2 oligodendrogliomas often have perinuclear halos on formalin-fixed, paraffin-embedded sections, but not on frozen sections. Note the neuron cell body and focus of calcification.

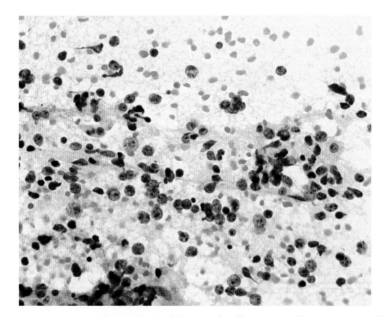

FIGURE 13.8 Intraoperative smears of low-grade oligodendrogliomas show uniformly round or almost round nuclei. Compare the sizes of the neoplastic nuclei with normal oligo-dendrocyte nuclei and red blood cells.

round, or almost round, nuclei with little atypia or pleomorphism. The intraoperative diagnosis of "low-grade infiltrating glioma" describes the behavior of all three of those neoplasms.

It is typically difficult to distinguish high-grade oligodendrogliomas from high-grade astrocytomas intraoperatively, thus warranting a diagnosis of "high-grade infiltrating glioma."

METASTATIC NEOPLASMS. The most common CNS neoplasms originate outside of the CNS (12,15). In adults, approximately 80% of metastases are found in the cerebral hemispheres, often at the interface of cortex and white matter. They may also involve the dura and leptomeninges. The most common type of metastatic neoplasm is carcinoma.

The cytologic and architectural features of metastatic carcinomas are similar to those of the respective primary neoplasms. Except for small cell variants, at least some cells of carcinomas are relatively large with nuclear diameters approximately three to five times (or more) that of red blood cells (RBCs) or the nuclei of normal lymphocytes or oligodendrocytes. Nuclei are atypical and pleomorphic, chromatin is often coarsely clumped, and nucleoli are often prominent. Mitotic figures are usually common and, in the brain, there is almost always tumor cell necrosis. In the CNS parenchyma, foci of carcinoma are usually well-circumscribed but are often multiple. Frozen sections often reveal glands or papillae. Not uncommonly, though, the frozen fragment of a parenchymal mass shows only a sheet of neoplastic epithelioid cells with indistinguishable cytoplasmic margins, and the differential diagnosis includes melanoma, lymphoma, and glioblastoma. If there is normal parenchyma in the section, a sharp border with the neoplasm suggests carcinoma instead of glioblastoma or lymphoma (e-Fig. 13.7). Smears almost always distinguish carcinoma from glioblastoma or lymphoma; preparations reveal polygonal cohesive cells instead of noncohesive lymphoid cells or glial cells with stellate cytoplasmic processes (Fig. 13.9, e-Fig. 13.8) Sometimes, even with good intraoperative preparations, it is not possible to distinguish a carcinoma from melanoma.

Lymphomas may occur as primary CNS neoplasms or be metastatic to the CNS. Primary lymphomas usually involve the parenchyma; metastatic neoplasms usually occur in the dura or leptomeninges, but may also occur in the parenchyma. In immunocompetent patients, primary neoplasms occur most commonly between 50 and 70 years. When clinical and radiographic features suggest that a CNS mass is a lymphoma, it is usually biopsied. In these cases, intraoperative consultation is used to confirm that a sample of the neoplasm has been obtained, and to determine what additional studies, such as flow cytometry, may be indicated before fixing the remaining specimen.

Approximately 95% of primary lymphomas are diffuse, large B-cell lymphomas composed of cells with pleomorphic nuclei, some with diameters approximately three to five times (or more) those of normal, mature

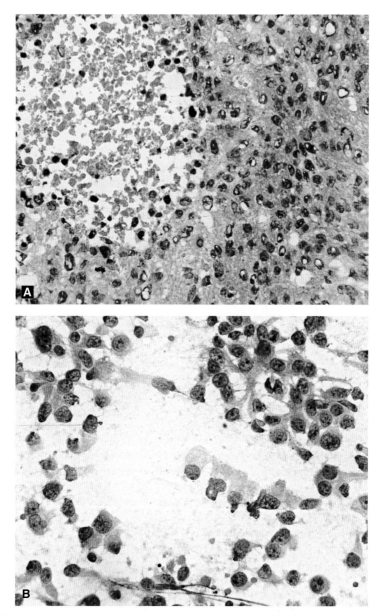

FIGURE 13.9 Intraoperative frozen section (A) and smear (B) of metastatic carcinoma. Sometimes, it is difficult to distinguish carcinoma from glioblastoma on frozen sections, but smears reveal the polygonal cells of carcinoma instead of the stellate cells of glioblastoma.

lymphocytes. Their chromatin is coarsely granular, often with several relatively large, pleomorphic granules and wide parachromatin spaces. Smears highlight the distinctive chromatin and often show lymphoglandular bodies; frozen sections often show a characteristic angiocentric

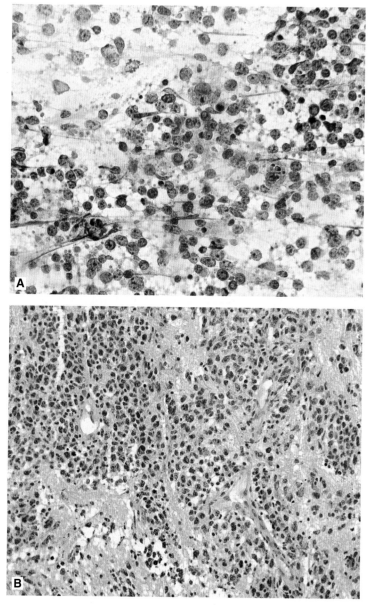

FIGURE 13.10 **A&B** Smears of CNS lymphomas show noncohesive cells with coarsely clumped chromatin; frozen sections show characteristic angiocentric architecture.

architecture (Fig. 13.10, e-Fig. 13.9). Sometimes, though, the angiocentric architecture is missing and the cytologic features are equivocal, and immunohistochemistry (or flow cytometry) is needed to confirm the diagnosis.

MENINGIOMA. Meningiomas are usually extraaxial, intradural neo-plasms that occur most commonly in adults between 50 and 70 years. They are generally well-circumscribed, but may extend into the brain or into dural, epidural, cranial, or extracranial tissue. They are graded by WHO as 1, 2, or 3 (15). Also according to WHO, there are thirteen histo-logic variants of meningiomas, the most common of which are meningothelial and transitional. The meningothelial and transitional vari-ants are usually grade 1 and are composed of cells with abundant cyto-plasm and monomorphic, round to oval nuclei with diameters approxi-mately 1.5 to 2.5 times the size of RBCs. Chromatin is often finely granular with wide parachromatin spaces and one or several small chromocenters; the nuclear membrane is often prominent. On sections, the cytoplasm of the neoplastic cells often appears syncytial and nuclei appear to stream or are arranged in whorls (e-Fig. 13.10).

Most of the time, the intraoperative diagnosis of meningioma is straightforward; head scans show an extraaxial mass and frozen sections are usually of good quality. Sometimes, though, neither the radiologist nor the surgeon is sure if a mass is extraaxial or intraaxial and, because of the epithelioid nature of the cells and freezing and cutting artifact, carcinoma becomes a consideration. Moreover, carcinomas sometimes metastasize to the dura. Cytologic preparations are often useful in these instances be-cause they reveal individual cells with relatively monomorphic nuclei and low N/C ratios (Fig. 13.11).

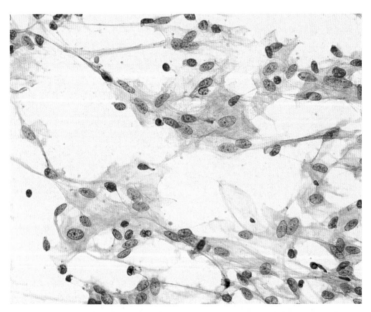

FIGURE 13.11 Smears of the common variants of meningiomas show epithelioid cells with monomorphic nuclei and low N/C ratios.

Frozen sections of some of the histologic variants of meningiomas, for instance, microcystic or clear cell meningiomas, may be particularly confusing. Sometimes, the meningothelial nature of the nuclei of the variants is apparent on smears. Nevertheless, familiarity with the histologic variation of meningiomas is helpful for intraoperative diagnosis of superficially located intracranial neoplasms.

Meningioma resections are the only neurosurgical procedures in which evaluation of margins is likely to be called for with any frequency. The presence of foci of "arachnoidal cap cell hyperplasia" on fragments of dura adjacent to the main tumor mass can present a challenge in this situation. When that arises, a diagnosis of "nests of arachnoidal epithelium present" may be warranted, followed up with a discussion with the surgeon regarding the difficulty of determining whether this represents isolated neoplastic rests or simply nodules of native tissue.

Two mesenchymal neoplasms of the meninges that are relatively uncommon—solitary fibrous tumor and hemangiopericytoma—may be difficult to differentiate from meningioma, intraoperatively. Solitary fibrous tumors are composed of spindle-shaped cells and contain abundant collagen and, on frozen sections and smears, resemble fibrous meningiomas. Hemangiopericytomas (WHO grades 2 or 3) are composed of cells with higher N/C ratios than the cells of the most common variants of meningiomas and they are arranged more haphazardly than the cells of most meningiomas (e-Fig. 13.11). In cases where distinction is difficult, the intraoperative report may indicate a differential diagnosis.

Supratentorial Neoplasms of the Cerebrum: Children and Young Adults

The most common neoplasms of the cerebrum in children and young adults are glial or mixed glial-neuronal neoplasms. The most common glial neoplasms are pilocytic and diffusely infiltrating astrocytomas. Pilocytic astrocytomas occur more frequently beneath the tentorium and are discussed with posterior fossa neoplasms. The most frequently occurring low-grade mixed glial-neuronal neoplasms are ganglion cell tumors, usually ganglioglioma.

Dysembryoplastic neuroepithelial tumors and pleomorphic xanthoastrocytomas (PXA) occur less frequently. PXAs are usually low grade (WHO grade 2) and are usually considered as glial, but they often contain cells that exhibit neuronal differentiation by immunohistochemistry.

Embryonal or "small blue cell" tumors are high grade, usually occur in younger children, and most exhibit neuroglial differentiation that can be detected immunohistochemically. The differential diagnosis for supratentorial embryonal neoplasms includes medulloepithelioma, primitive neuroectodermal tumor, ependymoblastoma, and atypical teratoid/rhabdoid tumor. In addition, choroid plexus carcinomas may have embryonal cytology.

The most common supratentorial neoplasm in children that is not glial or glial-neuronal is craniopharyngioma, which almost always occurs in the sellar region.

For the intraoperative diagnosis of supratentorial neoplasms in children, particularly low-grade neoplasms, it is useful to know clinical and radiographic data. However, even with that information, intraoperative diagnosis of a specific supratentorial glial or glial-neuronal neoplasm in a child or young adult is often difficult. The reasons for this are (i) some of the supratentorial neoplasms in this age group have similar clinical and radiographic characteristics; (ii) some have similar cytologic and architectural features; (iii) specific cytologic and architectural features that indicate the specific type of neoplasm, such as rhabdoid cells, dysplastic ganglion cells, or rosettes, may not appear on intraoperative preparations; (iv) specific cytologic features that indicate grade, like Rosenthal fibers or eosinophilic granular bodies, may not appear on intraoperative preparations; (v) several neoplasms in this group contain abundant extracellular matrix, leading to significant freezing artifact; and (vi) several neoplasms in this group contain abundant connective tissue, so cytologic preparations may be difficult to prepare or interpret. This difficulty with specificity means that often the intraoperative diagnosis of a supratentorial neoplasm in a child indicates a differential, for instance, "low-grade glioma," "low-grade neuroglial neoplasm," or "high-grade neuroectodermal neoplasm."

GANGLION CELL TUMORS. Ganglion cell tumors are either gangliocytomas, which are circumscribed neoplasms composed of relatively well-differentiated neuronal cells (usually ganglion cells), or much more commonly, gangliogliomas, with a glial component that is usually astrocytic. The ganglion cells in these neoplasms are cytologically and/or architecturally dysplastic, with features such as nuclear or cytoplasmic pleomorphism, binucleation, or abnormal clustering. Most ganglion cell tumors also contain eosinophilic granular bodies. Gangliocytomas and most gangliogliomas are WHO grade 1. Clinical and radiographic information may suggest the diagnosis of a ganglion cell tumor; they may be solid but often have a cyst and, on scans, often show contrast enhancement. They can occur anywhere in the brain but are most common in the temporal lobes, where they are often associated with epilepsy. Sections and smears are both useful for identifying, or at least suggesting a diagnosis of ganglioglioma intraoperatively (e-Fig. 13.12). Sections are useful because it is often easier to identify architectural dysplasia than cytologic dysplasia in the ganglionic component, and smears are useful for identifying the glial component.

DYSEMBRYOPLASTIC NEUROEPITHELIAL TUMOR. Dysembryoplastic neuroepithelial tumors (WHO grade 1) are rather well-demarcated lesions that are usually composed of glial cells that resemble oligodendrocytes and ganglion cells. Architecturally, in classical areas, bundles of axons are lined by oligodendrocyte-like cells and occur in an extracellular matrix in which ganglion cells appear to "float." Associated areas may not contain ganglion cells and, instead, resemble oligodendrogliomas, or show astrocytic morphology with long cytoplasmic processes. Because of the abundant matrix, frozen sections often exhibit severe artifact. Smears in classical cases usually contain oligodendrocyte-like cells with monomorphic, round nuclei with stippled chromatin. The key to intraoperative diagnosis is associating the finding of low-grade oligodendrocyte-like cells on smears with a highly characteristic clinical and radiographic presentation. The neoplasms are often in the cortex of the temporal lobes and associated with seizures, usually beginning before age 20 years, without other progressive neurologic deficits. On head scans, there is no mass effect, unless it is due to a cyst or peritumoral edema.

PLEOMORPHIC XANTHOASTROCYTOMA. PXAs (WHO grade 2) are composed of pleomorphic, sometimes bizarre astrocytic cells, some of which contain droplets of fat. Like ganglion cell tumors, PXAs also contain eosinophilic granular bodies and, also like ganglion cell tumors, are often located superficially in the temporal lobes, have a cyst, are contrast enhancing on scans, and lead to seizures. Intraoperative diagnosis is based on association of the radiographic findings with identification of very pleomorphic cells with fibrillar cytoplasmic processes along with abundant eosinophilic granular bodies, which typically indicate that the neoplasm is not high grade (e-Fig. 13.13).

Supratentorial Intraventricular Neoplasms

CNS neoplasms that may be located mostly in the lateral ventricles are ependymomas, subependymomas, neurocytomas, subependymal giant cell astrocytomas, choroid plexus papillomas or carcinomas, and meningiomas. Ependymomas occur mostly in children and young adults and are much more common in the posterior fossa and spinal cord. Subependymomas may occur in the lateral ventricles, but are more common in the fourth ventricle and, with ependymomas, will be discussed with posterior fossa neoplasms. Neurocytomas are composed of well-differentiated neural cells, and usually occur in the lateral ventricles of young adults. Choroid plexus neoplasms occur in the lateral ventricles of adults, but are far more common in children. Subependymal giant cell astrocytomas occur mostly in children with tuberous sclerosis. Intraventricular meningiomas are uncommon.

Sellar or hypothalamic/thalamic neoplasms may extend into the anterior or middle portion of the third ventricle, so pituitary adenomas, craniopharyngiomas, pilocytic astrocytomas, and germ cell tumors, usually germinoma, should be included in the differential diagnosis of a third ventricular mass. Similarly, pineal parenchymal neoplasms or germ cell tumors may involve the posterior third ventricle (17).

NEUROCYTOMA. Neurocytomas are circumscribed neoplasms (WHO grade 2) of well-differentiated neuronal cells that usually occur in the lateral ventricles near the foramina of Monro in young adults. Sometimes the neoplasms involve the third ventricle. In most cases, the cells are round to oval and have monomorphic nuclei that are round or almost round with diameters approximately 1.5 to 2 times that of RBCs with uniformly stippled chromatin. On frozen sections, the cytoplasm often appears syncytial, leading to a differential of "neurocytoma versus ependymoma" (Fig. 13.12). Intraoperative smears of neurocytomas show randomly arranged nuclei on a background composed predominantly of crushed granular cytoplasm and usually relatively few, if any, glial processes; smears of ependymomas usually show large numbers of cytoplasmic processes on a clear background (e-Fig. 13.14).

CHOROID PLEXUS NEOPLASMS. Choroid plexus neoplasms of the lateral ventricles occur most commonly in children. According to WHO (15), choroid plexus neoplasms are classified as papillomas, grade 1, atypical papillomas, grade 2, and carcinomas, grade 3. Approximately 80% of carcinomas occur in children. Intraoperative diagnosis of a choroid plexus neoplasm depends on the identification of papillae, which, although sometimes difficult to resolve on frozen sections, are usually easily observed on smears (e-Fig. 13.15). In children, ventricular papillary neoplasms are usually choroid plexus neoplasms. In adults, papillae with high-grade cytology usually represent metastatic carcinoma. Intraventricular neoplasms composed of papillae with low-grade cytology in adults are sometimes problematic, and definitive diagnosis requires immunohistochemistry and clinicopathologic correlation.

SUBEPENDYMAL GIANT CELL ASTROCYTOMA. Subependymal giant cell astrocytomas usually occur in the walls of the lateral ventricles of children or young adults with tuberous sclerosis. The neoplasms are well-demarcated, slowly growing, and classified as WHO grade 1. The neoplastic cells have different sizes and shapes but, characteristically, some are relatively large with abundant perinuclear cytoplasm and some, including the large cells, have long, fibrillar cytoplasmic processes. If intraoperative consultation is requested, frozen sections show large astrocyte-like cells with abundant perinuclear cytoplasm and smears highlight their fibrillar processes (Fig. 13.13, e-Fig. 13.16).

Sellar Region Neoplasms

The most common neoplasms of the sellar region of adults are pituitary adenomas and meningiomas. Carcinomas or lymphomas involve the sellar region far less frequently. Pilocytic astrocytomas and craniopharyngiomas are common sellar region neoplasms of children and young adults. Germ cell tumors, particularly germinomas, occur less frequently.

PITUITARY ADENOMA. Pituitary adenomas vary in size and circumscription. The neoplasms may be very small and confined to the sella, or they may be large, invasive lesions that involve the paranasal sinuses, the

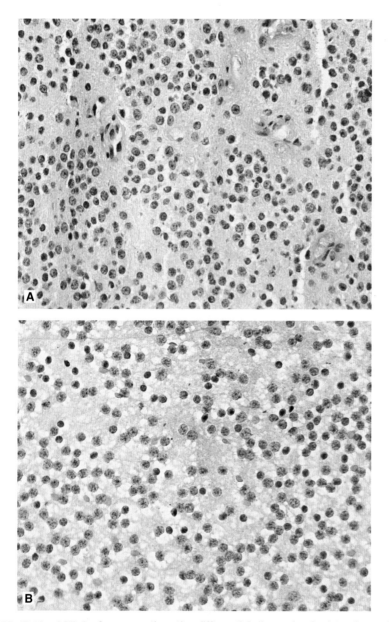

FIGURE 13.12 **A&B** On frozen section, the differential diagnosis of a lateral ventricular mass in a young adult may be neurocytoma vs ependymoma. Smears of most neurocytomas show individual nuclei with stippled chromatin on a background of crushed granular cytoplasm.

cavernous sinuses, or brain. Pituitary adenomas are composed of epithelial cells that appear round to oval or polygonal and, on sections, occur in sheets, sometimes with a sinusoidal arrangement, and sometimes with papillae or glandlike formations. Several neoplasms in the differential of

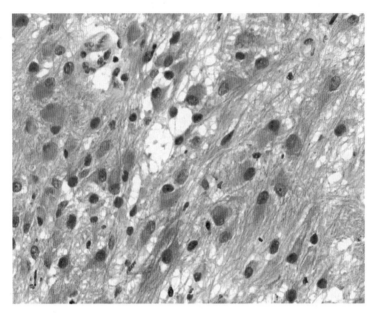

FIGURE 13.13 Frozen sections of subependymal giant cell astrocytomas show cells with abundant perinuclear cytoplasm and long, fibrillar cytoplasmic processes.

a sellar region mass in an adult are epithelial or epithelioid in nature and, because of frozen section artifact, intraoperative diagnosis with sections alone can be challenging. In this setting, cytologic smear preparations are often very helpful for diagnosis. For example, on frozen sections, nuclei of pituitary adenomas may appear unusually atypical and pleomorphic, suggesting the diagnosis of metastatic carcinoma, or indistinct cytoplasmic margins may suggest meningioma, but cytologic preparations will show cells with highly monomorphic nuclei with "salt and pepper" chromatin (Fig. 13.14).

Sometimes, during attempted resection of a very small adenoma, even one that does not appear on preoperative images, it is necessary to distinguish adenoma from normal anterior pituitary intraoperatively. In these instances, diagnosis using cytologic preparations alone may be difficult. Sections that reveal either the characteristic lobular architecture of normal anterior pituitary or its obliteration in an adenoma are often most helpful (e-Fig. 13.17).

In some cases, surgeons operating on a lesion in the sella may ask the pathologist to identify normal posterior pituitary. Only a very, very small fragment of tissue is submitted and, usually, a smear is the best intraoperative preparation. The posterior pituitary is composed of axons supported by specialized glial cells, and slide preparations reveal highly vascularized neuroglial tissue without glandular morphology.

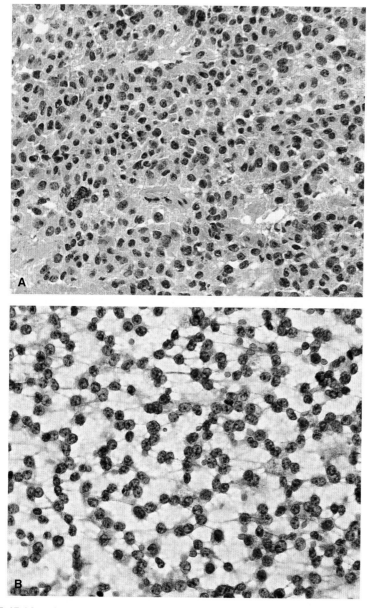

FIGURE 13.14 **A&B** Sometimes, nuclei of a pituitary adenoma appear pleomorphic on frozen sections; on cytologic preparations, they appear highly monomorphic.

CRANIOPHARYNGIOMA. Craniopharyngiomas are composed of squamous epithelial cells associated with connective tissue. Differences in the histology of the squamous component account for two variants: the adamantinomatous form that occurs in both children and adults and the papillary form that almost always occurs in adults. The papillary form is

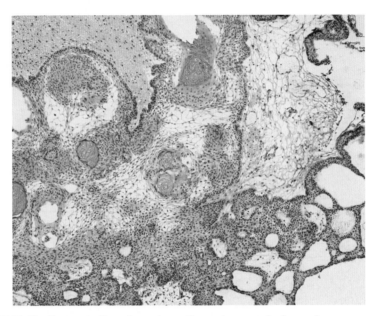

FIGURE 13.15 Frozen section of an adamantinomatous craniopharyngioma.

well-circumscribed but the adamantinomatous form less so, often involving nearby normal tissue; both are WHO grade 1. The adamantinomatous variant has loosely arranged connective tissue bordered by palisaded basaloid cells and then cells with more cytoplasm, which, in places, is splayed apart by extracellular fluid. Sometimes there are clusters of anuclear, highly keratinized cells. There may be cholesterol clefts, inflammatory cells, calcification, and ossification. Intraoperative diagnosis of adamantinomatous craniopharyngioma may be suggested by the gross observation of variegated cystic tissue. Frozen sections are usually of good quality (Fig. 13.15). Smears typically show fragmented, clumped tissue.

GERMINOMA. Intracranial germ cell tumors, most commonly germinomas, occur most frequently in the sellar and pineal regions in children and young adults. The neoplastic cells of germinomas are polygonal and relatively large with large, round to oval nuclei and, often, large nucleoli. Sometimes, the nuclei are highly atypical. Frozen sections show sheets or large clusters of cells separated by connective tissue septa containing lymphoid inflammatory cells (e-Fig. 13.18). Despite the connective tissue component, smears of germinomas often reveal small clusters and single neoplastic cells. The morphologic features of germinomas overlap with those of atypical teratoid/rhabdoid tumors, so, in young children, the intraoperative diagnosis may have to indicate a differential. Also, in older adults, a firm intraoperative diagnosis of germinoma is difficult because the morphologic features on frozen sections and smears resemble those of carcinomas and large cell lymphomas.

Pineal Region Neoplasms

A wide variety of lesions occurs in the pineal region, among them malformations, cysts, and neoplasms. The most common pineal region neoplasms are germ cell tumors, mostly germinomas; neoplasms of pineal parenchymal cells; and astrocytic neoplasms that vary in grade (18). In adults, ependymomas, meningiomas, and carcinomas occur less frequently in this region.

PINEAL PARENCHYMAL NEOPLASMS. Neoplasms of cells demonstrating pineal differentiation are classified as pineocytoma, WHO grade 1, pineal parenchymal tumor of intermediate differentiation, WHO grade 2 or 3, and pineoblastoma, WHO grade 4 (15). The neoplasms may occur at any age, but pineocytomas are far more common in adults, and pineoblastomas are far more common in children.

Pineocytomas are well-circumscribed neoplasms composed of cells with small round to oval nuclei with stippled chromatin and relatively abundant cytoplasm with short processes. Often, the cells form rosettes where nuclei surround aggregated cytoplasmic processes. On intraoperative frozen sections, the tumor cell cytoplasm appears syncytial and, because of the rosettes and low-grade cytology, the differential is usually with ependymoma. The two can usually be distinguished on smears: smears of pineocytomas are usually clumped because of a fibrovascular component, while smears of ependymomas almost always reveal cells with long, fibrillar processes.

Pineoblastomas are embryonal neoplasms composed of cells with scant, often indiscernible cytoplasm. Nuclei have diameters that are approximately two to three times that of RBCs and are round to oval or have irregular shapes with angulated borders. Chromatin is granular, packed or sometimes smudged, and mitotic figures are usually frequent. There is often tumor cell necrosis. Frozen sections show sheets of cells and smears show abundant single cells.

In general, pineoblastomas are distinguished from pineal parenchymal tumors of intermediate differentiation by mitotic activity and tumor cell necrosis, which usually depends on examination of formalin-fixed, paraffin-embedded sections of the entire specimen (e-Fig. 13.19). In adults, intraoperative preparations of pineoblastomas and pineal parenchymal tumors of intermediate differentiation often cannot be distinguished from those of metastatic small cell carcinoma with absolute certainty.

Posterior Fossa Neoplasms

The posterior cranial fossa contains the cerebellum, the brain stem (composed of the midbrain, pons, and medulla), and several proximal cranial nerve roots. Between the brain stem and the cerebellum is the fourth ventricle. Cerebrospinal fluid in the fourth ventricle enters the subarachnoid space through the foramina of Luschka and Magendie. The foramen of

Luschka is present at the cerebellopontine angles, along with the eighth cranial nerve.

In children, intracranial neoplasms occur in the posterior fossa as often as in the supratentorial compartment. The most common posterior fossa neoplasms in children are medulloblastomas, pilocytic astrocytomas, and ependymomas.

In adults, metastatic carcinomas are relatively common neoplasms in the posterior fossa, usually involving the cerebellar parenchyma. Ependymal neoplasms are also encountered in the posterior fossa of adults. Hemangioblastomas occur relatively infrequently. Choroid plexus neoplasms occur in the fourth ventricle, but are relatively uncommon.

The most common neoplasms in the cerebellopontine angle are schwannomas and meningiomas; only rarely do ependymomas or choroid plexus neoplasms occur in the cerebellopontine angle.

MEDULLOBLASTOMA. Medulloblastomas are embryonal neoplasms of the cerebellum that occur most commonly in children, but also rarely in adults. They are composed of primitive neuroectodermal cells that are invasive, and often shed into the CSF. They are classified as WHO grade 4. Cytoplasm is scant and nuclei are often round or oval to polygonal, but usually some have irregular shapes; diameters are approximately two to three times that of RBCs. Chromatin varies from coarsely granular with several chromocenters to closely packed; sometimes it appears smudged. There are usually mitotic figures. Sections show sheets of cells (Fig. 13.16),

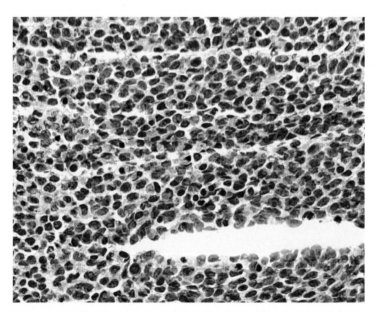

FIGURE 13.16   Intraoperative frozen section of a medulloblastoma showing relatively small cells with scant or indistinguishable cytoplasm.

sometimes with rosettes or nodular areas of more differentiated cells. Intraoperative smears show single cells and, sometimes, cells with nuclear molding (e-Fig. 13.20).

Medulloblastoma is by far the most common primitive neoplasm in the posterior fossa of children but, on intraoperative preparations, the differential may include atypical teratoid/rhabdoid tumor, and sometimes the diagnosis of "small cell neoplasm most consistent with medulloblastoma" is appropriate.

In adults, a neoplasm in the cerebellum composed of small, poorly differentiated cells is most likely metastatic carcinoma or, possibly, lymphoma. The finding of diffuse infiltration on frozen sections is more consistent with medulloblastoma than small cell carcinoma, but an intraoperative diagnosis of "small cell neoplasm: medulloblastoma versus metastatic carcinoma" may still be warranted. The finding of nuclear molding on smears militates against the diagnosis of lymphoma.

PILOCYTIC ASTROCYTOMA. Pilocytic astrocytomas are astrocytic neoplasms that are slowly growing, relatively well-circumscribed, and classified as WHO grade 1. They occur most frequently in children and young adults, and may occur anywhere in the CNS, but are particularly common in the optic pathways, the region of the third ventricle, and the cerebellum. Scans often show contrast enhancement and an associated cyst. Classical neoplasms are cytologically and architecturally biphasic with densely packed bipolar astrocytes and more stellate cells that are loosely arranged. Nuclei are round to oval or elliptical with diameters approximately 1.5 to 2 times RBCs with finely to coarsely granular chromatin and one or several chromocenters. Mitotic figures and tumor cell necrosis are uncommon. Sometimes, there are hyalinized vessels, Rosenthal fibers, and eosinophilic granular bodies. Both frozen sections and smears can contribute to intraoperative diagnosis. Smears show the overlapping, intersecting cytoplasmic processes of astrocytes, and sections reveal the biphasic architecture (Figs. 13.17, 13.18, e-Figs. 13.21, 13.22).

EPENDYMOMA. Ependymomas are composed of neoplastic cells that generally have long cytoplasmic processes and monomorphic, round to oval nuclei with diameters approximately 2 to 2.5 times that of RBCs and finely granular, evenly dispersed chromatin. The cell bodies are clustered, creating relatively anuclear areas composed mostly of cytoplasmic processes; the processes often radiate toward vessel walls, creating perivascular pseudorosettes. Infrequently, true ependymal rosettes are formed by columnar cells arranged around a central lumen. The neoplasms may be cystic, are usually well-circumscribed and are classified as WHO grade 2 or 3. Both frozen sections and smears are useful for intraoperative diagnosis. Smears reveal the cytoplasmic processes, and sections, the rosetted architecture (Fig. 13.19, e-Fig. 13.23).

It may be difficult though to distinguish pilocytic astrocytomas from low-grade ependymomas intraoperatively. Specifically, on frozen sections,

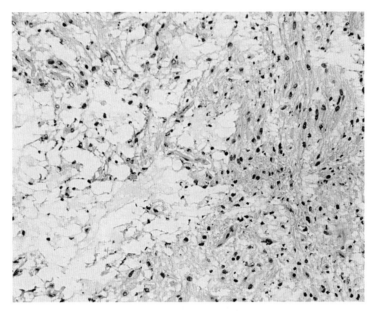

FIGURE 13.17   Frozen section of a pilocytic astrocytoma. Many pilocytic astrocytomas have biphasic architecture with both densely packed and loosely arranged astrocytes.

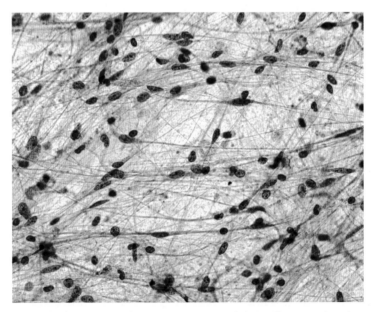

FIGURE 13.18   Smears of pilocytic astrocytomas reveal the stellate cytoplasmic processes of astrocytes.

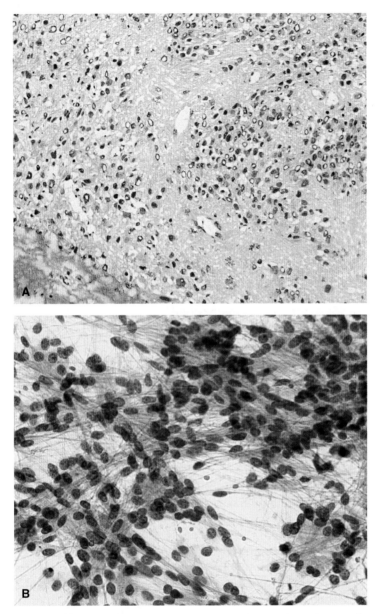

FIGURE 13.19 **A&B** Sections of most ependymomas show perivascular pseudorosettes; smears show cells with monomorphic nuclei and long, fibrillar cytoplasmic processes.

the densely packed areas of pilocytic astrocytomas, which are often perivascular, may resemble the rosettes of ependymomas. Moreover, pilocytic astrocytomas and ependymomas share radiographic features. Findings on smear preparations may help to distinguish the two: smears may reveal epithelioid cells with columnar cytoplasm or confirm the rosetted architecture of an ependymoma, or reveal an abundance of bipolar astrocytes in a pilocytic astrocytoma. Nevertheless, both neoplasms are relatively circumscribed, low-grade glial neoplasms, and an intraoperative diagnosis of "low-grade glial neoplasm: pilocytic astrocytoma versus ependymoma" is appropriate.

SUBEPENDYMOMA. Subependymomas are glial neoplasms that occur most commonly in the fourth ventricle of adults. The neoplasms are well-circumscribed, slowly growing (WHO grade 1), and often asymptomatic, so intraoperative diagnosis is infrequent. The tumor cells have highly fibrillar cytoplasmic processes and mostly small nuclei that are generally round to oval, but usually there are some nuclei that are relatively large and some with unusual shapes (19). Chromatin is finely granular and evenly dispersed, with small chromocenters. On intraoperative smears, variation in nuclear size and shape and fibrillar cytoplasm may raise the possibilities of pilocytic astrocytoma or diffusely infiltrating astrocytoma, but sections will show the characteristic ependymal architecture (Fig. 13.20).

HEMANGIOBLASTOMA. Hemangioblastomas are neoplasms that occur either sporadically or in patients with von Hippel-Lindau syndrome. Sporadic neoplasms occur most often in the cerebellum; von Hippel-Lindau–associated neoplasms are more likely to be multiple and also involve the brain stem and spinal cord. Hemangioblastomas are well-circumscribed, and often occur as a mural nodule associated with a cyst. The neoplastic cells are so-called stromal cells that occur among abundant, mostly thin-walled blood vessels. The stromal cells are round to oval or polygonal and relatively small with monomorphic, round to oval nuclei with diameters approximately one to two times that of RBCs. Sometimes there are rare larger, more atypical nuclei. N/C ratios are low because of abundant cytoplasm that is lightly eosinophilic and granular, foamy or clear. Hemangioblastomas are classified as WHO grade 1.

Because hemangioblastomas are invested by fibrovascular tissue and the stromal cells contain abundant lipid, intraoperative sections and smears are often of poor quality. Sometimes, though, the stromal cells can be recognized on at least one of the preparations and, in children, a definitive intraoperative diagnosis can made (Fig. 13.21, e-Fig. 13.24). In adults, it is usually not possible to rule out carcinoma intraoperatively, and a diagnosis of "clear cell neoplasm: hemangioblastoma versus metastatic carcinoma" is typically warranted.

SCHWANNOMA. Schwannomas are well-demarcated neoplasms of Schwann cells, and are classified as WHO grade 1. They are the most common neoplasms of the cerebellopontine angle, where they usually arise from the vestibular division of cranial nerve VIII. Many schwannomas exhibit biphasic cytology and architecture. In Antoni A areas, elongated spindle-shaped cells are densely packed and arranged in intersecting

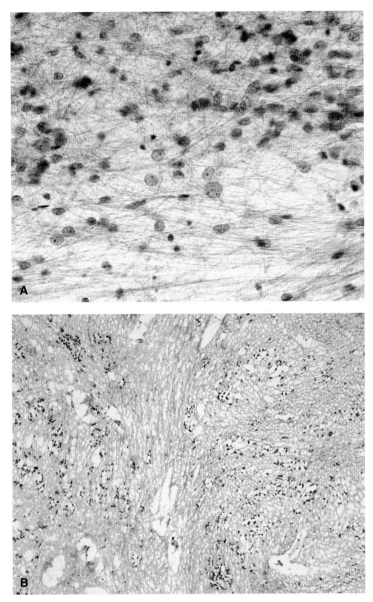

FIGURE 13.20 **A&B** Subependymomas are composed of cells with highly fibrillar cytoplasm that is apparent on intraoperative smears; frozen sections reveal their characteristic architecture.

fascicles. Antoni B areas are composed of loosely arranged cells with more round to oval nuclei and stubby, often indistinct cytoplasmic processes. Sometimes in the densely packed areas there are Verocay bodies, roughly parallel rows of nuclei alternating with anuclear areas. Sclerotic blood vessels are also common, and evidence of old hemorrhage (hemosiderin

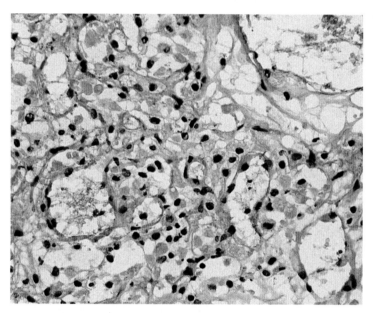

FIGURE 13.21 Hemangioblastomas are composed of neoplastic cells with eosinophilic, foamy, or clear cytoplasm and abundant, mostly thin-walled vessels.

deposits) may be observed. Frozen sections usually show the intersecting fascicles of neoplastic cells and at least some other characteristic features. Because of cell junctions, basement membrane, and intercellular collagen, smears show only clumps of neoplasm but, in the clumps, it is usually easy to recognize the fascicles of neoplastic cells (Fig. 13.22).

Sometimes, intraoperative preparations of a cerebellopontine angle neoplasm show only streaming spindle-shaped cells. In these cases, the diagnosis may be "low-grade neoplasm: schwannoma versus meningioma."

Spinal Region Neoplasms

Spinal canal neoplasms may be (i) intramedullary, that is, within the spinal cord parenchyma, (ii) extramedullary but intradural, or (iii) epidural. The types of neoplasms that occur most commonly in each of these locations are different, so radiographic localization is very helpful for intraoperative diagnosis. If the radiologist is uncertain of the localization, it is reasonable to ask the surgeon what the relationship of the neoplasm is to the meninges.

In children and adults, the intramedullary spinal neoplasms that are encountered most frequently are ependymomas, pilocytic astrocytomas, diffusely infiltrating astrocytomas, and hemangioblastomas. With the exception of myxopapillary ependymomas, these spinal cord neoplasms are histologically similar to the corresponding brain lesions already described.

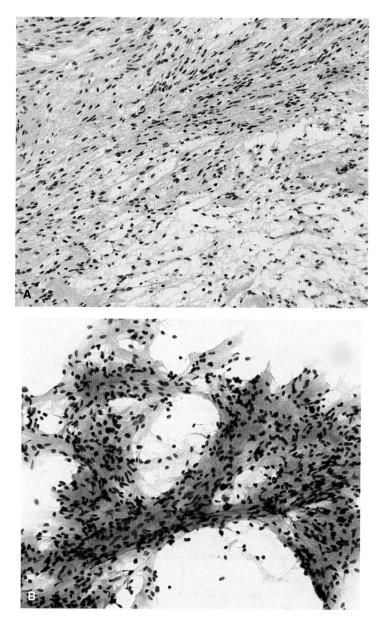

FIGURE 13.22 Packed cells in fascicles (Antoni A) adjacent to loosely arranged cells (Antoni B) on frozen section (A) of a schwannoma; a smear (B) highlights the fascicular architecture.

The extramedullary, intradural spinal neoplasms that are most common in adults are schwannomas and meningiomas. In children, schwannomas are most common (20). Sometimes, neurofibromas involve the spinal roots (e-Fig. 13.25).

Common epidural neoplasms in adults, often extending from nearby vertebrae, are carcinomas, lymphomas, and plasmacytomas.

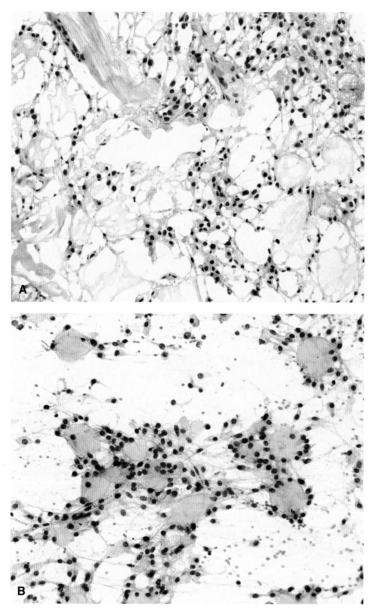

FIGURE 13.23   Intraoperative section (A) and smear (B) of a myxopapillary ependymoma of the cauda equina.

MYXOPAPILLARY EPENDYMOMA. Myxopapillary ependymomas occur almost exclusively in the cauda equina. They are usually well-circumscribed and are classified as WHO grade 1. The classical histology is that of small vessels surrounded by myxoid stroma and then layered cuboidal or columnar cells, as if the elongated cytoplasmic processes of a perivascular pseudorosette underwent degeneration. Usually, there are also areas where cells with intact processes are separated by myxoid stroma. Intraoperative sections may be difficult to interpret because of freezing artifact, but smears reveal cuboidal cells or cells with fibrillar processes with monomorphic, round to oval nuclei and myxoid stroma. Smears may show classical myxopapillary structures, structures without a central vessel, or just myxoid spheres (Fig. 13.23).

Telepathology in Intraoperative Diagnosis

It is often helpful to consult with an experienced neuropathologist when providing intraoperative consultation on neurosurgical specimens, although most institutions with neurosurgery services do not have a neuropathologist on staff. Advances in telepathology, including robotic microscopy, digital photography, and enhanced Internet access, now provide an opportunity to transmit images in real-time to a neuropathologist at a remote site. Horbinski et al. (21) recently reviewed the University of Pittsburgh experience using "teleneuropathology" for intraoperative consultations and reported diagnostic accuracy rates that were similar to those for conventional intraoperative consultation for most types of neoplasms, thus confirming the feasibility of this approach where sufficient resources are available to support it.

REFERENCES

1. Burger PC, Vogel FS. Frozen section interpretation in surgical neuropathology. I. Intracranial lesions. *Am J Surg Pathol.* 1977;1:323–347.
2. Burger PC, Vogel FS. Frozen section interpretation in surgical neuropathology. II. Intraspinal lesions. *Am J Surg Pathol.* 1978;2:81–95.
3. Burger PC. Use of cytological preparations in the frozen section diagnosis of central nervous system neoplasia. *Am J Surg Pathol.* 1985;9:344–354.
4. Cahill EM, Hidvegi DF. Crush preparations of lesions of the central nervous system. A useful adjunct to the frozen section. *Acta Cytol.* 1985;29:279–285.
5. Reyes MG, Homsi MF, McDonald LW, et al. Imprints, smears, and frozen sections of brain tumors. *Neurosurgery.* 1991;29:575–579.
6. Folkerth RD. Smears and frozen sections in the intraoperative diagnosis of central nervous system lesions. *Neurosurg Clin N Am.* 1994;5:1–18.
7. Brainard JA, Prayson RA, Barnett GH. Frozen section evaluation of stereotactic brain biopsies: diagnostic yield at the stereotactic target position in 188 cases. *Arch Pathol Lab Med.* 1997;121:481–484.
8. Firlik KS, Martinez AJ, Lunsford LD. Use of cytological preparations for the intraoperative diagnosis of stereotactically obtained brain biopsies: a 19-year experience and survey of neuropathologists. *J Neurosurg.* 1999;91:454–458.
9. Moss TH, Nicoll JAR, Ironside JW. *Intra-Operative Diagnosis of CNS Tumours.* London: Arnold; 1997.
10. Slowinski J, Harabin-Slowinska M, Mrowka R. Smear technique in the intra-operative brain tumor diagnosis: its advantages and limitations. *Neurol Res.* 1999;21:121–124.
11. Burger PC, Scheithauer BW, Vogel FS. *Surgical Pathology of the Nervous System and its Coverings.* 4th ed. New York: Churchill Livingstone; 2002.
12. Ironside JW, Moss TH, Louis DN, et al. *Diagnostic Pathology of Nervous System Tumours.* London: Churchill Livingstone; 2002.

13. Yachnis AT. Intraoperative consultation for nervous system lesions. *Semin Diagn Pathol.* 2002;19:192–206.
14. Joseph JT. *Diagnostic Neuropathology Smears.* Philadelphia: Lippincott Williams & Wilkins; 2007.
15. Louis DN, Ohgaki H, Wiestler OD, et al. *WHO Classification of Tumours of the Central Nervous System.* 4th ed. Lyon, France: International Agency for Research on Cancer; 2007.
16. Raisanen J, Goodman HS, Ghougassian DF, et al. Role of cytology in the intraoperative diagnosis of central demyelinating disease. *Acta Cytol.* 1998;42:907–912.
17. Suh DY, Mapstone T. Pediatric supratentorial intraventricular tumors. *Neurosurg Focus.* 2001;10:E4.
18. Drummond KJ, Rosenfeld JV. Pineal region tumours in childhood. A 30-year experience. *Childs Nerv Syst.* 1999;15:119–126.
19. Raisanen J, Burns DK, White CL. Cytology of subependymoma. *Acta Cytol.* 2003;47:518–520.
20. Rosemberg S, Fujiwara D. Epidemiology of pediatric tumors of the nervous system according to the WHO 2000 classification: a report of 1,195 cases from a single institution. *Childs Nerv Syst.* 2005;21:940–944.
21. Horbinski C, Fine JL, Medina-Flores R, et al. Telepathology for intraoperative neuropathologic consultations at an academic medical center: a 5-year report. *J Neuropathol Exp Neurol.* 2007;66:750–759.

INDEX